# PETE & TILLIE

## A REAL-LIFE NOVEL

(Almost) everything I needed to know
I learned from my patients

DENNIS GIESBRECHT, MD

Published by:

# FriesenPress

Suite 300 – 852 Fort Street
Victoria, BC, Canada V8W 1H8

www.friesenpress.com

Distributed to the trade by The Ingram Book Company

# PREFACE

I have been in medical practice for some forty years, and during that time I've dished out medical wisdom on a daily basis, some helpful, some hopeful, much of it ignored. I have endeavored to keep in mind that my practice was a service, and not just a livelihood. I have listened to the sorrows and suffering of thousands of people, many times with impatience. I should have listened more and advised less. People don't like a doctor who doesn't "do anything," and I have written hundreds of unnecessary prescriptions. I should have written fewer. Thomas Sydenham, a famous English physician, said, "The arrival in town of a good clown does more for the health of people than twenty asses laden with pills." I should have spread more humour and cheer. Time provides wisdom.

Nonetheless, I have enjoyed my years in medicine, and would like to think, that in the main, I've served God and my fellowman well. It has been an incredible journey. If you are entertained by my experiences, great. If it dispels some myths, wonderful. You might even carry away a few pointers to better health. This is, however, not a family health treatise. For that I'd suggest real face-to-face doctors. If you don't trust them, I can recommend a well-established, reliable quack – there are many right here in Manitoba.

Someone once said that the art of medicine is to amuse the patient while nature heals the disease. Others believe that doctors are able to put a scrambled egg back in the shell. The truth lies somewhere in between, probably closer to the first premise. I like what Cicero had to say: "In nothing do men more nearly approach the gods than in giving health to men."

The episodes recounted here are based on my medical practice that has now spanned four decades, although most come from the 80s and early 90s. Since those years there have been many advances in medicine, some of which are told here.

These accounts are based on actual patients, but the particulars have been combined, shuffled like a deck of cards, embellished, and modified. There is comedy and heartbreak, conditions familiar and obscure, even a little research interspersed with tales of the unbelievable and creative ways in which people abuse their bodies, and then demand that doctors reverse the damage. The vast majority of my patients came for routine physicals, had common illnesses, and were pleasant to deal with. Patients like that are wonderful, but they often make for dull stories. Hence, the characters in this book are a bit more unusual, bizarre, or difficult. And giving credit where credit is due – I have learned much from my patients – the art of medicine, patience, and compassion.

Now that I am in that "metallic" age – gold in my teeth, silver in my hair and lead in my pants, I am semi-retired and have become a recluse, slinking off to my computer in a basement corner to await the muses. My wife says it has come to throwing scraps of food down the stairs. What is it that compels one to write? Winston Churchill, a prolific writer, gave his reasons: "Writing a book is an adventure," he said. "It begins as an amusement, then it becomes a mistress, then a master, finally a tyrant." I think it is a little of all of those things. For one who detests paperwork on the job, this is a strange turn of events. I have many times questioned my audacity in writing this account, but I have been told that the ark was built by amateurs, the Titanic by professionals.

I have always been a prodigious reader, even as a child. Words fascinated me. A finely crafted story by Tolstoy or Steinbeck is a thing of beauty, akin to a Titian masterpiece or a Beethoven symphony. For me to indulge in the enterprise of writing is living a dream. A memoir was not a difficult choice – it was inevitable, except for the element of time. It was only the demands of family, practice, and community that kept this from happening sooner.

This book is about practicing medicine in a Mennonite town. Every resident is an expert. The remarkable thing about practicing here is that if you don't know what you're doing, someone else is sure to tell you. People are sophisticated and knowledgeable, naïve and ignorant, wretched, sweet, and infuriating, but always fascinating.

Winston Churchill also opined, "History will be kind to me – I intend to write it myself."

I am of the same mind. And so this story of my years in practice will reveal it to be a shamelessly brilliant career.

# Acknowledgements

I am indebted to a number of people who helped to bring this book to fruition: Dr. Marjorie Anderson, for expert counsel and content editing, Dr. Curtis Krahn, a long-time colleague, who reviewed the medical content, and Moira Neufeld, another friend and writer, who spent many hours on the final copyediting.

I also want to acknowledge my loving family, too numerous to mention individually, but who are supportive of whatever project absorbing my energy and ideas – and above all, deep gratitude to my incredible, long-suffering wife Rose, who read the manuscript numerous times, gave many useful suggestions, and provided much love and encouragement.

## Chapter 1
# A STUBBORN PLACENTA

The insistent jangle breaks through the thick fog of exhaustion. I sit up and fumble in the darkness for the phone.

"Hello?" I shake my head and a few more synapses begin firing. I turn the phone the right way up. "Hello?"

"Hi, Dennis. Jim here. Sorry to call you at this hour. I have a woman with a retained placenta who delivered an hour ago. We'll have to do a manual removal."

Several frontal-lobe circuits have reached operating temperature and the disagreeable prospect of getting out of a warm bed trickles into my consciousness. Several seconds of silence. Jim Sanderson, the local surgeon, is on the phone. "Dennis, are you there?"

"Yeah, I'm here," I respond. "I think I'm awake now. Retained placenta. What time is it, anyway?"

"It's three-fifteen. I called the OR staff, and they'll be ready in about twenty minutes."

"Okay, I'll be there."

"You have to go for surgery?" Rose murmurs from somewhere inside her pillow.

"Yeah." I slump back on to my pillow. "Stubborn placenta," in my best martyr voice. The only reply is a soft snuffling. I wriggle back under the covers. Why do people have babies at this obscene hour anyway? There is something perverse about a new birth, supposedly a joyful event, in the wee hours of the night when nobody wants to be there except mom, who, of course, would just like to get it over with. By this time I have already been in practice for several decades, but the night work never gets any easier.

Feeling irritated and abused, I stumble into the bathroom, pull on a pair of jeans and a shirt, slick down my disorderly hair, and splash some water on my face. I glance in the mirror – people should not be judged by their appearance at three in the morning. I make my way to the garage down the shadowy hallway, grabbing a parka from the hall closet. By the time I arrive at Bethesda hospital, my indomitable sense of duty has taken command, and I'm prepared for action. I change mechanically into the voluminous Christian Dior greens, wondering with some unease what I will encounter.

"Good morning," says Candace, the circulating nurse, one of those perpetually bubbly people. I must speak to her some time – such cheeriness seems wrong at this time of the night. I remembered being annoyed on more than one occasion by David Kroeker, a colleague from my first years of practice, who was defiantly upbeat at any hour of the day or night as if the intrusion were an adventure to be embraced, another jewel in his crown. To his credit, though, he had always been willing to help.

Candace has already set up the operating room, and is attaching the cardiac monitor and oximeter (blood oxygen monitor) to the patient.

"Morning," I grunt. "You're one of the lucky ones, too?"

"Yeah," she replies. "It doesn't get any easier, does it?" Candace is a dependable stalwart, an experienced RN who has worked many years on a rotation of scrub nurse, circulating nurse, and emergency call. It's reassuring to have her there in an emergency.

Jessica is a young mom who has just delivered a lovely baby girl, her second child. The newborn wailed raucously on arrival, highly annoyed at having been wrenched from her cozy environment, but now lies quietly in a bassinet in a corner of the room. Jessica's labor has not been as difficult as her firstborn, who had already blazed a trail using his little skull as a battering ram. Childbirth is an amazing cascade of events from conception to a completely dependent fetus, and finally, to a unique human life. The marvel is that of all the possible misadventures along the way, so few actually happen.

For Jessica, the mishap is an obstinate placenta – the pancake-like interface between mom and the fetus that supplies oxygen and nourishment. The placenta is stuck to the wall of the uterus like a barnacle on a ship's hull. With the placenta there, the uterus can't contract properly and shut off the large arteries that develop with pregnancy. A retained placenta can be a crisis because of the risk of hemorrhage. The patient can go into shock, and may even require emergency hysterectomy. The nurses on the ward had already tried nipple massage, and had Jessica empty her bladder. These measures sound like something out of Grandma's Compendium of Home Remedies, but may actually stimulate uterine contraction and expulsion of the placenta. This time they had not made any difference.

Jessica's complexion is ashen. She has lost between one and two liters of blood (out of a total of five), a dangerous amount. Her pulse rate is 110, too high, but her blood pressure is still normal at 115/75. She already has an oxytocin infusion to prod the uterus to contract and the torrent has slowed to a trickle.

"Hi, Dr. Giesbrecht," Jessica says with a weak smile. "Sorry to get you guys out in the middle of the night."

"Oh well," I say, "I had to get up to answer the phone anyway. Besides, there's not much you can do about a stubborn afterbirth, is there? How are you doing?"

"I'm very tired, and a little nervous."

"I'll give you a shot of my special homebrew, and you'll feel better."

I check the IV – 600 ccs of normal saline has infused so far, along with antibiotics – amoxicillin and metronidazole. This is an ideal case for propofol, an intravenous anesthetic drug that has recently come into general use. Propofol is short-acting, has a wide safety margin, and the patient recovers quickly with little nausea or hangover. I dial in Jessica's weight and the appropriate dose, and the electronic pump begins pushing a measured amount into her large-bore IV line.

"Is it starting to percolate up there?" I ask after twenty seconds of infusion.

"Oh, yeah, it is," she mumbles. "I'm feeling better... did you know you look like Robert Redfo...?" Her words trail off and her eyelids began to droop.

"Why, thank you," I reply, "How perceptive of you." She didn't hear my last words and wouldn't remember them in any case. I turn to Candace, "Did you hear that? Why is it that people only tell me stuff like that when they're inebriated or getting an anesthetic?"

"Hey," she shrugs. "Take it where you can get it."

Jessica begins to snore and shows no reaction when Candace preps her perineum with Betadine, an iodine-based antiseptic. I slow the infusion, adjusting the propofol dose periodically to keep Jessica at a safe anesthetic level – deep enough to keep her from feeling pain or moving, but not enough to drop her blood pressure, although every anesthetic lowers the blood pressure to some degree.

Jim has arrived. He scrubs quickly and dons a long rubber glove, known as a gauntlet, that extends to the elbow. (If your doctor ever brings out one of those during your physical, you should probably make a run for it.) He pushes his hand through the cervix into the uterus and unceremoniously begins ripping the placenta off the uterine wall chunk by chunk. Many procedures lead you to admire the surgeon's skill with scalpel and sutures. This is not one of them.

Jim is a man of few words. It's impossible to ruffle him. His stocky frame belies the deft smooth strokes with a scalpel. There are no wasted motions. He's supremely self-assured, a wonderful trait in a colleague – he assesses the situation, decides on the best course of action and moves ahead. He rarely second-guesses his decisions. For him, a bad outcome is just one of those things you can't always control. The right person in this crisis.

The bleeding is heavier again.

I press the monitor button to take her blood pressure. "Rats! Her BP is down to 80/50," I say calmly. I don't really feel that calm. "She's lost a lot of blood." I open up the IV to expand Jessica's blood volume and back off the propofol. "Are you nearly done? We may have to give her blood. In the meantime I'll switch to lactated Ringer's (to expand blood volume)."

"Yeah, a couple of minutes," Jim says. "Candace, have the lab bring up the O negative blood (emergency unmatched blood). We'll give her a unit or two if her blood pressure drops any more. Get the lab to cross-match her for three more units of blood." He glances in my direction. "Give her 250 micrograms of ergonovine?"

Ergonovine is an alkaloid derived from ergot, a fungus that infects plants of the grass family, specifically rye. In times past, it caused poisoning in cattle and humans eating infected grain, a condition commonly known as ergotism, or "St. Anthony's Fire," in reference to symptoms such as severe burning sensations in the limbs. Ergot alkaloids cause severely restricted circulation in blood vessels, sometimes leading to gangrene and limb amputations, and could cause convulsions or death due to inadequate brain circulation. Whole villages were sometimes affected by eating contaminated bread. Today ergonovine, used in controlled doses, is a valuable drug that persuades the uterine muscle to contract and stem the bleeding.

I take Jessica's blood pressure again – 65/40. "Houston, we have a problem," I say. "The blood pressure has dropped some more." The OR is eerily quiet. Candace looks at me apprehensively. I have never lost a patient like this, and don't intend to now, but with that amount of blood loss... Jim massages the boggy uterus between his hands to stimulate the musculature to contract. "I'll open up the IV a bit more. Get the ergonovine! Have them bring up the emergency blood stat!" In the meantime, I inject 25 mg ephedrine to contract her blood vessels and give her blood pressure a boost.

I draw the ergonovine into a small syringe and push it slowly into the intravenous line. Most of the placenta has been removed, so Jim quickly performs a D & C (scraping of the uterine wall) with a circular knife-like instrument to strip off any remaining placental tissue. Once the uterus is clean, the bleeding stops. The blood pressure rallies to 90/50. With the bleeding down to a trickle, and the small dose of ephedrine, the blood pressure returns to normal.

I heave a sigh of relief. That was too close for comfort!

I turn off the propofol and nitrous oxide, allowing Jessica to breathe pure oxygen. By the time she's transferred to the stretcher, she slurs, "Is it done already?"

Fortunately, Jessica doesn't require any transfusions. She remains stable, and will quickly make up the deficient hemoglobin. Every transfusion, no matter how closely it is matched to the patient's blood type will inevitably cause some antibody formation and a possible reaction should the patient require blood at a future time.

I walk into the doctor's change room and flop wearily onto the ancient orange vinyl couch.

"Well," says Jim, "she should be okay."

"I hope so. It was dicey there for a while. I don't know about you, but I've had my adrenalin rush for the day." I pull myself to my feet, remove my greens, and start to dress. "You know, I could have been a garbage collector. No stress. No responsibility. They're never called at night – you know, *wild party – emergency beer-bottle pickup on Reimer Avenue*. I don't think they need to submit a report at the end of the shift with the number of diapers or soup cans they collected. But no – I had to be a hero and go to medical school."

"Yeah," laughs Jim, "but somebody has to be the hero. I was going to be a teacher. Good pay, good pension plan, holidays at Christmas and spring break, and the summer off. So what are we doing here? My wife says I have no life."

"That's what Rose says, too. Maybe we can retire early and start our dream vocations – you can teach, and I'll collect garbage."

"We could," says Jim, "but I'm not qualified to do anything except cut. I'd have to go back to school. You'd have a real advantage – you could start your new career tomorrow. Or you might have to go to night school and get your PhD in waste management."

We laugh, more from relief than the lame humor. "Anyway," I say. "I guess this is not the time to wax philosophical. We have to be back here again in a couple of hours. Good night."

It's early January. The holidays are over and a long winter stretches ahead. I make my way into the frigid winter night, thinking about the night's events. I drive slowly back home on deserted streets. A few bright windows punctuate the dark streets – an insomniac watching television or a parent soothing a child's nightmare. Solitude and tranquility replace the frenzy of the hospital scene. There is a slight breeze and wisps of snow drift lazily across the road and swirl around the street lamps in little eddies.

I think about my conversation with Jim. Six kids later – I am still in Steinbach. It is now 1993, and I have already been in practice for 26 years.

In truth, I had intended to go into medical research. In the coming decades molecular biology would become cutting-edge science. I could have been happy cloistered in a lab. Or perhaps in a specialty like cardiology if research didn't work out. Above all, I had planned on not becoming a family practitioner. Dealing with ingrown toenails, hemorrhoids, and snotty screaming kids was way down on my list of things to do with my life. I had had no intention of settling in Steinbach, either. Well, okay... just a year or two to pay off student debts and buy some furniture. Oh, and feed and clothe several progeny.

Family practice is hard to beat as a fascinating occupation. Where else can you hear the latest gossip, recent fad diets, quack cures, or the best place to get your car repaired?

So Steinbach was where I began my medical practice. It is the principle settlement on the East Reserve, a tract of land on the east side of the Red River, founded in the late nineteenth century by Mennonites from the steppes of Ukraine.

My grandparents had emigrated from Ukraine back in the 1870's because of the uncertainty of government policies in Russia, particularly the question of exemption from military service. There were also internal problems within the Mennonite colonies of Russia – the more traditional element had a desire to distance themselves from other Mennonite groups, some of whom were embracing school reforms and new worship practices, like singing with musical notation. Some groups were seen as compromising their principles by becoming too cozy with government officials. There were constant struggles over land ownership. Increasing wealth among some Mennonites meant menial labor and little chance of financial advancement for others. Famine, persecution, and a loss of their traditional way of life forced later waves of emigration.

Dad recalled that my grandparents were not very articulate about their reasons for leaving Ukraine – it wasn't so much a deep-seated ideology as it was a fear of violence and the loss of their material and social way of life. The prospect of abundant farmland on the Canadian prairies was appealing. Grandpa and Grandma Giesbrecht, as with many of the 1870's migrants, were not without substantial resources to finance their emigration and begin farming in Manitoba. They eventually settled in the West Reserve, north of Plum Coulee and Winkler.

Steinbach was, from its inception, a Bible-believing, God-fearing community. Our forefathers had fought hard to maintain the living apart (*stillen im Lande*, quiet in the land) they thought necessary to protect their faith. They had, after all, wandered from Germany, Switzerland, and the Netherlands, through Prussia and Ukraine in search of that freedom. Since then we had changed, slowly drifting from our conservative past. Steinbach had successful businesses, money, and big homes, though prosperity and worldly lifestyles were not worn easily by everyone. To be the Automobile City and the Bible Belt at the same time often required a bit of creative theology. We told ourselves repeatedly that our motives were pure – it wasn't money that was evil, it was the love of money, and we certainly were not guilty of that. Lavish living was justified as the fruit of hard work and God's blessing.

We were often torn – some were in a rush to modernize and shed our Mennonite trappings, as if they were holding us back and making us objects of derision in the eyes of the world. We didn't always know how to make progress without abandoning the worthwhile doctrines of our Anabaptist faith.

I arrive at our home outside of town and drive down the long driveway with the headlights off – no point in waking anyone. I stop the car in front of the garage and get out. The winter sky is cloudless and studded with stars. The frosty silence is broken only by a gentle breeze whistling softly through the lifeless branches of the willow beside the house and the crunch of snow under my shoes. I stop to scan the heavens, a habit of many years, prompted by a fascination with astronomy. We are a mile from the light pollution of town, and the sky is black and brilliant. There's Sirius, the Dog Star, the brightest star in the winter sky, and Orion, the hunter. A little further north is another old friend, Pleiades, known as the Seven Sisters, a group of young and hot stars with a bluish twinkle. I watch for some celestial fireworks, perhaps a meteor or the northern lights, but the sky is quiet.

I feel small and insignificant under the sparkling canopy. Thirty minutes ago, the OR emergency had loomed so large and all-encompassing. To Jessica it was all that mattered right then, and we may well have saved her life, yet it was but one infinitesimal step in the eternal dance of the universe. If the cosmologists are right, all the elements making up every living thing on earth have come from the cataclysmic death throes of stars. It's a beautiful thought – life coming from the dying embers of heavenly spheres.

I'm profoundly grateful; I'm making a tiny difference. I have a fascinating profession, and as a bonus, they send me a cheque every two weeks. I have countless things to be thankful for, not the least of which is a warm bed. I begin to shiver as the cold penetrates my parka. I breathe some warmth into my gloved hand and decide to go indoors. I make a quick stop in the kitchen for a banana and a glass of milk to settle my stomach, and make my way as noiselessly as possible to the bedroom, and gingerly climb into bed so as not to disturb Rose – she has to be at work twenty miles away in St. Pierre by eight-thirty. I turn on the bedside light to read something supremely boring to wind down. An exhausted sleep comes eventually; the last I remember, the alarm clock reads 5 a.m.

Chapter 2
# NO CONCRETE RESULTS

My path to a medical career in Steinbach, Manitoba wasn't a single-minded pursuit – there were ambushes, twists, and dead-ends. Attending university seemed like the right thing to do following high school. My dad had been a high school teacher, and was one of the few Mennonites of the 1920's who had earned a university degree. Our home had a culture of education and personal growth. My parents never attempted to dictate my career path, but they did expect it would be something noble and pure, following God's direction. To their credit, Mom and Dad encouraged a university education. Many other Mennonites believed (and some still do) that it wasn't possible to pursue higher education without being corrupted and losing one's faith.

According to the cultural and religious ethic of my upbringing, life-altering decisions, indeed everything in life, was directed by God. I was positively uncertain about God's direction, however. There were no signs like white smoke from a chimney or skywriting: GET A MEDICAL DEGREE. Dad said that was because I hadn't been looking to God for direction, but at that stage I didn't really want any. I was repeatedly amazed how God seemingly directed people into foreign missions, teaching, or even making huge gobs of money. I would have been happy with *small* gobs of money, but I suppose I just wasn't "spiritual" enough. If my temperament was any indication, my career path should have been something science-related: biology, physics, perhaps mathematics. My interest in science had been fueled by a childhood fascination with nature and chemistry sets.

Medicine? Not a chance.

My elementary education took place in a one-room country school in the sheltered Mennonite farming heartland of southern Manitoba. Our church, school and practically every neighbour for miles around were Mennonite. It was like living in a protective embracing dome. As a child, I gawked at those other folks – a few *Enjlenda,* English people, in Plum Coulee and Winkler, but they were not allowed to contaminate us. Nobody told me these folks were evil and dangerous; I just *knew* they were. I was certain they all smoked, played cards, and didn't go to church. Such was the culture of my childhood.

I went to high school in Plum Coulee, Manitoba, a fact I keep to myself whenever possible. If that had guided my career path, I would be growing malting barley (it was okay to grow grain for brewing beer, but sinful to drink it) or selling hardware. Grade 12 had taken me to the Mennonite Collegiate Institute in Gretna, a venerable, cloistered asylum designed to direct raw, undisciplined youth down the road to the Promised Land. I had been raised with a strong sense of duty and moral obligation to heal the world. The Mennonite stock from whose loins I had been launched was known to be frugal, to have a Calvinist work ethic second to none and to be militantly non-resistant. We were lonely pilgrims on the narrow path to righteousness, had pretty much solved the scourges of war and sin, for ourselves at any rate, and were hard at work on overthrowing poverty. That didn't leave much territory for me to conquer. Nevertheless, I was determined to make some broad brush-strokes in history.

After high school, I entered United College, later to become the University of Winnipeg. I enrolled in the sciences – physics, chemistry, and math - with a healthy dollop of English literature and geography. I also took German, but was never sure why – perhaps because it was the path of least resistance – I had endured German through elementary and high school and in the view of many of our people, German was the only language God understood. Whenever anyone spoke about God or to God, it was in German. To my mind, German was stodgy and outmoded, and should have been relegated to our wandering past. As an impressionable seven-year-old, I had heard the nightly CBC broadcasts about World War II, had experienced food rationing, and seen the prisoners-of-war in our peaceful farming country. There was something sinister and repugnant about German – *Sieg Heil* and *Deutschland über alles* reverberated with the horrors of the war and the Nazi regime.

I had excellent grades at United College. I was a novice – I had no idea how little work was needed to pass courses in university. For my second year I enrolled at the University of Manitoba, and took a wider range of subjects, particularly physics, zoology, and mathematics. The sciences were rounded out with English literature and sociology. I had a vague notion of entering some area of scientific research, but as long as I had a few years of university ahead of me, I didn't have to burden my life with career decisions. My abilities in mathematics and physics caught the attention of a few professors, who suggested I take the Honors Math/Physics program. So in third year I was on the path to the stars. It was a heady atmosphere –perhaps I might one day explain the origins of the universe, or solve Fermat's last theorem.

One day after the first few weeks of classes, in a moment of epiphany, I looked around at my classmates – eccentric eggheads who became orgiastic on seeing a blackboard sprouting esoteric formulae. They had no life. I knew that because I had none. I had virtually dropped out of the social scene. Quantum mechanics and differential calculus became all-consuming, oozing from every pore. I asked myself if this was really what I wanted for the rest of my life. The next day I switched back to a regular science program, none the worse for my experience.

Third year. I became involved in various extra-curricular activities - football, curling, and playing in the University symphony orchestra, a loosely organized volunteer group. All of which is to say, less work and more fun. My marks collapsed like an undercooked soufflé.

I also discovered that I didn't need to abandon my spiritual upbringing completely – superficiality and a façade of piety would do nicely. Taking Christianity seriously was so demanding and restrictive. However, I fell in with the Intervarsity Christian Fellowship crowd – it was religious and many of the kids were Mennonite. I felt safe. My faith, though shallow, provided some boundaries. The female of the species provided diversions – I tried the dating game, taking nurses or fellow students to the symphony or live theater, but bars, movies and drinking were verboten on my list.

Finally, after four years, I was the proud owner of a Bachelor of Science degree.

Now what?

Enter my father. Dad was the only one of the Giesbrecht clan who had chosen not to farm for a living. He taught high school for many years before he took over the family farm. According to my dad, one could do no nobler thing in life than to serve in the teaching profession. "Give it a try," he urged. "Think of it this way, you can teach science and math, which you enjoy, and be an enormous influence on the lives of young people. What can be better than that?" I was vulnerable and defenseless. Saving the world would have to wait.

Four months at U of M summer school and presto! – I was a high school teacher. I spent a year in Stonewall collegiate, attempting to bring thirty-two intractable grade nines up to speed, including Pieter, a six-foot-two gangly teenager, who wrapped his long legs around his desk in the front row, stared at me from under a thick shock of blond hair, and dared me to teach him anything.

These kids had spent two years with George Bennett, a fixture in the school for three decades. He was a round, oily man; the sum of his waist and shoe size equaled his IQ, and if you put your ear close to his skull, you could hear the ocean. "Teaching is great," he boasted in the staff room. "I haven't read a book since Normal School (teacher training). I set up all my lessons during my first year of teaching." A self-made man who worshipped his creator.

I quickly discovered I had little patience with kids who didn't want to be there. The school system frowned upon Gestapo tactics – I was supposed to *motivate* kids to learn without the use of caning or thumbscrews.

George had endeared himself to students and parents alike by passing every student, including those with sadly deficient academic skills. Two of my fellow teachers and the principal in the high school were first-rate instructors, but ran into community discontent because they insisted on high standards and an end to the cronyism. They were fired. I beat the school board to it and resigned.

Other than organizing a sock drawer (which I have since forgotten how to do), I had not yet learned any useful skills. I landed in medical school almost by accident. I lived in a boarding house with several friends already enrolled in medicine, who apparently were thrilled to be there. I had a murky goal of a career in genetic research, more particularly molecular biology, and a medical degree seemed like a good start. As an added bonus, I would not have to make any major decisions for another four or five years. By graduation, the sun of enlightenment would have burned away the persistent fog and I would be able to see the road straight ahead.

Medical school was demanding. Volumes of material on anatomy, physiology, pharmacology; thousands of diseases, characteristics, causes, and cures. This was serious stuff – we had thirty hours a week in class, and many more on homework. It was an awful lot of effort just to avoid the workaday world, and I still wasn't convinced medicine was where my future lay. Then, several months into the first term, a curious thing happened. I became enamored of my studies and the prospect of an honorable career.

Anatomy was one of the major courses in first year – in addition to lectures, we spent several hours in the dissection lab every day. Dead bodies. Preserving fluids. Scalpels. What's not to love for any budding necromancer? Several in our group were personally acquainted with "embalming fluids," so our cadaver became affectionately known as Johnny Walker. Our troupe consisted of several males – a portly, self-assured Jew, a conservative Mennonite (me), a jovial West Indian, a standard Anglo-Saxon white, and a courageous female, who endured a great deal of good-natured abuse as one of the three (out of forty-eight students) women in our class. Our dissectee became like family, so much so that there was nothing left at the end of the year except a few desiccated bones and miscellaneous shriveled scraps, the kind of stuff Grandma would have used as soup stock.

Johnny had apparently died in prison after a skid-row life of alcohol and petty crime. He had no family, so in the academic equivalent of body snatching, he was pickled in formaldehyde, and shipped postage-paid to the medical school. Dissection of the human body is considered an essential part of a medical training, but it was outlawed for many centuries. The first known dissections were performed in Alexandria around 300 B.C. on criminals dead or alive.

Prior to being formally introduced to our marinated comrade, we were lectured on the sanctity of the human body by anatomist Dr. Franz Holman. "Dis iss not an animal," he said in his severe German accent, stabbing the air with a bony finger. "It iss a human body and ve must treat it viss respeckt." Holman was tall and skeletal with sunken eyes and hollow cheekbones, befitting someone who had spent his life with the dead. It was as though he had inhaled vast quantities of embalming fluid over the years, but the process was only partially successful.

I recall meeting Johnny for the first time. Dr. Holmann ushered us solemnly into the dissection lab. There were a dozen or so tables, each with a white sheet covering what was discernibly a human form. The pungent odor of formalin permeated the room, and for the next eight months would infuse our hair, skin, clothing, and the salami sandwiches we sometimes ate tableside.

Ralph pulled off the sheet. We stood there for a moment, not sure what to do. Most of us had never been exposed to death, and we were awed by the recognition that this was once a living, breathing individual. I hesitantly reached out and touched his fingers. They were cold and rigid. I shuddered at the thought – at one time, their warmth may have caressed a face, painted an exquisite canvas, or built a playhouse for an excited child, before their owner ended up in the back alley of life. Johnny's skin was a mushroom tone with an odd sheen, and his face was rugged and leathery as if he had spent his life in harsh sunlight. In spite of the repulsive color of death and the odor of formaldehyde, I couldn't help but wonder what we might have talked about had we met before his untimely death.

"Okay, who's going first?" asked Ralph, matter-of-factly. "We're supposed to start with the chest, right?"

"I'll do it," said Sidney. "What does the manual say? *Open the chest cavity cutting from the sternal notch to the abdominal wall.*" He resolutely grasped the scalpel and made a bold incision to expose the glistening white of the sternum underneath. Ralph took the saw and cut through the bone to expose the chest cavity. The lungs looked surprisingly dark, like a dirty bathroom sponge, the result of a life-long tobacco habit. Sidney pushed the lungs apart, and there lay the center of life, the heart, aorta, and the other major blood vessels.

And so it went from chest to abdomen to skull, from muscles to arteries, nerves, and organs. In addition to gross dissection, we spent hours peering through a microscope studying the astounding variety of specialized cell types and tissues that blended to produce an eye, an ear, or a kidney. The body is an intricate, artfully designed machine. The brain alone has 100 billion neurons, we were told, with up to 1000 trillion connecting fibers, known as synapses. This unbelievable intricacy may have been the result of Darwinian natural selection, but it hardly seemed possible.

It was not long into the year before the initial reverence and the heady aura of being in medical college had worn off.

"Listen, guys," Sidney said one day in a tone of conspiracy. "Tomorrow's anatomy lab – hang back a bit. Let Andrea get there first."

"What have you got in mind?" asked Ralph.

"Just wait and see."

Next day Andrea arrived at the dissection table, whisked off the sheet, and opened her anatomy text, as we watched from the doorway. She began reading the directions, absent-mindedly probing the rectus abdominus muscle, whereupon the withered and supposedly lifeless male appendage slowly began to rise. She recoiled, looked furtively about, and slapped the offending member. It started to rise again.

Sidney emerged from under an adjacent table. "Andrea, you're a hot chick. The guy is dead three months, and there's still a response." Sidney had been manipulating a thin wire threaded through the body of our very dead but suddenly amorous felon.

Some of our other antics were equally grotesque, like walking around the lab with a lab coat over one's head and a skull under one's arm. Was this behaviour a misguided attempt to deal with our own mortality? More likely, simple bravado. In the end, maturity, perhaps ennui, tempered the youthful exuberance and dissection lab become routine. After our final exams in year one, it was Sidney, the prankster, who delivered the eulogy and spoke in gratitude of the individuals like Johnny, who had unwittingly contributed to our medical education.

In third year, I made a name for myself in the research community – with my classmates, at any rate. We were required to complete a project to gain some insight into research methods. I was assigned to Dr. John McDermott from St. Boniface Hospital, who suggested that we attempt to add to the body of knowledge on renal calculi (kidney stones).

Kidney stones?

I was dismayed. Heart disease, maybe, or a cure for leukemia, but kidney stones? Could he have chosen anything less glamorous? "Wait a minute," I said, "You want me to make little concrete blocks using pee?"

"Yep. I know it sounds crazy, but we might just come up with something."

This was hardly the start of a brilliant career in medical research that I had envisioned. However, this idea came from my faculty advisor, a clinician of many years experience. Who was I to argue? If nothing else, I might garner the prize for most original presentation. Then again, I might follow Hennig Brand, a German of the 17th century, who spent years and his first wife's fortune in experimentation, convinced he could turn base metals and human urine into gold. He boiled down thousands of liters of urine and then refined the residue. Unsurprisingly, he found no gold, but did discover phosphorus in the effort.

Dr. McDermott sent me to the library to research kidney diseases, specifically to read an article suggesting that the chemistry of kidney stone formation in the body was akin to that of setting concrete.

"Obtain as many urine samples as you can from hospital patients who have a history of kidney stones," he said, "and an equal number of samples from those without any history as a control group. Use the urine from each to make a batch of concrete blocks and water for a third batch. You'll have to figure out some way to measure the quality of the finished product."

After checking hundreds of patient histories, I gathered forty urine specimens. Dr. McDermott found a small corner of the lab where I weighed cement, sand, and urine to the accompanying snickers of the lab techs. I poured the mixtures into three-inch cubes, each carefully labeled. One batch of blocks was allowed to cure for seven days, and another batch for three weeks. Good science should have controls, hence two more batches with water. I took each set of concrete blocks to the Engineering department at the University of Manitoba for testing.

"You want me to do what?" said Frank, a graduate engineering student. "Test concrete made with piss? You've got to be kidding!" He shook his head in disbelief. "I thought medicine was supposed to have all the bright guys."

"Hey, they laughed at Galileo too, you know; remember, he said the earth revolved around the sun? They laughed at Columbus. I know it sounds goofy, but that's my project. It was my faculty advisor's idea," I explained defensively.

"Okay," said Frank, "let's see what you've got." I looked around the room. There was a variety of bestial machines – a modern version of the medieval torture chamber. Frank placed each block in a device that slowly applied compression, while I recorded the pounds per square inch needed to make them crumble. The concrete made with water was stronger, but there was no significant difference between those made with urine from kidney-stone formers and those of non-stone formers.

"Ah," Frank said, "Now I know what happened when they built the foundation of my house."

I compensated for the lack of substance in my project with impressive statistics and graphs.

Dr. Daman was the reviewing professor. He was a brilliant physiologist who terrorized his classes with caustic questions that we could rarely answer to his satisfaction. He was famous for ignoring his own health and frequently had blood sugars of eighty, ten times normal. His parties were legendary, too – he and his students imbibed inspiring quantities of alcohol, and held a contest to see who could pee out the flames in the fireplace.

After my presentation, Dr. Daman said impassively, "Mr. Giesbrecht, there's a lot of flash and glitter here, but you really haven't got anything, have you?"

"No sir," I said boldly. "No concrete results." My classmates groaned. "But even in research you have to play the deck you've been dealt." My classmates applauded.

And with that, I secured a B grade, the end of my research career, and my place in medical history – with my classmates at any rate, who remembered me decades later as the researcher who made concrete out of piss.

After I finished my degree and residency in 1966, Steinbach, Manitoba became my bailiwick as a family practitioner. The realities of marriage and family put my previous ambitions of research and academia on hold, which time would prove to be a permanent condition.

## Chapter 3
# FREUDIAN SLIP

Lydia Heinrichs is in her late thirties, a handsome woman in a tailored navy suit and high heels. She has flawless chestnut hair tightly framing a patrician face. She exudes poise, culture, and money. Mrs. Heinrich's nine-year-old daughter Sylvia sits beside her – a prim lass in a flounced pink dress, her blond curls tied back with a pink ribbon. Most kids her age wear jeans and a t-shirt. She gives me a fleeting appraisal as I enter the examining room, then stares vacantly at the floor. Is this formal attire in respect of the occasion, or more likely, a sign of an anal-retentive, regimented family? I put that thought on hold – patients are not likely to appreciate an on-the-spot psychiatric evaluation before I've even talked to them.

Early on, people like Lydia intimidated me. Even now in the early 90s, 25 years into my career, I wonder why I'm being graced by her presence. I'm still not used to seeing the aristocracy of Steinbach society – they are reserved for my older and more respected colleagues. Seemingly, there are times I still haven't made the grade – certainly not compared with Dr. George Jamieson, the doyen of medicine in Steinbach. Mrs. Heinrichs probably can't get an appointment with George. He owns most of the noteworthy people in the community. Anyone

who ranks – business people, those with money or social standing would see George. He guards them jealously. If I see any of
them medically, it's only because it's an emergency or George
is overbooked.

Once or twice in the first years of practice, I had the temer-
ity to ask patients to come for a follow-up visit, and George
quickly corrected my waywardness. It was a lesson in medical
politics I didn't soon forget. Those first years were an education.
I had thought naively that doctors were motivated by altru-
ism, serving their patients and advancing the knowledge of
medicine. It was about that for George, certainly, but it was also
about status and ego. When I was hired, he emphasized that he
was too busy and needed help. Translated: I need help, but keep
your grubby hands off my patients.

Back then, my age was seen a handicap to some. Recent
training and youthful drive counted for little – most folks liked
their doctor to look worn and haggard – sure signs he was
dedicated and in demand. Being young, idealistic, and of an
academic bent, I focused on the science of medicine. I was a
professional, helping people by giving professional advice. I did
my job and tried to get it right the first time. Never mind all the
small talk – patients wanted facts. They wanted a cure for their
plantar warts and mortification (infection).

George was charming, a people person, concerned for his
patients, all of which compensated to a degree for his sometimes dubious medical knowledge. He was a demigod to his
patients, attending to their requests at any hour of the day or
night when he was home. He would take call for his obstetrical cases when he was in Winnipeg or even at the cottage, a
seventy-minute drive from town. David Kroeker or I invariably
delivered the baby – either George was not available, or if he did
race home (he thought he had a special relationship with the
constabulary, who would quickly realize the need for his heavy
foot) he missed the blessed event. That didn't seem to matter to

his patients – the important thing was that he was their doctor. Most weekends, the rest of us handled hospital rounds and new admissions. That, too, was okay with his patients – after all, he worked so hard, and deserved to get away. I never achieved that cult status.

In the late 60's and early 70's we were five physicians in Steinbach. There was an understanding that we looked after our patients twenty-four hours a day. That was the way country practice was done – take it or leave it. During those early years, we were truly general practitioners, providing cradle to celestial-transfer care. We were pediatricians, obstetricians, emergency medicine providers, anesthetists, cardiologists, psychiatrists, proctologists, and everything in between. We did, of course, refer people to specialists, but much less frequently than today. I even pulled an occasional abscessed tooth, and performed a few appendectomies and cholecystectomies under the tutelage of a colleague. My surgical career ended abruptly when a patient lost a toe due to my expertise with a scalpel. She proved to be a sweet, understanding, nine-toed woman.

"Hello, Mrs. Heinrichs," I say. "How are you?" I smile pleasantly at Sylvia and her mother.

"I'm fine, Dr. Giesbrecht," she said in a dulcet voice edged with condescension. No smile. "I'm here with Sylvia. I couldn't get an appointment with George." So she had wanted to see George Jamieson. Ah, well… second choice is good, too. "I want her to have a thorough examination. She is sick much too often."

"Hi, Sylvia. How are you?"

"She isn't very well," interjects her mother. "She has the sniffles, and an infected ear. She had a lot of pain yesterday, so I kept her home from school. She missed her piano lesson today."

I turn back to Sylvia. "Are you coughing? Do you have a fever?"

She glances briefly in my direction, but waits for her mother to respond. She gazes blankly at my diplomas from the University of Manitoba on the far wall.

"No, she hasn't had any cough or fever," Mrs. Heinrichs responds.

I see… Sylvia isn't allowed a mind of her own. Back to mother, "Is her appetite okay?"

"More or less normal."

"Has she had a lot of trouble in the past – you know, colds, flu, stomach aches?"

"She is sick too often, never very serious, but lots of stomach problems and colds."

I check Sylvia's ears and throat, and listen to her chest. There are no swollen lymph nodes and no fever. Her chest is clear. "She has a little congestion," I say, "and the eardrums look a bit dull, but there's no infection. All she needs at the moment is Tylenol and lots of fluids. Give it a day or two. If she has more problems, call me, or bring her back for another look." Would this meet with mother's approval, or is this too dismissive? Am I right in my assessment that she'll be okay with my not "doing something"?

"All right," she says with a tight-lipped smile, "We'll see how things go." I pass the test…for now. I do not suggest they come for a follow-up visit.

A month later, Lydia Heinrichs and Sylvia are on my list again. I must've done something right. I straighten my tie and brush a few flecks of lint from my collar. I open the door to the examining room. Lydia and her daughter are dressed for Princess Anne's wedding. I produce my most disarming smile. They sit glum and impassive.

"Hello, Mrs. Heinrichs," I beam. "How are things? Isn't it cold out there? That wind is just wicked."

"Sylvia has a lot of stomach aches."

Right. No small talk.

"Does she have any vomiting or diarrhea? Any fever?"

"No, none of that. She always has more pain in the morning before school. I've kept her home for two days now. And she missed her art class this afternoon. We need to do something about this." She looks at Sylvia with a faint, distant smile, and pats her hand. Sylvia pulls away and picks at the tassels of her silk scarf.

Sylvia's temperature is normal and she has minimal abdominal tenderness. She looks unhappy and resigned, a captive, like Rapunzel in the tower, but not ill. I take pains to do a thorough examination, mother watching my every move.

"There's not much to find," I say finally, "It may just be a mild viral illness. I think she'll be okay."

Mother waves a hand dismissing my opinion. "There has to be more than that," she says. Her voice takes on a hard edge, and her eyes narrow. "Just a virus? I don't think you're getting to the bottom of this."

I waver for a moment – I'm aware of the tension rising in my voice. "I really think that's all it is. There is no evidence of anything serious. But we should do some basic blood work – hemoglobin, white count, although I'm quite certain they'll be normal."

"Well, okay, we'll see," says Mrs. Heinrichs in a conciliatory tone. "Can she go to school?"

"Use your judgment," I reply, "but she seems fine. I think she could go to school tomorrow."

I see Sylvia and her mother again several weeks later. Sylvia has a sore throat and stomachache, and complaints that are unusual for a child of nine – headaches and fatigue. Physical examination doesn't reveal any abnormalities. Her blood tests from the previous visit are normal.

Two months pass and they are back for their fourth appointment. Sylvia has had another bout of stomach pain. I had expected them to be back in George Jamieson's fold long before this. I am still seeing this family, but I haven't helped them in any way.

"There's something really wrong with Sylvia," says Mrs. Heinrichs, in her usual brusque manner. "She is not doing well in school and she is disrespectful to the teachers. She has headaches, and she still wets the bed occasionally. I'm not pleased – you obviously haven't been able to find out what's wrong with her. I think she needs to see a specialist."

I agree. There has to be something more to this child's complaints. I will have to call on my psychoanalytical prowess, diagnostic skills honed to a razor-sharp edge. "Well, okay. Why don't we discuss this? Sylvia, do you mind going to the waiting room for a few minutes while I talk to your mother?" Mom raises her eyebrows in surprise, but nods at Sylvia, and her daughter flounces out of the room. My shirt collar seems too tight, and I can feel my palms begin to perspire. "You know, Mrs. Heinrichs," I continue. "Sylvia's problems are nonspecific – by that I mean they're vague and don't fit any definitive disease pattern. Every time you come, her complaints are different. I can get you a referral, but the specialist would need something more to go on. I have to be honest with you – I don't think there's anything wrong with your daughter." I take a deep breath, and march resolutely into the minefield. I know I'm right and this needs to be said. *Res ipsa loquitor* – the thing speaks for itself. "I, ah… I think it's her mother who has the problem."

Lydia Heinrichs looks at me as if I have just smacked her flawless face with a rectal glove. Her jaw drops. I wait for something vile to spew forth, but she sits in stunned silence, rooted to her chair.

"Sylvia's tense and unhappy," I continue, Freudian manual clutched to my bosom. I am picking up steam and gaining confidence with each word. I untangle my tongue from my tonsils and summon all the courage I have. Perhaps madness does run in my genome. "I may be way off base, but don't you think that you may be too rigid and demanding, and that's why she has all these problems? Does Sylvia really want to dress like that? Not many kids her age do." Lydia starts to tremble. She raises her gloved hand, but drops it again as I sally forth. "The music and art are wonderful, but do you ever let her do anything *she* wants to do? Maybe you need to loosen up. Show her some affection. Don't you think that might be part ... ?"

"You think *I'm* the problem?" Mrs. Heinrichs has recovered. It has taken rather a long time – I suppose I had the element of surprise on my side and she is unaccustomed to being lectured. "Sylvia's symptoms are my fault?" Her voice could melt your knickers. "I'll have you know I'm a good mother. She gets plenty of affection, and everything she wants."

I bite my lower lip, searching for the right words. "Maybe that's part of the problem," I say calmly, hoping to lower the decibel level. "I'm sure she has the best of everything, but perhaps those are all things *you* want her to have. She wants you, not the things you can buy her."

"I don't need to listen to this drivel. I'll take her to someone who knows what they're talking about." Her tone is best reserved for someone who has just signed his family over to Clifford Olsen. "I should have known better than to bring her to see you. You're an arrogant jerk." She grabs her purse, and stomps out of the office.

I sit for a moment and stare at the chart. I take off my glasses and rub my eyes wearily. This has not been my finest hour. I'm a trained professional, but when things bomb, I find myself second-guessing, doubts clambering all over my brain. I have committed psychiatric hari kari – this isn't how you win friends and influence people. I have based my assumptions on a few office visits – perhaps my analysis is way off the mark. Anything is possible when you don't know what you're talking about. Sometimes doctors need to speak less and listen more. Even if I am right, I could have used a better approach. Gentleness and compassion are as important as science and clinical acumen, but do not always come easily. One moment you're a professional bringing healing to the masses, enjoying respect and prestige, and the next, you're a slug under a rock.

I console myself with the thought that it was time to tell them the truth. Diplomacy has its limitations. Health and family are intimate parts of patients' lives, and there are bound to be emotional upheavals and hurt feelings when they are faced with the truth. She had it coming. Anyway, the die is cast – I can't undo what has happened. However, I determine to finish the afternoon with the utmost sensitivity and tact. Perhaps I should call her to apologize and offer her an appointment with another professional.

After the last patient of the day, some correspondence, and phone messages, I find my parka and walk to the parking lot. It is late January, the air fresh and clean after an afternoon snowfall. I brush the snow off the windshield of the Lincoln, and start for home. Every streetlamp, sign, and parked car wears a crown of feathery white.

I drive home slowly, turning over the contretemps with Lydia Heinrichs in my mind. I turn into the driveway, the fresh snow sparkling in the headlights like a vast carpet of diamonds. The sky behind the house is already blue-black, long ribbons of crimson, orange, and indigo where the sun passed minutes before. Venus is the only visible celestial body, glowing brightly in the west like a distant spotlight between wisps of cloud. Rose had already arrived home, and the windows of the house are bright and inviting.

I stop to shovel the brick walkway to the front door. I could never do that without wondering if I'll fall into a snowdrift with my first coronary. I comfort myself that my family history does not include heart disease, and that snow doesn't entirely deserve its reputation as an assassin. Still, I'm vaguely relieved I can walk into the house on my own steam.

"Hi, honey," I say as I walk in from my flirt with death by snowdrift. "Had a good day?"

"Not too bad," Rose replies. "The usual unreasonable families. How about you?"

"Well, pretty good, except for one outraged mother. I'll change and tell you all the gory details." The shirt and tie have to go – I can't relax still wearing professional trappings.

We sit down in the sunroom. I tell Rose about the afternoon's encounter with Mrs. Heinrichs. "It really bothers me when patients get upset. I guess that comes with the territory – you just can't please everybody. I suppose I had it coming – I was very blunt with the Empress. I hadn't helped her one iota, so I figured I had nothing to lose." I take a sip of tea and watch the snow swirling around the corner of the eaves. "But you know what really bothers me? I have a tendency to be too rigid and authoritarian with the kids, too."

Rose looks at me in astonishment. She puts down her cup. I sense immediately what is coming, but it's too late. "You're kidding! Dennis! A tendency? Haven't we had this conversation before?"

"Yeah…Yeah, I guess we have." I scowl and shake my head – I should have known better – one assault that afternoon should have sufficed. I hate when she is dead on like that, especially regarding my shortcomings. "I know, I know… I was a much better parent until I had kids. I am somewhat compulsive, I'll admit that. I have to lighten up, but it's hard to let some things slide."

"A lot of the things we get uptight about are not that important," Rose counters. "You know, like, will it matter in five years what color they dyed their hair? The kids only have one childhood."

"You're right! You're absolutely right. Sometimes you want so badly for your kids to do the right things and live for God and all that, you get yourself in a knot about stuff that isn't really important. You think if the outward things are there, like they don't smoke or do drugs, then their hearts must be right."

"We just have to keep on guiding them and praying for them, and stop worrying about all the little nonessentials."

"Yeah. Sometimes I wonder if I should be in medicine. I'm too impatient. I don't always have the empathy I should have. Maybe I'd be better hidden in a lab somewhere. Dealing with people's lives day after day doesn't come easily for me."

"Don't be so hard on yourself – every doctor has cases that go wrong. If you really have doubts, we can talk about it later. You'll probably have a much better day tomorrow."

"Yeah, I hope so," I nod. "Anyway, this discussion is giving me a headache. I think I'll slink off to the computer."

Our family totals six – Scott and Jodi, and four older children from my previous marriage. Brent, Kim, Jann, and Carla are on their own by this time, working or in school.

Scott is our youngest son, the fifth Wunderkind in the line of succession, a bright lad of fifteen, with dark eyes and luxurious wavy hair if left to nature, but now unrecognizable with dreadlocks. The dreads had followed blue and orange hair, and preceded tattoos, none of which had been sanctioned by anyone in authority, least of all his parents. We decide Scott had a creative bent, which will eventually evolve into something more mainstream like architecture or engineering. We still had some serious delusions about being in control. "A child isn't happy with nothing to ignore," wrote Ogden Nash, "and that's what parents were created for." The worst waste of breath, other than playing the bagpipes, is advising a teenager. He had announced on his thirteenth birthday that he was now old enough to make his own decisions. This began the Seven Year's War. He wanted to do the right thing, but his parents were so archaic and unreasonable, it just couldn't always be done. Teenagers are an affliction, but there has to be some penalty for sex.

Jodi is eleven, the youngest. She has inherited her mother's russet eyes and dark hair. She's petite and pretty. A sweet child, but with an adder's tongue, sharp and sardonic. Instead of the requisite doll or teddy bear, she takes a book to bed with her every night. Our kids are bright, but not prodigies. Prodigies are youngsters who know how to go to their psychiatrist all by themselves.

I haven't seen Mrs. Heinrichs or her daughter for a year or so. After the previous flameout, I presume they are seeing the royal physician, so I'm astonished to see her name on the list again this afternoon. I'm nervous and edgy. Why are they here again? The threat of a lawsuit? Do I apologize, ignore the past encounter, or launch a counteroffensive? I decide to let her set the tone. When her appointment time arrives, she is sitting in my office, sans Sylvia. She is as attractive and smartly dressed as always, but in jeans and sweater. There are even a few strands of hair out of place. She's relaxed and smiling. The frosty condescension has seemingly melted away. She tells me she has come for a checkup. Who or what is responsible for this personality transplant?

"Dr. Giesbrecht," Lydia says, "Before we get started, I'd like to talk to you about our last visit. Remember when Sylvia and I were here? I'm sure you haven't forgotten. I was really steamed when we left your office. I thought you were an arrogant creep, and told people that. I want to apologize. Thank you for what you said that day. It got me thinking. My husband and I sat down one day soon after and took stock of our parenting. We *were* much too rigid and demanding. My expectations and rules were so onerous, it was no wonder Sylvia was having problems. We made some changes, and she is doing much better. Our family is miles ahead of where we were."

"Wow," I say. My heart slows twenty beats per minute. I feel a surge of self-confidence. "I accept the apology, but I know you were just trying to manage your family as you thought best."

"Yes, but we were way off course."

"I'm humbled," I continue. "I felt very bad that day after you left. The diagnosis may have been right, but I was hurtful. When I thought about my own family, I realized I was too uptight and rigid myself. You know, like, physician heal thyself? Anyway, I'm glad Sylvia is doing well. Thank you for sharing that. Can you tell me what changed?"

"Well, we're spending more time with our kids. We got rid of most of the rules – kept just a few essentials. Sylvia decided she didn't like art classes. She's doing piano and playing ringette, can you believe it? And by the way, she wears jeans like the other kids."

"No more stomach pains or headaches?"

"No, she's been very well."

I have a momentary flush of vindication. "That's great," I say. "You have made my day. I'm happy things worked out that way. Anyway, are you having some health problems?"

"Well, nothing serious, I guess – I'm not sleeping as well as I used to. And my eyes feel a little sore."

I begin my examination systematically as I had been trained – start with the head and neck, then the lungs, heart, abdomen and extremities. I was thankful we were practicing modern patient examination techniques, unlike Hippocratic physicians who smelled and tasted urine, sweat, earwax, and pus. One really had to possess a burning desire to serve mankind.

When I first entered the room, I had noticed, Lydia was flushed and looking a little bug-eyed. "Lydia, please follow the light." I alternately raise and lower the otoscope. Her eyes follow, but I see what I was looking for – the eyelids are a little slow to follow – lid lag, showing white sclera above the pupil. I take her hands, and hold them out in front of her. She has a fine tremor, and her palms are damp. Her heart is racing along at ninety beats per minute, high for an adult at rest, like a car in neutral with a foot on the accelerator. "Have you lost any weight?" I ask.

"Yes, as a matter of fact, I did lose a few pounds, but my appetite is good."

"Any shortness of breath or leg swelling?"

"No, not really," she answers.

"Do you feel hot in a room where others seem to be comfortable?"

"Yes, but I thought it was menopause. My periods have been sporadic the last six months."

"Well, it could be menopause, although you are a bit young for that. I think you have an overactive thyroid. It's as though your thermostat is set too high. You also have what we call exophthalmus. That means your eyes become painful and bulge a bit – that comes with hyperthyroidism. We'll get some blood tests to check your thyroid level."

I palpate her neck again, and ask her to swallow. The thyroid gland moves under my fingers, and I can feel a subtle enlargement.

The rest of the exam is normal. "Okay, here's the requisition. After the blood tests have been taken, start these prescriptions. One is for propranolol – it's a beta-blocker that partially blocks the effect of too much thyroid hormone. It will slow your heart rate and help with the nervousness and tremor. The other is propylthiouracil, a drug that directly cuts the production of thyroid hormone. We'll start with a low dose and see how it goes. Come back in two weeks – by that time the medications should be working – it takes a week or two until the propylthiouracil kicks in."

Mrs. Heinrichs is back in two weeks. "I'm feeling much better," she says.

"The nervousness and palpitations are gone?" I ask.

"Yes, and no more menopause." Her tremor is gone and the heart rate has slowed to a respectable seventy beats per minute.

"Good. See these tests? The thyroid hormone or T3 was high, and the TSH, or thyroid-stimulating hormone is low.

TSH is the pituitary gland or command-center hormone that controls the production of thyroid. Right now your thermostat seems to be set at a normal level, but in a couple of weeks, we'll do the blood tests again, and see if we have to adjust the dose."

"My husband was wondering whether I should see a specialist."

"As a matter of fact you should," I reply. "There's no rush, things are stable now, but we'll get you an appointment with Dr. McAdams. He may suggest you stay on these medications, or he may suggest radioactive iodine treatment. That knocks out some of the thyroxin-producing capacity of the gland."

Dr. McAdams orders a thyroid scan to make sure the over-active hormone production is not due to an isolated thyroid nodule that could be malignant. He suggests Mrs. Heinrichs take the radioactive iodine to knock out some of the thyroid gland. As frequently happens, the treatment destroys too much thyroid tissue, and Lydia requires replacement therapy for the rest of her life. In the ensuing years, she does well, requiring only routine monitoring.

I hadn't seen Sylvia for a number of years, either. Then one day a pretty teen dressed in jeans and t-shirt shows up in my office. I recognize her as the girl with the pink frills and stom-achaches. She is poised and well spoken like her mother.

"Hi, Sylvia," I say. "It's nice to see you again. Your mom tells me you're doing very well."

"Yes. Things are good."

"Great. That's nice to hear. What can I do for you?"

"I'd like birth control pills."

"Oh… okay." I say. This always poses a dilemma. In the 70's, the pill became popular, but attitudes were still very con-servative, and the idea of giving them to an unmarried female was tantamount to encouraging her to have premarital sex. The conservatives said handing out contraceptives was wrong, and encouraged teenage promiscuity. The liberal side of the debate wanted doctors to honor these requests to prevent unwanted pregnancies and dangerous abortions.

"Are you sexually active? Sorry to be so nosy, but I have to ask these questions."

"No, but my boyfriend and I have talked about it."

"Have you talked to your mom about this?"

"Yes, I have," she replies, matter of factly. "She said I should wait until I'm married. Mom says that we shouldn't have sex before marriage. I think that's old fashioned. I told her we would probably do it anyway. She said to think carefully about it, but the decision was up to me." Amazing – an enlightened mother and daughter who have actually discussed a taboo subject.

"Well, I think your mother is a wise woman. Are you sure you are ready for this? Don't get pressured into something you might regret."

"I've thought a lot about it. I'm not sure, but I know I don't want to get pregnant."

"Okay, I won't tell your mom you're starting birth control. I think it's better if you talk to her yourself. I'll give you three months worth of samples. If you change your mind about the pills, throw them out. If not, come back in three months, and if everything is okay, I'll give you a prescription for a year. At the end of that time, I'll insist on a complete physical and Pap test before I renew the prescription. Sounds fair?"

I give Sylvia the samples and explained their use. I never see her again. She may have changed her mind, or seen another doctor.

I continued to see Lydia Heinrichs for routine medical care for several more years until the family moves to Alberta, the promised land of oil and money. I had started badly with Lydia, but our relationship ended well. Lydia took the trouble to call and thank me for her family's care during the previous ten years. It was gratifying to hear from her – patients rarely did that.

**Chapter 4**

# SONS, WHORES,
# AND BANKERS

"Your tired, your poor, your huddled masses," as Emma Lazarus once said, not to mention the hypochondriacs, drug-abusers, and transients who had worn out the patience of the experienced physicians – those people were my province as a new family doctor. It was a proving ground for a neophyte's listening skills, caring attitude, and clinical expertise. Some of these odd characters were still in my care many years later. In truth, I liked the down-and-outers – they were simple folk who appreciated their doctors and thought we were gods. Patients like that were a rare and prized commodity. The common folk were less intimidating – a refreshing change from the pretensions and demands of some of the well-off.

In those days, what the doctor said was rarely questioned. I was a guru of truth and wisdom. We were respected – nurses stood up when we walked onto the ward! And I always wore a suit and tie as part of the image.

When I stopped to think about it, I couldn't believe I had the audacity to tell people, rich or poor, what to do, especially in life-and-death situations. People actually changed their occupation or their lifestyle based on my counsel! What if my advice was way off? I felt a measure of comfort when I remembered the countless people who unfailingly ignored my advice. Medicine was definitely simpler in those early days – fewer drugs and therapies, lower public expectations, and less pressure on physicians to produce results.

Whatever the case, Helen Boyko was one of those common folk. She was a widow from Sandridge, a little village in the southeastern hinterlands of Manitoba. She always seemed genuinely glad to see me, and was always grateful for my efforts to keep her ramshackle, fixer-upper body going. She believed that my advice was nothing less than sanctified wisdom, bless her heart. I was one of the few people she trusted. The fact that it was my job to look after her health didn't matter to her, as long as someone listened.

Helen was squat, two spade-handles in the beam, and walked with a distinctive waddle – the consequence of stubby legs, arthritic hips, and a sixty-year love affair with fatback (salt pork belly). She was shabby and smelled of mothballs and garlic. She usually purchased her wardrobe from the Self-Help store on Bag Day, when an entire shopping bag stuffed with second hand clothing could be had for seven dollars.

Fast forward to the 90's. It's one of Helen's monthly appointments. Daphne, our friendly and helpful receptionist, eagerly awaits her visits and each new wardrobe malfunction. Daphne dresses with a great sense of style, and always marvels at Helen's bizarre creations. On this occasion, Helen is decked out in a purple coat that clashes royally with her pea-green felt hat. She wears pants, multihued fortrels topped by a brown sweater pocked with black stitches that prevented torn loops from unraveling the entire garment. The accompanying bouquet is full-bodied garlic, with notes of five-dollar perfume and Irish Spring.

Carolyn shows Helen into the examining room. Carolyn is the RN in our corner of the building. She offers telephone advice, gives the shots, and gets me off the hook when I'm late or called away on emergencies. "I like Helen," she says. "She's colorful and down-to-earth. She says it like it is."

"Good afternoon, Mrs. Boyko," I say, with my best smile. "How are you?"

"No good," she says, shaking her head. She settles the hat on her lap. I glance at her greasy hair – the hat wasn't really that bad. "Two day I didn' get out of bed."

"So what was the problem? Why couldn't you get out of bed?"

"So sick. Fever, headache. I cough and cough."

"Why didn't you come in to see me?"

She has that patented look of disgust that I had come to know well. Thankfully, thus far it had never been directed at me. She speaks slowly when angry, her words barely audible, and her face expressionless, but with menacing intensity.

"Alex wouldn't take," she mutters. "No time for his mother. He don' care I die. But he have time to go to pub with that woman. She just sit around and eat my food. I tell her get job."

"Who's that woman?" I ask. A new member of the cast.

"Martha!" she spits out. "Alex' girlfriend. She live our place. Bitch!"

I would love to meet this enchantress. However, it's probably an appropriate time to change the subject. I get up from the desk and motion Helen to the examining table. "We'll check your blood sugar, too," I say. "Have you been taking your pills for diabetes?"

"No pills. Alex wouldn' get. He say he too busy, but I hear them in bedroom. They just fool around and wait for me to die. They want my money. I give to hospital and Christmas Cheer. They don't know where I give money."

I try to dispel the images scrolling through my mind – Alex and Martha in flagrante delicto – the strongest argument I'd heard yet for kids not living with their parents.

"You know, Helen, maybe you'll just have to get used to having Martha around. Perhaps if you'll talk to them and work something out, you can all get along. I could talk to your son, but it's better if you do. He is forty years old, right? You can't tell him what to do anymore." Heck, I couldn't tell my fifteen-year-old what to do anymore.

"Whore!" she says. If there really is an 'evil eye,' I saw it that day. Helen waves a gnarled fist in my face. "If my husband living, he use shotgun."

"Well, okay," I say quickly. "Let's check you over. I'll help you get on the table." I examine Helen's chest and abdomen. There are a few crepitations and rhonchi, the harsh sounds of inflammation and possible fluid in the bases of her lungs. And her liver is obviously launching a formal protest. I can feel the edge of her liver four or five centimeters below the ribs – hepatomegaly, an enlarged liver – due to cirrhosis.

"Helen, have you been drinking?"

Her eyes widen in surprise with a hint of admiration at my detective work. "I have lil' drink sometime. How you know?"

I didn't know for sure, but it was a pretty safe bet. She's had problems with alcohol for many years, insulting her liver with cheap whiskey and homemade firewater. Past admonitions had met with limited success. I had ordered an x-ray of her abdomen – it showed an enlarged liver, but no other abnormalities. An x-ray was crude by today's standards, but it was all we had. The lack of sophisticated testing that is standard now, like ultrasound and CT scans, forced us to rely on a thorough physical examination and good diagnostic skills.

I make a point of examining her abdomen on every visit. She is convinced I can tell exactly how much alcohol she has consumed.

"Your liver is sick. You have to stop drinking. It makes your diabetes worse, too."

"I won't do any more. Just lil' drink for Ukraine Christmas? Maybe for wedding." She holds up her hand, measuring a stiff tipple between thumb and index finger.

"Okay, for Ukrainian Christmas. Anyway, you have a bit of pneumonia in your lungs; I can hear some crackling and wheezing, but nothing serious. I'll give you a prescription for antibiotics. Come back in four or five days and we'll check your chest again… Helen, you know you can come see me any time if you need something. I'm sure your son will bring you."

She gets up to go. She fumbles in her purse and produces a fat wad of bills. There is more to this woman than good looks! She extracts a hundred-dollar bill and deftly stuffs it into my jacket pocket. "Here, you take. You work hard. Buy wife nice present."

"Helen, that's very nice of you, but I'm sorry, I can't take that. The government pays me to look after you, and I can't take money from patients." I give the bill back to her.

"Just take – nobody find out." She jams the bill into the other pocket.

"I'm sorry," I say again, handing the bill back to her. "I can't take your money. Besides, you shouldn't be carrying all that cash around with you."

"Alex and that woman – I go away, they look in my room."

"Why don't you keep your money in the bank? It will be much safer there."

"No, my son get." The evil eye is reemerging. "The bank all crooks."

"Okay," I sigh. "Here's your prescription. See you in a week."

I come back to the room after seeing the next patient and rummage in my desk drawer for a prescription pad. There is the hundred-dollar bill. I take the pad and quickly close the drawer.

"Daphne, did Mrs. Boyko come back into the office?" I ask.

"Yes, she said she had left her gloves in there. I offered to get them for her, but she said she could get them herself."

I recount the story later at the supper table. "If you don't know what to do with the money," Scott says quickly, "I'll take it. I need money to buy baseball cards."

"Don't you have a few thousand sports cards by now?" Rose asks. "Why do you need more? They cost a lot of money."

"Mom! There are lots of cards I don't have. I have hardly any NFL or NBA cards. Why do people collect things? Why do you buy more jewelry every time you go shopping? I know those cards will be worth a lot of money someday. I'm not a complete idiot!"

"No," Jodi retorts. "You're right, some parts are missing."

Scott smacks her on the shoulder and the battle is on.

"C'mon, you two. Settle down! Anyway, Scott, thousands of people are collecting cards – they may not be as valuable as you think. And I can't keep the money, it's unethical."

"If people want to give you money, that's not ethical?" Jodi turns up her nose. "If somebody gave me money, I'd take it. Who is this weird lady, anyway?"

"Well, it doesn't matter who she is," I continue. I was careful when relating experiences not to use patients' names. "Anyway, I'm a doctor and the government pays me to look after patients, so it's not right to accept this money."

"Okay," says Scott, "She's not paying you. She's just showing her appreciation. If you don't feel right about it, we'll take the money." I am blessed with helpful and supportive children.

"Appreciation is fine," I counter. "Maybe a blueberry pie or flowers occasionally, but not money. I have to give it back."

"Okay, but can I have thirty bucks to buy some cards?"

"Oh, by the way," Rose says, "Jodi and I are going to pick up our puppy this evening, remember? I wasn't so sure at first, but now I'm excited."

I had forgotten. We had decided that we should get a dog for Jodi and Scott. It had been a major debate. Who would look after the feeding and grooming? Who would take him out for his bowel and bladder functions? Where would the dog go when we were away? We had never talked this much about having another child, although that would have taken divine intervention since Rose's tying off. We'd had a mutt when I was growing up, and I thought our kids should have the experience of a neglected pet, too.

Kim had shared her expertise on the choice of breed. Kim was the oldest of four daughters, a gentle and compassionate girl, who had a warm spot in her heart for all fauna on planet earth. She was in Alberta at the time, working at a resort. Eventually she would train as a vet assistant, a career that suited her eminently. At various times in her life she had owned hamsters, horses, a three-legged cat, an assortment of dogs, a one-eyed fish, and gerbils. Many were skid-row animals missing various body parts, and often came from animal shelters. She had provided good care, shots, and whatever else was needed to nurse them back to health, and she had acquired a prodigious amount of animal knowledge, particularly about dogs. "You should get a Bichon," she had advised. "They're affectionate, intelligent dogs, and make good family pets. They don't bark much and they don't shed." The decision was made.

Jodi was given the privilege of naming the new family member, and promptly christened him Mozart. The name had more to do with whimsy than music appreciation. Mozart was still at the dog breeder's for two weeks of potty training. He proved to be an intelligent pooch, and apart from a few anointings of the family room rug and little brown mementos scattered about the house, soon learned his toilette. He had this melt-your-heart trick of hiding his face with his paws when yelled at for various transgressions.

One of our first acts of cowardice was to have Mozart robbed of his masculinity. In spite of this brutality to his little body, he would clumsily hump whatever anatomical parts of a visiting canine were near at hand, even the occasional human leg, evidence of residual hormones or hard-wired neural circuits.

I had done a little research. The Bichon Frise was first bred in the Mediterranean region as a lap dog for French royalty. (Bichon Frise literally means "curly lap dog.") My choice would not have been a Bichon. Perhaps something halfway between a white powder-puff and a macho, show-em-who's-boss Doberman, but the choice was not mine to make.

The week following Mozart's arrival, the lovable lady from Sandridge was back to see me. I produce the hundred-dollar bill.

"No, I won't take," she says. "That for you."

"Mrs. Boyko, I simply can't accept this – it would be dishonest. You have to take it back. Give it to the hospital, or the Red Cross, or wherever you want."

She studies my face for a moment, and slowly puts the cash back into her purse. But at the end of the afternoon, the money is back in my desk – only this time there are two hundred-dollar bills. How did she manage to do that? Daphne has no idea either. I decide something needs to be done.

"Mrs. Boyko, listen! If you keep on doing that," I begin gruffly on her next appointment, "I'll have to give the money back to your son, or you'll have to see another doc..."

"I can't come see you? Just let me die?" The emerging look on her face has so far been reserved for sons, whores, and bankers. I'm about to join their ranks.

"You won't die," I quickly respond. "There are other doctors who would see you. Mrs. Boyko, I'm serious! I'll be happy to look after you, but you have to stop giving me money!"

She thinks for a moment – the wheels are turning slowly. "Okay, no money," she says.

The money stops coming. I check her liver every visit, and every visit she promises not to drink anymore. She brings wild blueberries, dill pickles, and paska at Easter, mostly for me, sometimes for Daphne and Carolyn. Accepting home produce, we decide, does not violate any code of ethics.

"She's strange," says Daphne, "but she's a sweet old thing."

Nothing unusual happens to Helen for several years. Then one day in late September I receive a call from her. She is very ill, she tells me. Her son is in Kenora, trucking, and she can't get anyone to take her to the hospital. She implores me to come to her house and gives me what sounds like explicit directions from Sarto, a hamlet about ten miles from Steinbach. I assure her I will come that day after office hours.

I did make some house calls, almost exclusively to elderly folk who had difficulty getting around. We didn't do that a lot, though – most people in the community had extended family in the area available for transport, and almost everyone had a car – this was, after all, the Automobile City. House calls were not very useful – they were time-consuming and little could be done at the home. Invariably the patient would have to come to hospital for tests or treatment anyway. I decided I would enjoy a drive in the country, a pleasant break from routine.

I pass through the metropolis of Sarto – four or five homes, one convenience store, and two Orthodox churches, one Ukrainian, one Greek, across the road from each other. The churches are small iconic buildings with modest onion domes. They always strike me as incongruous in such a tiny community, with bush and prairie for miles around.

But then we lived in Steinbach with twenty-three churches, most of them Mennonite. If one denomination baptized by dunking and the other by sprinkling, we needed two churches. If one church used musical instruments, and another didn't, we would need four. If one dunked and used musical instruments, that would call for another one or two. Many churches had a history that dated back to Ukraine, and some of these divisions remained entrenched in Canada. Some church splits were based on loyalties to strong, charismatic leaders. Some wished to

47

remain conservative in customs, dress, and interpretation of the Scriptures. Whatever the reasons, we apparently needed them all and each had their own corner on the truth.

I drive through Sarto and turn south as directed. I'm on a dirt road, well-traveled at first, but after a mile it fades into ruts trailing through tall grass and scrub, as if civilization was a continent away. A copse of poplar, alder, and saskatoon bushes presses in on both sides. The birch are turning a brilliant yellow and the dogwood bright scarlet. I stop the Suburban and roll down the window to drink in the fall air – warm, mellow, and pure.

A bird flies across the trail and disappears into the undergrowth – long tail, brown back, plain-white chest – it must be a black-billed cuckoo. I haven't seen one of those in years. I should have kept my binoculars in the vehicle. I seldom indulge my interest in the avian world any more; there doesn't seem to be time. My astronomical telescope would often sit untouched for many months at a time.

I sometimes resented the demands on my time, but medicine was the path I had chosen. When the calls came, I had to go. I would hear from my associates after any attempt to protect my time. Family and pastimes were okay, but heaven forbid they interfere with patient duties. If you're not willing to make those sacrifices, I was admonished, you shouldn't be in medicine.

The beauty and solitude are revitalizing, but I have a patient to see, and dinner will be waiting at home. I drive on, the bush hemming me from both sides, then after another mile, the trail runs across a gravel road. Turn east, I had been told – there is a farmyard with an old windmill on the corner. No farmyard, no windmill, but I turn east anyway, and after a mile come upon evidence of human habitation.

I drive down the narrow dirt driveway to ask directions. On the left is a ragged file of poplar and Manitoba maple; most have long ago given up the ghost – broken limbs and white trunks trail long shards of bark. On the right is a building, unpainted gray and swaybacked like an aging nag. I'm not sure whether it's a house or barn, perhaps both. There are several old implements, one a horse-drawn mower, rusted and almost hidden by shoulder-high nettles and ragweed. I sit for a moment wondering which end of the building to approach for signs of life, when a dog bursts from behind the building, baying furiously. I open the car door and begin to get out, but abruptly change my mind as the huge animal hurtles toward me, displaying an inspiring set of canines. I'm not about to surrender a mouthful of my gastrocnemius to the dog, but as I jump back into the vehicle, a couple emerges from the building.

"Elvis!" the shorter of the two bellows, waving a pitchfork. "G'wan! Git!" Elvis cowers and creeps away, slavering, his upper lip curled in a sneer.

The couple advances, or more properly, moseys toward the car. I get out again. Dogpatch with Lil' Abner and Mammy Yokum! The male is a vast, ungainly man with a shock of black hair, wearing coveralls with one strap unfastened and dangling down to his waist. He has a child-like, open expression. The female, who must be his mother, is half his size. She has a dirty Allis Chalmers cap covering most of her gray hair, a mud-brown dress, and rubber boots. The corncob pipe is missing from the picture. Mammy clutches a pitchfork, combat-ready.

The giant holds out his hand. "My name Ivan. I'm twenty-six."

"Ivan, shudup." She smacks his arm and turns to me. "What do you want?"

"I'm looking for Mrs. Helen Boyko," I say. "Can you tell me where she lives?"

"What do you want her for?"

"I'm Dr. Giesbrecht from Steinbach. Mrs. Boyko is a patient of mine – she phoned me to come and see her."

"We have cows and pigs," Ivan says, and gestures excitedly toward the building.

"Ivan, shudup." Mammy smacks Ivan's arm again, but his grin doesn't fade. She turns back to me. "Never heard of you. You really a doctor?"

"Yes, I've been in Steinbach for many years."

"I'm twenty-six," Ivan said. "We have a TV..."

"Ivan, git in the house."

"Issat your car?" he says. "I like your car."

Mammy waves the pitchfork in Ivan's face and he retreats. "Mrs. Boyko lives on this road – a mile east on the left."

"Thank you very much," I say. "Goodbye."

Ivan is back. "Can I ride in your car?"

"Ivan!" Mammy bellows. "Git in the house."

I would have loved to have a tour of the establishment, perhaps with Ivan as guide. They might have offered me a swig of Kickapoo Joy Juice. I marvel as I drive off the yard – a cultural remnant of a past generation living just a few miles away from town.

I find Mrs. Boyko's place as Mammy has directed. The "whore," Martha, greets me at the door. The house is old, but the interior spartan and clean. There is a heavy pall of garlic and Lysol in the air – no bacteria will survive here. Martha, the girlfriend, has obviously taken charge of infection control. Out of the corner of my eye, I see the closed door to another bedroom – the images are resurfacing – I quickly follow Martha into Helen's bedroom.

Helen Boyko is lying on a large bed that nearly fills the room. There is a small bedside table with her medications, a purse, and a picture of a middle-aged, balding male – I supposed it to be her late no-nonsense, shotgun-wielding husband.

"Hello, Dr. Giesbrecht," she says weakly. "Thank you, you come. Very sick."

Helen is indeed very ill. She moans in pain as I examine her bloated abdomen. She has had a small umbilical hernia for many years, but it has never caused any symptoms and she has repeatedly refused surgery. Now the bulge is large and tender, like a ripe purple plum. She had begun vomiting. It's evident the hernia is incarcerated with abdominal contents, probably a loop of bowel. The blood supply is compromised and we could be dealing with a length of dead intestine. This is now much more serious than a garden-variety rupture.

"Mrs. Boyko, we have to get you to hospital right away. You'll need an operation, but I think we can fix this."

"I die," she whispers. "No operation."

"You'll be fine. Dr. Sanderson is very good, and I'll be there to put you to sleep. We'll take good care of you. This can be fixed. Okay? I'll have the surgeon see you as soon as you get to Steinbach. If I can use your phone, we'll get the ambulance to pick you up."

I drive back home, and have supper before the hospital phones. Mrs. Boyko has arrived, and I call Jim Sanderson to see her.

He calls back after thirty minutes. "I agree," he says, "The hernia is incarcerated, and we'll probably have to resect the bowel. We'll be set to go at eight."

When Jim incises the skin over the bulge, a loop of small bowel pops out, an angry blue-black. He untwists the bowel and enlarges the opening to allow the blood flow to return, but the intestine remains a mottled cyanotic blue. It's too late – a ten-inch section of bowel will have to be resected before the hernia can be repaired.

Helen Boyko has a difficult post-operative course. She is 80 years of age with liver failure, diabetes, and heart disease. And as frequently happened in those days, especially in people with poor nutrition or cancer, Helen suffers a dehiscence a week after her surgery when the wound opens in spite of several stay sutures (large nylon or silk sutures outside the wound) and a tight abdominal binder. It was not unusual to have a patient literally 'spill their guts' when the sutures gave way about a week after surgery, because they weakened so quickly. For many years, so-called catgut (actually sheep intestine) or chromic sutures (catgut treated with chromium salts to slow the absorption) were used. These sutures lasted 7 to 10 days. Fortunately, synthetic suture material (like Dexon) would soon be coming into use – it's much stronger and takes 10 to 12 weeks to dissolve, so eviscerations become rare.

Helen rallies enough to go home, but comes back within a few days, obviously on her last legs.

"I die," she announces again, and this time I know she is right. Her health travelogue with me has spanned a period of twenty-two years. "Father Sidorski come see me, and he say I go to heaven. He say he pray God give me clean heart. I give him money for the church." I look at her in surprise – she had always vilified the Reverend as just another crook. There is nothing like death staring you in the face to focus your investment strategy.

"Well, Helen, your heart is weak, and your liver and kidneys aren't working very well anymore. There isn't much more that we can do."

"I ready. Father pray for me. He say I have to forgive Alex and that woman."

"Did you tell them that?"

"I tell Alex I forgive, but no money. I give to Christmas Cheer."

She struggles for breath, and every sentence is an effort.

"Did you forgive Martha, too?" I ask gently.

There's a pause as she gazes out of the window of her hospital room. Her answer is almost inaudible. "I forgive."

Helen dies several days later with Alex and Martha at her side. I walked into Helen's room; they are each holding one of her hands in theirs. I walk to the nursing desk to complete the death certificate. Laura, the head nurse for the medical ward, hands me an envelope, crudely labeled, 'Dokter Gesbrect.' In it are two crisp hundred-dollar bills. I smile. Helen Boyko has had the last word after all.

## Chapter 5
# TOURNIQUETS AND OTHER MIRACULOUS CURES

Friday at last. It has been a long day and a grueling week. I have seen the last patient and completed all the charts. I can ease back on the throttle. I turn off the lights, but the curse of modern civilization interrupts my escape. I'm sorely tempted to ignore the phone, but decide it may be something fantastic; perchance a Revenue Canada tax error and they owe me money! It turns out to be a new admission, so I take a quick trip to the hospital before heading home.

It's already dark when I walk out to the parking lot. A north wind has sprung up. The cold brilliance of the moon rising above the dark church silhouette to the east heralds a frigid night. I start the car, then spend several minutes scraping frost off the windshield.

The inevitable ravages of aging are evident as I walk along the hall of the medical ward, irreverently known as the departure lounge – the average age of the antediluvians hovers around 80 and my own groupies, about 85. There are all the usual alluring hospital smells of Dettol (disinfectant), hospital meals, bedpans, and fetid illness. I remember hospital smells from an èarlier age

55

when chloroform or ether permeated everything. Some patients are here for treatment and will go home in a week or two, but many are awaiting placement in a nursing home or other long-term facility.

Some years back, 9 AM was to be an inviolable time of day – patient activities were briefly suspended for the funeral announcements on local radio. If their own name didn't come up, they would sigh with relief and carry on with their day, whatever that was confined to a hospital bed. Beginning early in my tenure in Steinbach, I slowly acquired elderly folks in my practice – I was in demand for my bedside *Plautdietsch*.

Mr. Peter Petkau is the new admission, an eighty-eight year old, brought in by his wife. The ER admitting physician had charted under Reason for Admission, 'Failure to cope.' Actually, it's his wife who has the failure. She is simply overwhelmed with his care and doesn't know where else to turn. Mr. Petkau is beyond looking after himself, what with dementia, heart disease, and diabetes. He has also had a prostatectomy, in order to relieve his urinary obstruction. I scan Peter Petkau's history and preliminary lab results, when Laura, the head nurse, calls, "Dr. Giesbrecht, come to Mr. Petkau's room. You have to see this."

The smell of age hits me like a tsunami as I walk into the room – yeast, urine, and Corynebacterium (body-odor bacteria). Life is not always pretty at the best of times, particularly near the end of the line. The nursing staff has not yet had a chance to sanitize; tomorrow the room will smell clean and clinical. While helping the old gentleman undress, Laura had been surprised to see a swollen penis. On closer examination, she had seen the ends of a shoestring protruding from the edematous tissue. Mr. Petkau's dingus had been unceremoniously throttled.

"Where's his wife," I ask.

"She's around the ward somewhere doing her Christian duty, visiting patients," answers Laura.

Mrs. Petkau is a kindly, gregarious person, who loves to compare notes with fellow pilgrims. It doesn't matter that she doesn't know them all. It's fair game to walk into any room to discover who was there, and inquire as to their health. Many years ago, this behavior was not uncommon among older Mennonites. Privacy was not an issue. It was their duty to bring cheer and friendly gossip to one and all. Laura scours the ward and soon brings Mrs. Petkau back to her husband's room.

"*Mrs. Petkau, wua'room es sein Pessat auf je'bunge?* Why is his penis tied off like that?" I ask.

"*Doa wia de Tiet äwa en Je'lakj. Doat wia mie soo enn'oolet. Ekj muss de Tiet äwa wausche.* He was dribbling all the time. I was so tired of doing laundry."

"This is a first for me." Laura shakes her head in disbelief.

"Mrs. Petkau, using a tie like that is very dangerous," I scold gently, continuing in Plautdietsch. "The cord cuts off the blood supply, and the penis could become gangrenous and might have to be amputated."

"*Oba en Glommskopp,* I'm such a cottage-cheese head (dunce)." She lowers her head. "I didn't know that. I just wanted to stop the mess. I untied it three or four times a day to let him pee. I thought that would be okay."

Laura unties the tourniquet.

"That's incredible, but I think he will be okay," I say to Laura. "We'll see if there is any infection in his prostate or bladder. Let's put in a catheter for the time being. We'll have to start placement papers – I don't think he can go home again. In the meantime, he'll have to stay in hospital so we can give him proper care."

The endangered appendage survives the assault and does not fall off, but Mr. Petkau required a catheter for the rest of his days.

The weekend progresses uneventfully. I make rounds on Saturday and Sunday before church. My patients, including

Peter Petkau, are doing well. Sunday afternoon and time for some reading in the sunroom.

Our domicile had been built on six acres of prairie a few years earlier. It's a two-story house with a reclaimed brick exterior, and a windowed turret like a medieval castle that encloses the dining room downstairs and Jodi's bedroom upstairs. The house is inviting and open, but with enough space for individual privacy. The entrance is large with a full view of the family room – leather couches, a wood-burning fireplace, oak bookshelves. We insist on burning wood – we enjoy the smell of wood smoke, the crackle and warmth of smoldering birch logs. Several Dali prints hang in the family room, the artistic musings of his tortured mind somewhat at odds with the orderliness of the home.

Off the family room to the right is the sunroom with two walls of windows and a few live plants. It's is a great spot to unwind, sip a java and look out over the garden and beyond to a field of alfalfa, and the rambling border of evergreens, hawthorn, and willow surrounding the golf course. Except for one neighbor, there are no houses to be seen; a tranquil island of green in summer and white in winter. Outdoors we can hear the muted roar of traffic and see the city lights beyond the line of trees. The sounds of civilization are nearer overhead – single-engine aircraft on take-off or landing from the airstrip a half-mile to the northwest.

Open to the left are the kitchen and eating area, the heart of the home where family congregates. We love to entertain, and Rose has developed a reputation as an exceptional hostess and chef.

From the entrance, a corridor to the right leads to the library with a green couch, the leather creased and worn, a large window, and oak bookshelves lining the walls. Rose and I have a mutual love affair with books. A story told by Margaret Lawrence or John Steinbeck is a treasured thing, but we have a need to possess the book itself in order to truly own it. My books do not go easily to the hospital book sale, a fate reserved for outdated university texts. Our tastes are diverse; Rose reads Anne Perry or Maeve Binchy or an occasional "you gotta read this one" recommendation from me, like *The Life of Pi* or *The Russländer*. I buy *A Short History of Nearly Everything* or books by Frank McCourt and Ian McEwan. We've accumulated many books neither of us has read, but will "some day" before our vision fails or someone hauls us off to the Creaky Bones Rest Home.

The phone rings and Rose answers. "Honey, it's for you. It's the hospital."

"I have to go for surgery at 3:30," I say when I get back to my book.

"What's the surgery?".

"It's a patient of mine in hospital. He was just admitted on Friday. You know, the guy with the shoelace on his John Thomas? Apparently, he has an acute abdomen now. I knew he had gallstones, but they hadn't bothered him for years, so we decided that at his age and state of health, we would wait and see."

"John Thomas?" said Rose. "Where'd you get that?"

"That's British slang for penis. The leading man in *Lady Chatterley's Lover* gave his appendage that name."

Rose giggled. "John Thomas. Anyway, now you have an emergency?"

"Yeah, I guess so. Sorry, that's the way it goes. The on-call doctor saw him yesterday, and thought it was cholecystitis (inflamed gallbladder), but Mr. Petkau was distended and vomiting, so Jim was called in."

3 P.M. I drive down Loewen Boulevard past a cemetery, three churches (one Catholic), and the Steinbach Family Medical Center, deep in thought, wondering how Mr. Petkau will handle the surgical assault. It's a grey, menacing day in early April with a bitter north wind driving sleet that scours our faces like sandpaper. Winter won't yield to spring without a skirmish.

There are dirty black heaps of snow on the north side of buildings and windbreaks – the last vestiges of winter. The streets are wet and grimy from melting snow and a season's worth of sand and salt.

Peter Petkau is a high risk, but there's a possibility of infarcted bowel (dead bowel from blocked blood supply), so Jim feels we had no choice. Anesthesia in an elderly frail person is like building a house of cards – you flub one, and the whole structure comes down. The human body has amazing resilience, but in an octogenarian, it doesn't take much to trigger a landslide.

I administer the drugs very gingerly – intravenous thiopental, a rapidly acting barbiturate used for many years to induce anesthesia, and Halothane, an inhalational gas to keep the patient asleep. This is still the early days of rural surgery and anesthesia. The first anesthetics I administered were somewhat primitive by modern standards. I did use intubation (a tube for ventilation placed in the trachea) and Halothane. The only tools I had were a stethoscope, a blood pressure machine, and my eyes and ears. Cardiac monitors had not yet arrived in the OR.

Mr. Petkau handles the anesthetic surprisingly well. As Jim had suspected, the bowel is obstructed – the cause: gallstone ileus. A huge two by five centimeter stone is blocking the ileum, part of the small intestine. The bile duct from the gallbladder to the duodenum is usually the size of a thermometer, so nothing but the tiniest stones are able to pass. With chronic inflammation, an abnormal connection had formed between the gallbladder and the small bowel, and the stone eroded through the walls of the gallbladder and the bowel and passed into the gut. A bowel resection needs to be done together with cholecystectomy, removal of the gallbladder.

I phone Rose after two hours into the operation, "Everyone's there?"

"Yes, the kids are all here. When will you be home?"

"I'll likely be another two hours. It's not going so well. Serious case. I'll tell you about it later."

"Okay," Rose says, "I think we'll eat at six – see you later."

"Yeah, I guess so. I'll let you know if I can't make it home by seven."

The repair is more difficult because of adhesions and scarring from previous surgery. Mr. Petkau survives the assault to his frail body, but he will have a stormy post-operative course.

Rose was unfazed by the disruptions. As an RN, she understood the demands – the missed family meals, ball games, and concerts. They were an annoyance, but part of the package. A ruptured appendix or a newborn waited for no man. Sainthood came at a price. It wasn't easy to get together as a family. The older kids were working or in school, and my schedule hijacked many events. I finally make it home by eight.

"Nice of you to stop by," says Rose. "Your man is doing okay?"

"Stable for the moment, but he's very sick."

"Well, you're not on call next weekend. Maybe we'll have better luck."

"Yeah," I sigh ruefully, "I hope so."

I sit down to warmed-up steak and scalloped potatoes. "Sorry, guys," I say. "That's the price we pay – sacrifice for the good of others."

"Yes, dad," says Jann. "We're very proud to have a great humanitarian for a father. It's people like you that make our country great." Jann is adopted and provided a marvelous change from the dreary family DNA. She laughs easily and provides a provocative, irreverent edge to every conversation. Jann is part Jewish – something she uncovered in her search for her biological parentage, and explains why she is never at a loss for words. "How much will you get paid for the afternoon?"

"Not enough. There is no compensation for missing time with my wonderful children. Money isn't everything, you know."

"It's not everything, but it's right up there with oxygen," Jann replies.

Jann lived in Winnipeg and worked for an investment company. Brent was the eldest. He was in university working toward a teaching degree, his wife Glenda training as an occupational therapist. Kim lived in Alberta. Carla was the youngest of the four, a slim blonde, enthusiastic about everything, and given to a theatrical take on life. She was studying at Caronport Bible College in Saskatchewan. We knew better, we told her repeatedly – the real agenda was finding a husband. This took much time and effort – we saw little of her for four or five years. And to prove us right, she did eventually marry a tall, rugged American she met at Caronport.

Early on, family relationships had been difficult. Divorce and remarriage had created an emotional cauldron. It took time to assuage the guilt, forgive, and cultivate trust. Wounds healed, only to open and fester from time to time. The older kids came for visits, weekends, and vacations, but a blended family was never easy.

I finish my warmed-over meal, and sit down in the family room with a cup of coffee.

"I got to drive my boss's Porsche this week," says Jann. "He asked me to pick up a birthday present for his wife, a ten-thousand-dollar necklace. He doesn't make a million a month for nothing."

"Wow," I say. "Talk about filthy rich. Someone has said common sense among men of fortune is rare."

"Yeah, well… Sam just fired his best friend because he thought his friend was making too much money. He's a real sweetheart. But it is kind of fun shopping with his money."

"Well, Jann," says Brent. "Maybe you can sneak in some shopping of your own – you're probably running perilously low on purses and shoes."

"You can never have too many."

"So have you started observing all the Jewish festivals?" I ask. I get up to add a few more logs to the fireplace. The papery birch crackles as it catches fire and flickering shadows dance like shadowy spirits around the room. It was cozy and convivial – just the ticket after a stressful afternoon. Yet I can't quite relax – my patient is in trouble, and I will be called back.

"Yeah, but I was raised Mennonite, so I get a double blessing."

"Hey, Jann, why don't Jewish mothers drink?" I ask.

"Okay, I'll bite. Why?"

"Alcohol interferes with their suffering."

"Oh, Father. Careful. Just remember we're the ones who'll choose your nursing home."

The call comes at eleven that evening. I drive to the hospital and walked down the hall of the surgery floor. Ten or twelve people are gathered in the hallway outside Mr. Petkau's room. Jim Sanderson is waiting for me at the desk.

"It doesn't look good," Jim says. "His breathing is labored, he's cyanotic, and his blood pressure has dropped. He's probably had a pulmonary embolism (a clot in a blood vessel in the lung). I gave him some heparin preop, but I guess it wasn't enough."

I walk into Mr. Petkau's room. His wife is at his side, holding his hand, and a daughter is standing at the foot of the bed, handkerchief in hand. Mr. Petkau is dusky and sweating. He struggles for air despite the oxygen mask. The monitor shows a regular heart rhythm, but his blood pressure is 70 over 45. I listen to all quadrants of his lungs. He has some air entry everywhere, but there's a lot of harsh wheezing.

"We got a portable chest x-ray," says Jim at the desk, "but it was more or less normal. That's often the case with early pulmonary embolism. The blood gases show low O2 and low CO2, which could be PE. Should we start him on heparin (anticoagulant) or send him in?" This was before thrombolysis (clot-busting drugs) came into general use.

"I don't think he has much of a chance regardless of what we do," I say. "Let's see what the family says."

I wade into the knot of family members and explain Mr. Petkau's situation. "Your dad is very sick as you can see. There is only a slim chance that he will make it, regardless of what we do. He's old and has many health problems. We could try anticoagulation, you know, a blood thinning drug. Or we can transfer him to Winnipeg – he's really too sick for that, and there probably isn't much they can do either."

"You're thinking of giving him blood thinners like they use for heart disease?" says Alvin, one of the sons. "What are the chances that will do any good?"

"Well, he's likely past the point where it will help, but we can try. It might prevent further clots, but there is a risk of bleeding or stroke with that drug."

Alvin turned to his siblings. "What do you think? Dad has had a long life, and he's ready to go. I don't think he would want anything done just to prolong his life."

"I agree," says Sharon, a daughter. "I think we should let him die in peace." There were nods around the family circle. "We'll see what mom says. Is he getting something for pain? We don't want him to suffer."

"Yes, we are giving him small doses of morphine just to keep him comfortable."

Sharon comes back to the desk after a short family conference. "We're all agreed that nothing more should be done. He's had so many health problems, and this might only prolong his life for a few days, right?" I nod. "He's had a good life. Thank you so much for his care."

I'm relieved by their decision. With common sense and an unshakable faith, the family accepts death as part of life – in this case, a long life, well-lived and well-loved.

I think back to Gus, a 52-year-old man without the comfort of faith and a caring family. He suffered from obesity, diabetes, heart disease and a constant battle with the demon rum. I had by turns warned and cajoled him to change his lifestyle, but he thought himself invincible or just couldn't be bothered. Before long, he had developed congestive heart failure, which responded for a time to medication. Gus saw a number of specialists, but made no substantive changes in his lifestyle. A day before his death, he lay in Steinbach hospital bed with end-stage cardiac disease. His options were gone. I had consulted the cardiologists one final time. They had little to offer. If we pushed his drugs any more, his blood pressure would drop into his shoes, and if we backed off, his lungs would fill with breath-choking fluid. He had what we sometimes referred to in training as GRAFOB (Grim Reaper at Foot of Bed).

Gus struggled for air, and his face was florid. Between gasps he pleaded, "Dr. Giesbrecht, you have to do something. I can't breathe! Please! I don't want to die."

"I'm so sorry, Gus," I said. "There is nothing more we can do. Your heart is too far gone." He looked at me for a long moment – his face reflecting anger and despair. He closed his eyes, as if waiting for me to disappear. "I don't know what else to say – are you ready to go? Would you like to talk to the chaplain?" He cursed and refused any talk about spiritual matters. He died the next day, obdurate and bitter.

Mr. Petkau dies peacefully just after midnight, his family by his side. I'm thankful for a family with a comforting faith and the wisdom to know when to let go.

When I get home, Rose has gone to bed and the house is dark. I shed my clothes and slip quietly into bed. After mulling over the day's events, I finally fall into an exhausted slumber.

It's still dark when Rose wakes me. She has already bathed. The stupor of inadequate sleep begins to lift gradually, like a mist on a cold spring morning warmed by the sun. I ease into the bathtub. The water is warm and soothing. I can afford a few moments of relaxation before the rush of the day.

"So, how's your patient?" asks Rose.

"He didn't make it. Just too much for a wornout body to handle."

"Well, at that stage it's probably a good thing he could go."

I watch Rose applying mascara to her dark eyelashes. "The metamorphosis is unfolding once more before my very eyes."

"What do you mean – metamorphosis?"

"Well, you know... when a caterpillar emerges from its cocoon as a beautiful butterfly?"

She laughs. "That's not very flattering – the butterfly part is okay, but the caterpillar? Anyway, cosmetics are God's gift to women."

"And women are God's gift to men. I love you either way, with or without make-up."

"But it's a little easier with, right?" Rose asks. She has moved on to the curling iron.

"Well, okay, maybe a little, but all you're doing is enhancing the innate attractiveness. Besides, it's the inner beauty that counts."

"Yeah, right! When a man spots a gorgeous figure, it's just the inner beauty he sees, right?"

"Of course," I counter. "That's all we're looking for."

Rose did have inner beauty – a generous nature, a love for others, honesty, a sense of humor. The external was there, too – guileless, burnt-almond eyes, hair the color of umber, a slender nose, and a flawless chin – finely chiseled features from a long line of Gallic ancestors. I especially loved her French eyes, romantic and mysterious. Mine were a tedious German blue.

"Anyway," I continue. "What are you doing tonight?"

"There's parent-teacher night at the Junior High. I didn't know anything about it until I cleaned out Jodi's backpack yesterday. There were a few petrified sandwiches and a note she got two weeks ago about parent-teacher interviews. We should go, we missed the last one. Her teachers will think we don't care about our children's education. We *do* care, don't we?"

"Well, yes, of course we do, but you'll have to represent us," I protested. "I've got school board… I guess I could be at the interviews until seven-fifteen. Where did Jodi get that messy streak, anyway? It must be your side of the family."

"No, it wasn't my side," Rose said. "When I was a kid, my room was always neat as a pin. Anyway, I'll have to nag Jodi to clean up, it's like a landfill in there, four inches of stuff on the carpet."

Heredity is what sets parents wondering about each other.

# Chapter 6
# A MATTER OF PERSPECTIVE

"I've been taking Gravol for bedtime, but it doesn't always help," Rose says one evening. "Could you find me something else at the office?" She has been having abdominal pain, heartburn, and nausea intermittently for several years.

"I can bring you some omeprazole," I suggest, "Maybe that will help."

"Omeprazole? Is that something new?"

"Yeah, relatively new. It's one of a newer class of drugs than the H2 blockers. They are called proton-pump inhibitors – they block the stomach cells from producing acid."

"Okay, whatever, as long as it helps. I wake up at night a lot because of indigestion. I'm getting fever, or hot flashes. That's probably the onset of menopause."

"Hot flashes? Well, just think of them as power surges. Or perhaps life's next phase of wisdom and serenity."

Rose snorted derisively.

"Anyway, you probably should have the stomach problem checked out. I'll get Jim to set you up for an S & D (stomach and duodenum x-ray) as soon as possible, so hopefully we'll find out what's going on."

An S & D was the gold standard for many years. Today gastroscopy to examine the stomach and duodenum directly and take biopsies is the accepted investigation, and is much superior. A widely-held belief is that ulcers are caused by stress and poor diet, but in most cases those are negligible factors. A major advance has been the discovery that a bacterium, Helicobacter pylori, caused the majority of peptic ulcers and a course of antibiotics usually eliminates the problem. This was finally accepted as standard therapy around 1990, despite the fact that back in the 1920's some researchers thought that a bacterium was associated with ulcers and gastric cancer. In fact, in 1968 Lykoudis, a Greek physician was fined 4,000 drachmas for treating his patients with antibiotics. It just goes to show that doctors sometimes take a long time to get it.

The morning after Rose has her S & D, I go to the x-ray department to talk to Dr. Mel Levitt, the radiologist who comes from Winnipeg on a daily basis to interpret our x-rays. Waiting for a written report would take a few days. I can't wait that long.

"Good morning, Mel. Got a minute?" I ask. He is seated in a small room in a hidden corner of the hospital, a bank of x-ray lights in front of him, dictating. "Have you seen Rose's x-rays? What do you think?"

"Good morning. I was going to give you a call. The S & D itself looks okay, but there is something else that's a little worrisome."

"Really? So what are you saying?"

Mel rummages through the pile of x-rays on the counter and pulls out one of the films. "It's an incidental finding. I was surprised to see it. Here, can you see that?" He points to a faint translucent spot on the liver.

"Yeah, I can see that. So what do you think it is – a tumor?"

"Well, it's a fairly large solitary nodule – about a centimeter in diameter. It could just be a benign cyst or even an artifact on the x-ray, although it doesn't really look like either."

I didn't want to ask the obvious question, but I had to know. "You think that could be a cancer? Like a metastatic lesion?"

Mel nodded, without looking up.

"Really? From where?" I couldn't believe what I was hearing.

"Possibly bowel, ovary, maybe kidney."

"Oh man, you're not kidding, are you?" I say, gripping the edge of the desk. I bit my lower lip. The implications are beginning to sink in. "So what do we do now?"

"Your wife needs a CT scan. I do radiology at Victoria hospital. I'll see what I can arrange, maybe for the end of the week."

I stand a moment beside his desk absorbing this information. Suddenly I feel as if I'm in a huge void, and the bright lights are crushing my brain. "Thank you," I say finally. "I really appreciate that. You're here tomorrow? I'll check with you then about the appointment."

I leave the x-ray department in a daze.

A hundred sinister possibilities whirl through my mind like the highlights of a movie preview. I go to the doctor's lounge and sink into the corner sofa. I cover my face with my hands, uncertain about the next move. It's astonishing how our perspective on life can change so drastically in a moment, as if the heart of our wonderfully complete life had suddenly been ripped out. This happens to other people, not to a doctor's wife. Metastatic cancer! Mel said it didn't really look like anything else.

After a few minutes, I phone the office to cancel my morning's appointments. Then I call Rose at work. "Honey, I'm coming to have coffee with you. Do you have time? I have a free morning."

"A free morning?" she says. "Great, how did that happen?"

"Oh, the staff messed up. I'll be at your office in an hour. Is that okay?"

"Sure. I don't have any appointments until the afternoon. The paperwork can wait."

I make my rounds in a stupor. "Mrs. Suderman is doing better," says Laura. "But she's still short of breath and her blood pressure is a little high. Should we increase her diuretic?" She pauses. "Dr. Giesbrecht, are you all right?"

"What? Sorry. Yes, increase the furosemide to 80 mg a day. Is there anything urgent? I'll be in later if you need me."

I drive the twenty-five miles to St. Pierre where Rose works, oblivious to the highway traffic. It was a dazzling early spring day, full of energy and promise. A green tinge was beginning to infuse the shaggy brown remnants of winter along the roadside. It is early spring, but I hardly noticed.

"Hi, sweetie," Rose says when I walked in the door. "This is a nice surprise." Her desk is tidy - just a telephone, a photograph of our family, and patient charts in orderly stacks.

"Hi. Ready for a break?"

Rose worked as a home-care coordinator in the neighboring municipalities, which included several villages and towns. The health offices were in the basement floor of the local hospital that should have had DNR (do not resuscitate) written above the entrance. The hospital was antiquated and had seen white metal beds come and go. In winter, the steam heating pipes hissed and clanked in protest. The window caulking was crumbling, and during a vicious winter storm, miniature snowdrifts formed on the sill. One memorable weekend the ceiling tiles directly above Rose's desk gave way from a slow leak in the bedpan flushing facility. Fortunately the sewage did not damage any files or equipment. "I've always told you I have a shitty job," she had said with a laugh.

Rose is in good spirits. Maybe it would be a mistake to tell her. I could tell her the x-ray was poor quality and she needed a CT scan. But I knew when the probing began, I could not lie to her.

"Should we go to the restaurant?" she asks eagerly.

"Sure, anywhere is fine."

"Okay, I'll just tell Ginette that I'll be out for a while."

"So you're having a good day?" I ask. "You are always so methodical and organized."

"Yeah, as long as I can keep up with the paperwork. No major headaches so far. I'm seeing a problem family this afternoon, so we'll see what happens."

We settle into a booth in the small main-street café, one of only two restaurants in town, and order coffee. Jumbled chatter drifts from three or four tables, punctuated by the discordant squeal of the café door. "Is everything okay? Rose asks after several minutes. "You're very quiet."

I blink several times and rub my eyes. "Honey, I talked to Mel Levitt this morning, and he showed me the films of your S & D." Rose put down her cup.

"Oh, oh," she says, "*That's* why you're here. Not good?"

"The stomach and duodenum part is fine, but there's a spot on your liver."

"Oh, my word. It's cancer." Her face is impassive – she felt things deeply, but was always in control.

"Mel doesn't know for sure what it is. I asked him what he thought, and he said it could be benign, or even an artifact, but it could also be metastatic cancer. He's arranging a CT scan. It should happen within a week."

There, it's out. Rose is silent. I take her hand and squeeze it. Neither of us speaks for a time, unsure of what to say. I feel my eyes misting. My mind is numb. Rose gazes out of the small café window and studies the traffic.

"Well, you just never know, do you?" she says finally.

"I know it sounds grim," I reply, "but let's not jump to conclusions just yet." Easy to say, trying to convince myself.

"So where is this thing exactly? What does it look like?"

"It's in the right lobe of the liver – a round spot about a centimeter in diameter. It's easy to see, but it could just be an artifact."

"Artifact – you mean a flaw in the film?" Rose says. "That's not very likely, is it? I mean, Dr. Levitt says it's probably cancer. If it's in the liver, it's not usually the primary. So if it has already metastasized from elsewhere, that's doesn't sound too good. Where could it come from?"

"Well, from bowel, ovary, or kidney. I don't know, let's see what the CT scan shows."

"I can't believe it. I thought my upset stomach was just indigestion or gallbladder, or whatever. But cancer..."

My coffee sits on the table, lukewarm and untouched. Rose has a few sips, but for a hard-core addict, used to ten or twelve cups a day, very little has disappeared. We fall silent again, absorbed in our thoughts.

"Should we go?" Rose says, matter-of-factly. "I've got lots of work to do. My high maintenance family is coming at one, and I have to get all my documentation in order."

"Okay. Are you sure you'll be okay? Would you rather come home? Your wretched family can wait."

"I'll be okay. How about you?"

"I haven't canceled my afternoon appointments," I reply. "I guess it's better if we go back to work. There's nothing we can do right now, anyway. I'll try and get home a little earlier."

"Okay, I'll be home around five thirty."

I cancel a few appointments and try to concentrate on patient problems, but my inner turmoil intrudes at every opportunity. I'm done at six. The paperwork will have to wait.

Rose is already home. "I'll make some tea," she says. Cola was the usual happy hour beverage, but today a soothing cup of Lipton's finest seems more healing.

I pull off my jacket and tie, and throw them on the sofa. We sit down on the sunroom couch.

"How are you doing?" I ask. I search her eyes.

"I'm okay. I've been praying. I know God is in charge, and whatever happens is fine. It'll have to be. The good thing is if I die now, I won't have to worry about getting Alzheimer's."

"You're awfully cavalier about this. You kinda sound like it's all over. You're only forty-five. I don't want you to cash in your chips just yet. I want to grow old and crabby with you. We're talking as if this is cancer for sure and you're on your deathbed. It's just a spot – it might be nothing."

I have a fleeting graveyard thought: Mercutio in Shakespeare's *Romeo and Juliet* describes his wound after being sliced open with a sword, "'Tis not as deep as a well, nor as wide as a church door, but 'tis enough, t'will do."

"I know, it might not be cancer," Rose says. "I have faith that God will do what's best for us. But you're right. Let's talk about other things."

"Okay," I say with a deliberate effort. "Let's see… Did you see the tulips by the side of the house are coming up? A bit of color will be so pleasant after all the snow and muck."

"I noticed. I put in a whole pile of bulbs last fall, so they should look good. …I hope you keep up the yard after I'm gone." Rose teases. "When you remarry, the blonde floozy can help you with the flower beds, if you tell her which end of the hoe to use."

"Can we do some interviews soon? I hate to leave this too long. Maybe an ad in the paper? I'd like someone with money."

"Don't worry. I've picked someone for you."

"Great. Is she past eighty?"

"Yeah, but she's blonde and she has money."

"Oh, good," I say. "If she has enough, the money should last longer than she does." We laughed and for a moment, the pain is gone. "But do you mind hanging around a few more years? I really want to spend the rest of my days with you. It's great to find that special person you want to annoy for the rest of your life. Tell you what – some of Regehr's tomato juice will fix you right up."

Regehr was a local legend, a healer who for a 'donation' gave cancer patients tomato juice with a secret ingredient. He could produce testimonials from far and wide about the cancer-busting properties of his concoction.

"Are we telling anyone about the liver thing?" asks Rose.

"Let's wait until you have the CT scan. Then we can share this with our family and friends." We tell no one, not even the kids. We're not about to decant our troubles just yet, but it's hard to remain silent.

The week is hell. Our conversation inevitably comes back to the same topic no matter how much we tried to avoid it. Work is a blessing – it forces me to think about something else, if only for a few minutes at a time. We go about our activities as usual, but everything seems surreal – this monstrous thing has trespassed into our comfortable world. We dutifully attend Jodi's band concert at the Junior High. Tuesday is school board meeting. I enjoy the thrust and parry of debate, and the mael-strom in my brain calms briefly, but nothing seems to be of any consequence. Harold Kliewer is on a rant about busing in-town students – his pet project. He says some kids might have to walk a mile to school, I remember that, but his arguments leave me utterly cold. The teachers were demanding a sixteen percent pay increase and we're offering zero – both stupid, indefen-sible positions, but my indifference cannot be measured by any instrument yet devised.

It's remarkable how little the usual preoccupations of life matter. Everything that concerns our lives – our spacious home, the gardens, our travels, our self-absorbed lifestyle seem trifling and ephemeral.

The kids do matter. We discuss what will happen to Scott and Jodi if Rose died. Scott is in grade ten, and will soon be on his own. Jodi is just entering her teens and needs her mother to guide her through those turbulent years. We talk about their guardians if I were to die too. The four older kids are on their own, and less of a concern.

We repeat all the assurances of love. We tell ourselves repeatedly we are making too much of this dreaded thing. Surely, it is inconsequential; somehow we'll wake up and live happily ever after. We sleep fitfully, and leave for work in the mornings feeling like we have been sucked into a black hole from which there's no escape.

Humor works for short periods. Rose says we had better order the raisin buns and cheese, and I volunteer to call Don Cherry to speak at the funeral. My wife has always lived by the Biblical injunction, go forth and shop. However, even shopping, usually better than a month's worth of Prozac, doesn't cut it.

This is a Herculean struggle for me. Rose is the wind beneath my wings, my best friend. She's my confidante, my psychotherapist, the foil I need to test my ideas and counter-balance wayward tendencies. How will I survive without her? I knew I would, everybody does somehow. Life is supposed to have happy endings. We find a measure of contentment, and suddenly it's snatched away by some stygian nightmare or God's capriciousness. I wish for a stethoscope on God's heart – does he really know what he's doing? I become angry, but ultimately I know that's okay – He can handle that. God doesn't promise unending bliss, only constancy and caring.

By the second week, I sleep out of sheer exhaustion. For the first time in my life, I look forward to sleep, freeing me from the tyranny of thought for a few hours. The practice has always been a challenge, but now it's grueling. My patients deserve good care and I can't let my personal problems get in the way.

I keep reassuring Rose (and myself) that it is, after all, just an x-ray image we are dealing with. There isn't yet any proof of something serious. Maybe it was a bad x-ray, or an isolated lesion that can be removed, and she will be fine. My experience as a physician keeps getting in the way like a black, towering cloud that blocks the sun. What are the chances – a spot like that doesn't just show up, and in the liver, it's invariably a grave sign.

Dr. Levitt makes an appointment for a CT scan within two weeks of that fateful Monday. We drive to Victoria Hospital in Winnipeg in contemplative silence, and after a short wait, Rose has her CT scan. Mel Levitt is there to meet us. "Are you guys okay?" We nod numbly. "Hang around after the scan. I'll have a look at the films and let you know."

Rose and I sit in the waiting room, watching the constant flow of humanity swirling in and out of the bowels of the hospital. I wonder what poignant stories of tragedy and triumph these people could tell, many likely much worse than ours.

Mel emerges after a long twenty minutes. I jump up. "I looked at the scan. There is nothing there," he says matter-of-factly.

"Nothing there?" I repeat, unbelieving. "You mean the CT is normal?"

"There is no sign of a tumor. The CT is normal. I got out the x-rays from last week and I have no idea what that was."

"There's no cancer," Rose says quietly to herself, not quite sure of what she has heard.

"Nothing," says Mel. "I'm surprised, to tell you the truth."

"Was that spot just an artifact, or what?" I ask. The oppressive weight on my shoulders has already lifted.

"I guess it was," says Mel. "I really don't know for sure."

"Isn't that something?" I say. "Thank you so much for getting this done so quickly. We really appreciate it."

It's a marvelous drive home. I don't remember now if the sun was out, but it was an astonishingly bright day. We stop at Robin's Donuts. The lukewarm coffee was superb and even the smoke-cured doughnuts are an epicurean delight.

"Shoot," I say, greedily inhaling the polluted air. "The floozy will have to wait."

"I guess so," laughs Rose. "You're stuck with me. No blonde, no money."

That evening we sit down with our Cokes in the sunroom – Rose's diet, and my regular. The yard looks spectacular through the windows, though the lawn is just beginning to green. Early shoots of daylilies and peonies are pushing their way through the debris of last summer. Signs of growth and promise are everywhere.

"Isn't this whole thing amazing?" I marvel. "What was that all about, anyway? Was it just a smudge on the x-ray? Or was there really a cancer and God took it away? Whatever it was, it's a miracle. It's just unbelievable!"

"Well, I believe it," says Rose. "And you know what? It's gone, and I feel great, and I don't care what it was."

We drink our elixirs with light hearts. We watch as a hummingbird zips about, searching for the feeder it frequented the previous summer. It hovers briefly in front of the window as if to say: "Get with it, you lazy bum! I'm starving out here."

"I'll have to put up the hummingbird feeder," I say. "I guess I should do that this evening. And start on the flowerbeds."

We determine that we will reorder life's priorities, love generously, speak gently, and live simply. Material things will matter less. Life is good, and we will make it better. Although bad habits soon began trickling back, crossing that dark valley has made a difference.

# CHAPTER 7
# THE LANGUAGE OF
# MY ANCESTORS

Now hospital admissions for children are rare in rural hospitals. However, back in the 70's there were a remarkable number of kids in the hospital with minor ailments. Ninety percent of those admissions were ear infections, croup, and gastroenteritis, the majority of them viral illnesses. Our hospital had a thriving pediatric wing, complete with croup tents, where we regularly steamed small children like so many Christmas puddings. Now these illnesses are usually looked after at home. Parents are more knowledgeable, and many have pediatricians, along with the family doctor, caring for their kids

I wasn't in practice very long before I was forced to dig deep into my meager knowledge of German. Low German, that is. *Plautdiestsch*. The language of our Dutch/German/Flemish/ Swiss ancestors. As a child, I had been reviled by Grandpa Giesbrecht for an unpardonable sin – the inability to speak Low German. *Fedaumje Enjlenda* (damn Englishman), he would say. I had slowly acquired a smattering of *Plautdietsch* listening to aunts, uncles, and grandparents, with enough subliminal exposure to become reasonably fluent. *Plautdietsch* was somewhat of an anomaly in my own family, used among my siblings and friends as a novelty – *Schietstremp*, shit stocking, had way more conviction than scaredy-cat or sissy. It had actually come easily once I was forced to use it. In *Plautdietsch*, there was no tact or sophistication – medical terms were colorful, primitive, and earthy. It was amazing how many words were onomatopoeic – the sound mimics the meaning of the word.

Jakie Siemens was a four-year-old who had the extraordinary propensity of coming down with 'Friday flu' until the nursing staff cottoned on to the fact that mom and dad partied on weekends and either couldn't find or couldn't afford babysitters, what with the cost of beer and cigarettes. Kids could really cramp one's style. Mom reported all manner of critical fevers, coughs, and abdominal pains, which healed miraculously once the child was immersed in the healing waters at Bethesda hospital.

However, children whose parents cry wolf do occasionally become genuinely ill. On an early April weekend, Jakie is deposited in the hospital with diarrhea and dehydration – serious and decidedly messy, but not life threatening. Dr. Kroeker is away for the weekend, so I'm called to look after the young lad. I have not encountered his parents myself and know the family only by reputation. They never appear during his hospital stay – weekends can be hectic socially.

Of greater concern than the diarrhea are Jakie's bruises and painful arm, which sets off alarm bells in my head. The nurses have been told he fell down the stairs at home. He has bruising of his arms and abdomen and a large hematoma on one side of his face. X-rays reveal a greenstick fracture of the humerus. The bone in a young child buckles like a green tree branch, hence the name. Jakie screams whenever the nurses approach or I attempt to examine him. After his arm is stabilized in a cast and he receives a bit of TLC from the nursing staff, he is a different boy, although he still has an ill-tempered colon.

Jakie wakes up early Sunday morning, crawls out of bed, and trundles down the hall to the nursing station, peering around the corner of the desk.

Laura is charting at the desk. "Good morning, Jakie. Is there something you want? Do you want breakfast?"

He shuffles awkwardly to her chair. He bends his head and whispers, "Somebody shit in my pants."

Laura smiles sympathetically. "Somebody shit in your pants? Jakie, that's terrible. Who could have done that? Let's go clean you up, okay?" Jakie takes her hand and happily trots down the hall to the bathroom. He confides that when he grows up, he wants to be a "chicken-plucker like my dad."

Monday brings a surprising twist – Children's Aid has decided to intervene and place Jakie in foster care once he is discharged. They have been monitoring the family – there had been a prior incident of abuse of an older sibling, now in a foster home. I check Jakie again and make meticulous notes – this has all the earmarks of an impending court case. Jakie is discharged from hospital to the care of a foster mom. The parents are AWOL.

My premonition is right. The parents seek to regain custody of Jakie. As the attending physician, I am summoned to testify in court on behalf of Children's Aid Society.

Testifying is a detestable duty. I would rather have a Revenue Canada audit. A colonoscopy or root canal would be more entertaining. Being grilled by an adversarial lawyer or posing as an expert witness is not my idea of fulfillment. Frequently the case is remanded, or our testimony is not required, all of which adds up to a wasted day and needless angst.

I am to appear in Winnipeg at 11:00 AM, so I book off the morning. I consoled myself that a small measure of martyrdom will look good on my final résumé. I arrive at the Law Courts building, and I'm shown into an antechamber to await my turn to testify. It's a long, narrow room with wooden benches like church pews along the walls. Several people conversing animatedly in Plautdietch are already seated in the room, a male in overalls and plaid shirt, and two women in long skirts, kerchiefs, and white socks. I surmise they must be Jakie Siemens's parents. The other woman appears to be an aunt. There is a lull in the conversation as they size up the newcomer.

"*Kjans du dissem, waut nü 'nenn kaum?* Do you know the guy who just came in?" asks Mr. Siemens.

I study the portraits of Queens Counsel justices on the mahogany-paneled wall.

"*Nä, eck kjan am nich,*" one woman replies. "*Hee ess soo oopjedonnat – en Haulsbaunt en schmocka suit, hee woat woll nijch aun onse sied senne. Hee woat woll eene fonn dee onnopprejchtije Off'cot senne.* No, I don't know him. He is so dressed up ('thundered up'), with suit and tie – he probably isn't on our side. He's probably one of those crooked lawyers."

"*Am lattet soos en Enjlanda,*" the husband says. "*Oba hee haft korte Hoa soos en Russ.* He looks like an Englishman, but he has short hair like a Russian."

"*Nah,*" asks Mrs. Siemens after a moment, "*waut meen jie, woo waut dit gone?* Well, what do you think, how will this (case) go?"

"*Ech jleew nich sea goot. Ellre habe weinijch too saje disse Doag.* I don't think it will go very well. Parents don't have much say these days."

"*Wie habe aul en Stoot jewacht. Waut ess de Tiet?* We have already waited quite a while. What is the time?"

"*Doat ess haulf twalw.* It's eleven thirty," I offer, looking at my watch and watching them out of the corner of my eye. They recoil as if the late Onkel Diedrich has just transpired through the wall. An uneasy silence falls over the room as they fix their gaze on the floor.

I'm called shortly. I'm pleasantly surprised – the questions are straightforward and to the point. There is no cross-examination and I'm excused in fifteen minutes. A month passes and we get word from Children's Aid – the boy will stay in a foster home. Apparently, Jakie's health improves remarkably after that. He is not seen in our hospital again.

Although my *Plautdietsch* was somewhat suspect, it proved useful early in my practice. Two of the patients I encountered in my first year were a young married couple who had recently emigrated from Mexico. They had virtually no knowledge of English. I was a greenhorn with a medical degree, a head full of ideals, and no experience.

Peter and Elizabeth are seated in my office, holding hands nervously. They have the blush of youth and innocence. They are open and sincere, but with the deferential manner of those in the presence of authority. That's *me*! Whatever their problem, it seems of immense magnitude. Peter has been chosen as the spokesperson and quickly comes to the point, "*Docta Giesbrecht, wie sendt jroots befreet. Wie sendt uns sea goot. Wie hann but nu bloos jekust. Doa mut noch irjentwaut meija senna.* Dr. Giesbrecht, we just got married. We love each other very much. So far we have kissed many times, but we think there must be something more."

I stare at them, momentarily at a loss for words. "*Woo lang seen jie befreet?* How long did you say you were married?" I ask, leaning forward in my chair, wondering if my hearing is deficient.

"*Twee Wäakj.* Two weeks," Elizabeth says.

I'm dumbfounded. I can't believe we're having this conversation. Wouldn't they just naturally find out somehow? When I was 11, I had sat at the feet of my older cousin Dave, who described in graphic detail the unbelievable things that men and women did to one another. Then my education expanded exponentially, when in a dusty corner of a second-floor closet, I found an ancient health text that had illustrations on anatomy and bodily functions. Doesn't everyone get their information from the same reliable sources – the gutter or the schoolyard, or watching cattle on the farm? This couple had never asked and no one had told them? When they canoodled, wouldn't certain natural phenomena just begin to happen?

I would have to call on the language of my ancestors. I had learned enough to get by: "*Pesskjneppel*, penis", and "*daut jeit doa 'neen*, that goes in there, and then you just… well… move." I fumble in Low German for a few minutes, their faces still blank. My artistic skills were not up to even the standards of public washroom graffiti, but I would have to try. I draw a crude diagram on a prescription pad. It's a case of "adult content – viewer discretion advised." I explain the technique as best I can in Low German.

A look of wonderment spreads over their faces. "*Oh, soo schauft daut. Wie wiste nuscht doa fonn. Wie senn sea dankboa.* Oh, that's the way it works. We had no idea. We're very thankful," Peter says.

I'm tempted to add, "Try it a few times, and let me know what you think," but decide prurience would be unprofessional. I watch them leave, hand in hand, wondering how long it will take them to get home.

A family is an entity composed of children, men, women, an occasional animal, and the common cold. Kids invariably hate being in the doctor's office. They are ill and already in a foul mood, so an adult male who administers needles and other forms of torture is not a beloved father figure. Again, the situation calls for an assortment of *Plautdietsch* and English.

Katie Dueck, a young mom, is dressed in conservative Mennonite style with a dark skirt and blouse. Katie brings with her the usual suspects – a family with pinkeye, painful ears, and a rash – four kids, one an infant. Katie's hair is pinned back in an enormous braid that circled her head like a coiled python. She has a sallow face with no make-up. Folks like this are considered lower caste Mennonite society, often looked down upon by the rest of God's elect. Medical care is a challenge because of their ignorance and primitive ideas about medicine. For many of them, regular bathing, deodorants, and toothbrushes are foreign concepts. Katie's English is poor, so we conversed in a blend of mangled English and Low German. She looks a trifle harried. "Can you "sheck" the boys once? Herman is so scratchy."

"Sure, I can do that," I say fearlessly. Herman sprints out of the door and down the hall with Mom in hot pursuit. Meanwhile, Menno discovers the cabinet beside the sink, and pinches his finger in a vaginal speculum. Maria, the three-year-old is wailing her heart out when Mom temporarily abandons her. She has the fundamentals of a cute toddler, with long curly hair and a button nose peppered with freckles, but as Mark Twain said, "A soiled child with a neglected nose cannot conscientiously be regarded as a thing of beauty." Annie just sits there and watches in bewilderment.

Finally, everyone is rounded up. Mom has cleaned Maria's encrustments and is consoling her on her lap. The boys are sitting quietly on the floor, awaiting their turn. Menno has sore eyes, Maria has sore ears, and Herman has a rash.

I summon my courage and approached Maria with the otoscope. She begins howling again, her body flailing in her mother's arms. My attempt to get near her is like trying to examine a wounded badger. Katie says helpfully, *"Wan dü nijch jescheit best, dan waut dän Dokta dei ne Nootel jäwe.* If you don't behave, the doctor will give you a needle." I cringe, and mumble some soothing words, which are completely lost in the maelstrom. I call Carolyn for help. She pins Maria's head in her armpit, grabs two limbs, mother immobilizes the other two, while I manage a three-second look into Maria's ears. Katie sets Maria down, and sinks heavily into the office chair, beads of perspiration on her forehead.

One of Maria's eardrums is dull and slightly red – a sign of middle ear fluid, common in young children with colds. The Eustachian tube is tiny and blocks easily in infancy. I explained to Mom that this is likely a virus causing some congestion, that we will do a throat swab, and I'll see the kids again if they get worse. I explain that the majority of earaches can be managed with Tylenol and watchful waiting.

"Not penicillin?"

Everybody knew about penicillin. In the first decades after the advent of antibiotics, penicillin was the miracle drug, and to most people, the term was generic for any antibiotic. There were only a few – penicillin, chloramphenicol, then sulfa drugs. In fact, medicine was decidedly simpler – digitalis and quinidine fixed most cardiac problems, aspirin and acetaminophen controlled arthritis and headaches, phenytoin (Dilantin) treated seizures, and methyldopa and diuretics were used for hypertension. Early editions of the doctor's bible on drugs, *Compendium on Pharmaceuticals and Specialties,* was a like a pamphlet compared to the massive tome of today.

"No, no penicillin." I repeat the instructions.

"Okay, Herman has a rash? Let's have a look."

Herman is happy for the attention. He willingly peels off his plaid shirt and overalls. This is easy – there are dozens of tiny blebs, many of them in straight lines, and scratch marks over his waist, elbows and hands.

"That's scabies. It's a tiny mite that burrows under the skin, and causes severe itching, especially at night. A lot of the redness and crusting is from scratching. Herman, you can put your clothes back on." He points to his ears. "Sure. I'll look in your ears, too."

"What I should do?" asks Katie. She drops her hands in her lap and shakes her head. Things are not going well. One child isn't getting any treatment, and the second has blood-sucking *Ojesseffa,* insects.

"Well, I'll give you some lotion with permithrin. You have to apply it to every inch of skin from the neck down. Leave it on overnight, and wash it off in the morning. You'll have to treat all the kids. You'll also have to wash all their clothing and linens in hot water, and put them in the dryer to kill the mites. Vacuum all the bedding, furniture, and rugs, and throw the bag away. Then in a week you'll have to treat all the kids overnight again." I repeat all the instructions in Low German as best I can.

"That's terrible much work," Katie groans. "We got no washing machine or dryer."

"No dryer. Okay, you could take all the clothing, put it in a plastic bag, and put it in the deep freeze for a day – that will usually kill the mites, too."

"Got no deep freeze."

"Well, maybe you have a friend or relative who has a dryer."

"I'll see," says Katie wearily, having already discarded that piece of advice.

It's Menno's turn. He's six with an attitude. "Can you sit up there, Menno," I say cheerily, indicating the examining table. I'm determined to help this family if it takes me all afternoon.

"No!" He refuses to move.

Mom tries pleading and threats to no avail. Carolyn has a small stash of lollipops, but Menno can't be bought. I decide to try the direct approach – Menno simply needs to see who is in charge. I grab him under the armpits and swing him over to the table. He hauls back and aims a vicious kick at my oysters. It's a glancing blow, but enough to stop me in my tracks. I stagger and the room starts to go black, but somehow I manage to keep my grip on Menno and to place him on the table. I brush away a few tears and straighten up with great care.

"Menno!" says mom reprovingly. "Be good boy. Not very nice."

My sentiments are remarkably similar. However, Menno had got his licks in and now decides to cooperate. I'm not about to push my luck and look only at his eyes. One is slightly red, with some greenish discharge.

"He has pinkeye." More bad news. "Wash the eye four or five times a day with clear, warm water, and then put in eye drops. I'll give you a prescription. You have to use a separate washcloth and towel, and be very careful – it may spread to the other kids. Bring him back in two or three days if it isn't clearing up."

"Penicillin?" asks Katie. Her face brightens momentarily.

"No, penicillin won't help. There is some antibiotic in the eye drops."

Katie leaves with her kids following dutifully down the hallway like a brood of ducklings crossing the highway. I drop into my chair, and massage my tender groin.

The next patient is a woman of eighty-seven – she should be easy – all I have to do was stay out of range of her cane.

## Chapter 8
# BIG JIM AND THE TWINS

It is six-thirty. The last patient has been seen and the phone messages answered, including a quick call to Resthaven Nursing Home to rescue a woman with a life-threatening case of constipation. The clinic is quiet except for the chatter of stragglers in the hallway comparing illnesses and sharing advice. I have finished an exhausting day sorting through a typical inventory of human woes.

In a rare fit of devotion to duty, (and pleading from patients for completed forms) I tackle some correspondence. Every profession has its curse. No, it's not difficult patients. It's paperwork. I selected two charts from the ever-present pile on my desk – an insurance form and a request for sick time. One or two pieces of dreaded paper work a day – that way officialdom gets its pound of flesh, but the stack, of course, never disappears completely. With each passing year, the tentacles of a giant bureaucracy made up of individuals, insurance companies, and government becomes more strangling. Unfettered bureaucracy brings out the beast in otherwise caring, rational physicians.

I pull the top chart – an insurance request for Metro Stadnyk's family. The company is requesting another report of all his past history – illnesses, hospitals, treatments, referrals, outcomes.

I assure them that Mr. Stadnyk is indeed deceased, that I have supplied all the evidence required, including another copy of the death certificate after they lost the first one, and that after six months the family is hiring a lawyer to end the insurance company's delaying tactics. Writing that letter feels really good – cathartic and satisfying.

Another chart is a request for a letter to an employer authorizing sick time. Trouble is, the employee likely had the flu right enough, but waited until he was back to work to request a note. I hate that – it puts me in a bind. It's usually a cold or back strain without seeking medical advice, then a request for time off after the fact. Oh, well, it would be boring if people always used common sense. I developed a sure-fire pass-the-buck approach – write a note to the employer explaining that the patient has probably had the ailment in question, but was seen only after return to work. The rest of the charts will have to wait for another day.

The short ride home is already liberating, like walking onto a sun-dappled tropical beach. Home for some peace and unmedical conversation. The days are longer now, the air less biting. In the long stretch of turf between the road and the house, the luminous pale-green of late May is emerging from the unsightly remnants of last fall. The last of the snow has retreated to the lee of the willow hedge on the north. I walk into the garden. The earth is beginning to stir, but will need some supervision and guidance. We have three acres of lawn, flowerbeds, and trees, a spread appropriate only for those with an unquenchable love of gardening, or dementia. "You don't have to be crazy to do this," I tell visitors, "but it helps." I have a weakness for water features: a fountain, fishpond, and a large pool with a waterfall and lilies. Tropical water lilies are a favorite – exotic, requiring special care and expertise. After the daily flow of ailing humanity, I'm always eager to get into my grunge-encrusted Levis and rotting sneakers. It's a creative, rejuvenating thing: planting a shrub, trimming a tree, cutting off a diseased branch, changing the landscape one small corner at a time, like refining subtle features on a canvas. It isn't just restorative for the garden, it's healing for me as well. And an amputated limb, or diseased perennial are simply dumped at the nearest landfill – no intensive care units or burial permits.

Fortunately, Rose is as deranged as I when it comes to gardening, and looks after a dozen flowerbeds. Our vegetable garden is trifling by comparison – a dozen tomato plants, a few cucumbers and squash. Vegetables are an afterthought – cabbage and turnips aren't that glamorous.

The ground is soft, and spongy ice still covers the lily pond. I'll have to wait another week or two for the backyard rejuvenation clinic to begin.

I walk into the house and give Rose a playful hug and kiss. "Hi, honey, what's for supper?"

"One of your favorites," Rose replies. "*Klopps* with egg noodles and *Ssipplefa*, hamburgers with noodles and onion gravy."

"Bravo! You've evolved into a true blue Mennonite and a domestic goddess to boot." *Klopps* and *Ssiplefat* – Mennonite comfort food – a bit of a stretch from French cuisine, but adequate to provide the calories necessary to till the soil, worship the Lord, and make more little Mennonites. "Don't you feel fortunate to have signed on with a superior culture?"

"Yeah, right! If the cornerstone of your culture is *Ssiplefat*, it's a bit lame. Anyway, I'll let you take out the garbage while I get the food on the table."

Rose is always "letting" me do stuff, like, "I'll let you vacuum the main floor, while I dust the upstairs." Or a special privileges from a few years back, "I'll let you change Jodi's diaper, while I finish the laundry."

We sit down to supper. "Jodi, is it your turn to say grace?"

She scowls, but launches mechanically at top speed into the singsong:

God is great, God is good.

Let us thank Him for our food.

By His hand, we all are fed – give us Lord, our daily bread.

Amen.

I barely have time to bow my head, let alone think thankful thoughts – though I'm always thankful for *Klopps* and *Ssiplefat*. "Okay," I protest, "Another land-speed record. Do you even think about what you're praying?"

"You could say a prayer of your own instead of the same old thing," Rose adds. "Saying grace is just thanking God for our daily provision."

Jodi pokes around her noodles searching for maggots. "Do I have to eat this stuff? It's gross."

"Careful," says Rose. "I have a recipe for broccoli casserole and I'm not afraid to use it."

"So much for thankfulness," I say. "This is good stuff – it'll make you grow big and strong."

"Dad!"

"Well, eat some noodles with butter if you like," Rose says.

"Can I put Velveeta on them?"

"Sure, go ahead. You should eat some meat and carrots, too. So, Scott, how was school today?"

"Fine."

"Did you learn anything interesting?"

"Nope."

Jodi slathers her noodles with great gobs of cheese. Rose has a determined look on her face – we are going to have a pleasant family meal, including genuine conversation. She organizes the contents of her plate into ethnic neighborhoods while she plans her next topic.

"How was your day, Jodi?"

"Okay."

"Anything happen in school?"

"Mom!"

Rose keeps poking at her food. Jodi grabs Rose's plate. "Mom, why do you always do that?" She rapidly rearranges the noodles, meatballs and carrots, and hands the plate back to Rose. "Here, it's all organized. Now you can eat."

After a momentary flash of anger, Rose laughs. "Okay, okay. Dennis, how was your day?"

"Fine."

"All your cases went well?"

"Yeah."

I had to illuminate the path for crabby, wayward people all day. I'm fervently dissecting my meatballs, with *Ssipplefat* caressing my palate and salvaging my precipitously low blood cholesterol. And there is no stress in the vicinity of *Klopps* and *Ssipplefat* (and strawberry-rhubarb pie).

"Boy, you guys are great company," says Rose. "Can't we have a nice discussion at supper time once in a while?"

"Then tell us about your day," Scott retorts without looking up.

"Okay, I will!" Rose replies. "I saw a very interesting woman on a home visit. She lives in a little farmhouse on the edge of Winnipeg. She could have written the book on obsessive-compulsive disorders. Everything is lined up in her pantry and fridge, with the tallest items at the back and spaced the same distance apart. Even the hangers in her closet are exactly one inch apart."

"So, why did you have to see her?" asks Scott, between mouthfuls. Grandma love this boy. He eats anything.

"Well, she was driving her husband nuts with her constant cleaning and polishing. It took her an hour to polish the kettle, another hour to clean her glasses with Kleenex and a toothpick. Her husband was starving because she needed four hours to make a simple meal and clean up the dishes. We suggested they use paper plates and TV dinners. Can you imagine a person like that?"

"Mom!" says Jodi. "Who loads the dishwasher so each compartment has a daddy knife, a mommy fork, and children spoons?"

Rose smiles. "Well, I'm just trying to make housework less boring."

I quickly change the subject to divert the kids from bringing up *my* compulsions. Just because I sort my M & M's before I eat them doesn't mean I'm not sane and balanced. "Where is Mozart? He's usually patrolling the table hoping for a tidbit." I get up for a glass of ice water from the fridge dispenser.

"Oh," says Rose, "he's in his kennel in the laundry room. He had his haircut today. I told the dog groomer to cut his hair short, but she pretty much shaved him. He's embarrassed about his nudity and won't come out."

"Weird dog," I say.

"That's not so weird," Scott says. "Would you come out of the bathroom if somebody shaved off all your hair?" I choke on a mouthful of noodles. Everyone laughs. At last the kids are enjoying mealtime.

"We'll have to get him a little sweater," responds Jodi. "Then he won't be naked."

"Good idea!" Rose agrees. "Tomorrow I'll see if the pet shop has one. I had to bring his dish to the kennel so he would eat."

The sweater had solved the problem. Mozart emerged from his self-imposed exile only while wearing the garment until his hair grew in. We could always tell when he was himself – any handclap or toss of his chew toy would send him off on a frenzied race through the house, around furniture, through the dining room, all the while growling ferociously – like he'd been given an overdose of amphetamines. This was apparently a characteristic behavior of his breed, known informally as the 'Bichon Buzz.'

Mozart loved people and the moment strangers came in the door, he would wag his tail furiously and sniff everything within reach. A watchdog he was not – any intruder would be greeted: "Welcome, thieves, help yourselves. Just let me smell your pants and you can take whatever you want." Mozie, as he came to be known, adored Rose and followed her everywhere. Mornings when I emerged from the bedroom, Mozie would be waiting at the door, looking past me as if to say: 'Please, get out of the way and allow me a glimpse of my beloved queen.'

The telephone rings. "Dad," calls Jodi. "It's for you."

It's Myrna, an RN from the emergency department, "Dr. Giesbrecht, there's a Mr. Ivan Hanchuk here with an itchy rash."

"Great," I say. "Let me guess – he's had it for two weeks."

"Yeah, how did you know that? He says it's really bothering him today, and he hasn't had time to come in before."

"So where's the rash?"

"He won't tell me."

"Oh, there. Maybe he has the carnal flu (gonorrhea)."

"What?" asked Myrna. "I don't think it's the flu."

"Sorry. Just kidding. He could have come to the office during the day. Two weeks, and now it's an emergency." I sigh loudly for dramatic effect. "Okay, tell him I'll be there shortly."

"What's the problem?" asks Rose.

"Some guy with a rash. I'll be back soon. I might as well do it now and maybe I can have dessert in peace."

Still chafing, I drive to the hospital in the Jeep Cherokee we had recently acquired. Although a bonus in winter, four-wheel power was not the sole reason we bought a Jeep. I'm in mid-life (okay, a bit beyond) and my youth is fading. My usual sedans were dreary and uncool. I needed something sexier. I couldn't afford a Harley *and* a car. The kids thought the Jeep was way more hip – a Lincoln Continental has very little cachet on the schoolyard.

I work unsuccessfully on my attitude. Isn't Ivan Hanchuk just typical? Have people no consideration? I'll have to give this ingrate my patented spiel on respect for other people's time and the proper use of our precious health care dollars. I work hard and deserve a little quality time with my family. My righteous indignation has reached a fever pitch. By the time I drive into the outskirts of town, I have my lecture well rehearsed.

I'm going over the speed limit, a bad habit of many years. Periodically I would get a ticket, which would for a short time temper my need for speed. I wouldn't dream of helping myself to money that I hadn't earned or walking out of a store with a CD in my pocket, but speeding? That wasn't really breaking the law, especially when I was racing to save another life.

I'm about to move on to another of the many injustices I suffer each day, when I spot a police cruiser partly hidden on a side street, lying in wait for his unsuspecting quarry, like a hunter in a blind waiting to blast a hapless duck out of the sky. The red cherry bursts into life as I whiz by. I continue driving the two blocks to the back entrance of the hospital, with the officer in hot pursuit, lights flashing. Doesn't the RCMP have better things to do than to hassle upstanding, law-abiding citizens? I wave my stethoscope as I jump out of my car, race to the emergency department and disappear behind the curtain where Ivan Hanchuk is waiting. I'm breathless from the thrill of the chase. The officer follows me into the hospital and walks up to the desk.

"Was that Dr. Giesbrecht?" he asks Myrna.

"Yes, it was."

"Did you call him to come to the emergency department?"

"Yes, I did – there's a patient waiting for him."

I listen from behind the curtain, wondering if he will ask the next logical question: is this really an emergency? No more questions. The officer turns on his heel and walks back to his cruiser.

My frustration has dissolved, but my pulse is still racing. I have taken on the highwayman and won. This time.

"Hello, Mr. Hanchuk, how are you?" I say amiably. "Nice to see you. What seems to be the problem?"

"I'm glad you came, doc. Sorry about the time, but Big Jim and the Twins are driving me crazy."

He points to his crotch.

"Big Jim and the Twins?" I guffaw, hanging onto the examining table. "A rash?" I break up again. "Well, let's have a look," I say when I have recovered. "Are you a trucker, by any chance?"

"Yeah." He looks up in surprise. "How did you know? I drive long distance." He drops his pants to show me the fiery contagion on his privates. The scrotum looks extraordinarily prickly and distressing.

"I thought so," I say. "The Twins have a fungus." I chortle again. This rash seems to be an occupational hazard for long-distance truckers. The long hours of sitting contribute to the problem, together with tight skivvies and jeans. "We can fix that – at least for a while. Wash the area frequently and dry well. You need more air to keep the area dry – using boxer shorts and loose-fitting lightweight pants might help. I'll give you some anti-fungal crème to use a couple of times a day." I was about to suggest a small fan mounted under the dashboard aimed at the strategic area, but decide that this is probably a bit over the top.

"Thank you so much," he says. "Sorry again about the time, but when you're on the truck for days, keeping appointments is very difficult."

"Sure, any time, Ivan. Glad to help. By the way, don't you have a family doctor? You should have a physical to make sure everything is okay. Rashes like that are sometimes the first sign of diabetes."

"I don't really have a family doctor. I don't think I have diabetes. There's nothing like that in our family, but I'll have a checkup sometime."

My little homily never even comes to mind.

I drive more slowly on the way home. My conscience pricks me; it can be such a hindrance. Being in possession of a Mennonite conscience is a formidable thing not to be trifled with. I will have to work either on my conscience or my behavior, but I can't decide which would be easier. The two are probably closely linked, but anesthetizing my conscience any further would not be a good thing. I got away without a speeding ticket, but this had not been an emergency, and I had abused my position.

Scott and Jodi have already scattered when I get home. They are impatient and have things to do. As always, when meals are interrupted, Rose has saved a cup of tea to keep me company. I tell her the whole sordid tale.

"Wouldn't it be better just to stick to the speed limit?" she says. "And maybe you should review your Hippocratic Oath."

The Hippocratic Oath? She is right of course, and irritatingly logical to boot. With a wife, who needs a conscience? My wife has not an ounce of hypocrisy in her body – I totally hate that in a person.

The Hippocratic Oath. Medical ethics – do no harm, patient confidentiality, teach the art and healing of medicine, benefit the sick without intent of personal gain – all wonderful things. Never mind that Hippocrates recommended never using a knife! "There is nothing in there about speeding or thumbing your nose at the RCMP," I say. "But you're right, that was kinda dumb."

Doctors really do care about their patients. When I started practice, I wasn't sure it would really be like that. We do the best we can for our patients, of course. We might even care about them in a professional way. But I soon realized that patients make or break our days. We think about, talk about, dream about our patients. We worry about them 60 hours a week, and often when we shouldn't. Like when the kids want to go for ice cream. Or when certain marital opportunities present themselves. Romance is decidedly less so when you can't get a patient's bowel obstruction off your mind.

As doctors we do, of course, lead electrifying lives – every day filled with drama, romance, and adrenalin-fueled life-and-death decisions. Nowadays we see it regularly on ER, or Grey's Anatomy. There is also an astonishing amount of sex in medicine. Well…on TV, anyway.

"Honey," I say as Rose and I relax with Earl Grey, "do you ever get irritated with the questions people ask?"

"What kind of questions?"

"Oh, you know. You meet a casual acquaintance, and the small talk begins: 'Lots of sick people? I hear there's lots of flu going around,' or your dad's all-time favourite, 'Is the hospital full?'"

"Yes, I know," Rose replies. "I get asked those questions too. Like… 'I could never be a nurse. How can you take all that blood and vomit, and…?' Usually accompanied by a shudder."

"Another one, 'I guess it's hard being a doctor, but it must be very rewarding.' Someday I'll put an item in the Carillon News":

For the reader who has always wondered, but was afraid to ask, here are the answers to the top questions people ask doctors:

1. Yes, there are lots of sick people.
2. Yes, there's lots of flu going around.
3. Yes, the hospital is full.
4. Yes, it's very hard being a doctor, but
5. Yes, it's very rewarding.
6. No, you never get used to getting up at night.
7. If any of these things ever change, I will
    put another notice in this paper.

"Why are you so crabby," asks Rose. "Are you off your prescription drugs again?" She laughs maniacally. "People are just trying to be friendly. Most people are very grateful for what we do. By the way, I forgot to tell you – we're going to a birthday party for my mom on Saturday. It's going to be supper at the Bright Pearl restaurant."

"Rats," I say. "That's our only night off this week."

"Well, I know, we have too many things on the go, but family is important, too."

"Yes, but with your five sisters and five brothers, and your mom and dad, that averages to one birthday per month, and then all the other things your family celebrates."

"We don't go to nearly all of them. When was the last birthday we attended?"

"I don't remember," I whine. "But it can't be that long ago. Your family gets together for something almost every weekend. You can go if you want, I think I'll stay home."

A cold front has suddenly moved in – probably climate change. I catch the body language too – grim face, eyes straight ahead.

I read something about the female brain – the wiring for communication is better than in the male brain. As a matter of fact, in the male embryo, a blast of testosterone nukes the communication center. A woman uses an average of 20,000 words a day, a male, 7,000. Rose didn't need nearly that many to let me know I was in deep doodoo.

I have my shortcomings. Rose does too, but they are trivial compared to mine. We occasionally have arguments that dissolve into charged silences that may last several days, like the Cold War with occasional disarmament talks.

"Fine, go ahead." Rose gets up and walks to the kitchen.

"Anger is just misdirected passion," I yell after her. She ignores me. I pale at the word *fine* – it's something women use to end an argument when they are right and you need to shut up;

and *go ahead* – this is a dare, not permission – do it at your peril. I should know by now, don't speak unless you can improve on silence. I had better buy a gift, perhaps flowers or lingerie. Or chocolates – they're better because no one gets upset if you buy extra large. Chocolate does have many redeeming qualities.

Really, I like women better than men. Men are okay – if you want a good laugh or an informed discussion about the Blue Jays or a late model Ferrari, it'll have to be a guy. But women are gentler, more mysterious, look better, and smell nicer. They also drive us nuts, and bring doctors more business.

I think about our squabble over families. After Rose's brush with cancer, we were determined to restructure our priorities. With the pressures of practice and community responsibilities, it wasn't always easy to stop and smell the Roses. Or spend time with the kids. Or... go to family birthdays.

On the subject of families, I was blown away by Rose's family tree. They were Lesages – the Wise Ones. I keep forgetting that. Someone had traced her family back to three brothers who were the confreres of Samuel de Champlain, the Father of New France, then back all the way to 1066, the Battle of Hastings.

My immediate family was more simple – ah... make that uncomplicated. My parents had passed away some years ago. I had an older brother, who was a retired electrical engineer, a sister who was a schoolteacher, and a handicapped sister with hydrocephalus living in a nursing home. My oldest sister was also handicapped with very poor eyesight and hearing. All lived in Winnipeg. A younger brother lived in Montreal with his wife, both psychiatrists. The Manitoba connection would see each other once or twice a year if we were lucky – at Christmas, and whenever long absence prompted contact.

My mother was a Dyck by birth. The Dyck family tree were direct descendants of Sir Anthony Van Dyck, the foremost seventeenth century Flemish painter, a very talented, handsome, and debonair man, who was knighted and appointed court painter by Charles I of England. Well, okay... all the above is true except the part about Mom's family being his descendants. With a twinkle in her eye, she loved to tell me the nobility version of our ancestry. I eventually discovered this story was totally in jest.

Grandpa Dyck's first wife died and left him with nine children. His second marriage to my mom's mother resulted in another twelve children. When Grandpa Dyck passed away, Grandma remarried after several years. Her second husband, Grandpa Warkentin brought another six children from another marriage into the hopper. Family gatherings were mind-boggling. Mom had brothers and sisters, stepbrothers and stepsisters, half-brothers and half-sisters, with all their spouses and children. The family soon rivaled the entire population of Lichtenstein.

Dad's family consisted of one brother and seven sisters – most were farmers who lived within a few miles of the home-stead. Dad's mother was a woman of mercurial moods: cold, grim, and manipulative. She was adept at playing one child against another, vilifying on one hand, and handing out lavish gifts to favorites on the other. Grandpa was defeated and bitter. I was terrified of both. In spite of this, there were many functions, or more correctly, dysfunctions that we celebrated – Christmas, Easter, *Himmelfoat* (Ascension), Thanksgiving. Grandma's birthday, and Grandpa's birthday, even after he had passed away. At these gatherings, vast quantities of weapon's-grade rations were consumed – roast chicken, *bobbat,* (a stuffing of sweet dough fortified with raisins and prunes), *holupshie,* (cabbage rolls filled with ground pork and rice), and *rollkuake* and *rebues,* (deep-fried puff pastry and watermelon) – and the list goes on. Food was up there on the Mennonite manifesto of life, right after attending church.

It is now several months after our argument about families. By this time, I have been to several birthday parties, and learned just how important families are.

I'm greeted by the jarring sound of the telephone as I walk in the door after clinic hours. It's downright annoying – you can't get away from Alexander Graham Bell's irksome invention unless you're a hermit in the wilds of southeastern Manitoba.

"Dennis, the phone is for you – it's the hospital," says Rose.

"I talked to them just before I left the office, like ten minutes ago."

"Well, ER wants to talk you again."

"Hi, Dr. Giesbrecht." Myrna is on duty again. "Mr. Hanchuk is here. He says you are his doctor and he needs to see you."

"Oh, really? The only time I've seen him was a few months ago with a rash. What's his problem today?"

"He can't hear. He says his ear is plugged."

"Let me guess – he's had it for two weeks. Only five days? Okay, whatever. I'll be there shortly."

Ivan Hanchuk has impacted cerumen (earwax) which is easily flushed out with our little water cannon. "Ivan, you can't make it to the clinic for these things?" I ask. Again, I chicken out on the sermon.

"I'm on the road a lot, and when I get home, there are so many things to look after, I just don't have time for appointments. But I haven't forgotten – sometime I'll come for a physical."

I'm not convinced. He has likely settled into a habit, as some do, of using the system when it suited his timetable. Ivan was only mildly annoying compared to the hockey players who suffer a laceration, continue the game to its conclusion, and then bend the elbow at the local tonsil-washing emporium with their buddies before arriving in ER at 1 AM for suturing.

Nine months later, I have another call from ER, this time just before I leave the house for work in the morning.

Cathy, another RN, is on the phone. "There's a Mr. Hanchuk here. His wife says you are his doctor. He doesn't look so good. He's very lethargic, short of breath, and seems dehydrated."

"Okay, I'll be there in a few minutes."

I arrive in ER and Cathy briefs me, "He's in room 3. His blood pressure is low, and he's a little confused." This time Mr. Hanchuk seems truly ill.

Ivan's wife is at his side in the examining room. She anxiously jumps up, her brow furrowed. Ivan is lying on a stretcher mumbling incoherently between labored breaths. He looks flushed. "Hi, Mrs. Hanchuk," I say. "Your husband looks very sick. What's the story?"

"Dr. Giesbrecht, thanks so much for coming. He came home from a trip yesterday with a big boil on his leg," she answers. "He was very tired, so I sent him to bed with some Tylenol. This morning he started vomiting and his breathing was funny."

"Was he very thirsty or peeing a lot?"

"Yeah, I guess he was, come to think of it."

I do a quick examination. He is breathing heavily, but his lungs are clear. His breath has the telltale sickly-sweet smell of ketones, produced when the body is unable to use glucose for fuel because of a lack of insulin, and burns muscle and fat instead. This produces fatty acids, which are oxidized into ketones. Ivan's tongue is dry and the skin on his arms and abdomen does not spring back when pinched – a sign of dehydration. I pull the trouser legs up to reveal a bulging furuncle just below his knee, with a large area of swollen, angry skin around it. The infection has likely developed because of diabetes, and may have precipitated the crisis.

"Your husband has diabetes. He's probably had it for a while, but now he has something we call ketoacidosis or diabetic shock. That's why he has this strange breathing. We'll get some tests done, and start him on fluids and insulin."

"Oh my," she says, her eyes wide. "I told him the last time he was home he should go for a checkup. He wasn't feeling good, but he said he would be okay."

Ivan's blood sugar is 56 mcg per milliliter, nine times the normal level. His serum potassium and sodium are both low – evidence of dehydration and metabolic imbalance.

Ivan has likely had diabetes for some time, if I think back to his fungal rash. Infections are more common in diabetes because of the high blood sugar levels. We start him on intravenous fluids, and a slow infusion of insulin. His blood sugars are monitored every hour, but the insulin resistance would not break until he had received 270 units of IV insulin. I order a gram of Cloxacillin every six hours for the infection. The most likely organism would be staph, at that time still sensitive to the penicillin family of antibiotics.

I go back to see him just before office hours in the afternoon, and again at 6 p.m. "Hi, Mr. Hanchuk, how are you doing? You're looking a lot better. You were a very sweet man this morning."

"Hi, doc. Yeah, I'm starting to feel better." He looks comfortable now. The labored breathing is gone, and his skin has lost most of the wrinkled, flabby appearance. His last blood sugar is 15.

"Okay," I say. "We're going to stop the intravenous insulin, and start you on injections of long-acting insulin. We'll keep the IV for now. In the meantime, we have to open that boil on your leg. I'll put some freezing in the area, although it doesn't take very well with infection, so you'll have some pain. We don't want to use a general anesthetic right now, okay?"

"Sure, I'm tough, go ahead."

Laura brings a small tray with instruments. I draw up 5 ccs. of xylocaine in a syringe and inject over the white bulge. There's a small area of necrosis where the abscess is ready to rupture, so the incision causes only mild discomfort. I cut an X into the abscess and a small volcano of pus erupts from the wound. The painful part is irrigating to remove as much pus as possible and then inserting a long packing strip into the wound to keep it from closing before it healed.

Ivan's leg heals well on antibiotics and good diabetic control, but it takes several weeks. His sugars hover between 6 and 9 on metformin and a twice-daily dose of insulin. He continues trucking, but manages to maintain regular clinic visits. Surprise – Ivan turns out to be a model patient.

The diabetic crisis finally got his attention – he attends a diabetic teaching clinic, learns to monitor his own blood sugars at home, and takes meticulous care of his health. His ongoing care becomes routine, the way it should be when people take their health seriously.

## Chapter 9
# THE CASE OF THE WANDERING MAMMARY

"We'll look after your things while you see the doctor," Carolyn says. Emma trundles slowly behind her down the hall of the clinic.

"No! I'll keep my stuff. Somebody will steal it."

"Nobody is going to steal your stuff, Mrs. Smith. It will be quite safe."

"I'll look after it. Don't call me Mrs. Smith. I'm no Mrs." Emma follows into the examining room, formidable in her enormous trench coat surrounded by five or six shopping bags.

"Okay, Emma," replies Carolyn. "Have a seat. What do you want to see the doctor about?"

"Got a rash on my ass."

"Oh," Carolyn says in surprise. "Okay... Dr. Giesbrecht will be with you shortly."

Carolyn catches me coming out of the supply room. "Emma Smith is here – you know, the bag lady? She has a rash on her butt. Well... that's not exactly the word she used. She's certainly a crotchety old thing."

With her lifestyle, Emma was something of a celebrity in town back in the 70's. Steinbach seemed an unlikely setting for someone living on the street, but perhaps there was less competition than in the big city. No doubt she had a history, but she was not about to divulge any of it.

Emma always made a fashion statement – her mousy grey hair had not had the benefit of shampoo or a comb for many moons. She wore an ankle-length, grimy blue coat, winter and summer – it was easier to wear it than to carry it – and it bulged oddly with her belongings. She was on the downhill side of sixty, and her face was blotched and leathery like an over-cooked pizza, likely a result of long hours of exposure to cigarette smoke and the elements. A furrowed brow guarded her steely eyes. Emma habitually arrived at the clinic without an appointment, and expected to be seen immediately, as though she had difficulty fitting us into her busy schedule. I had made her acquaintance early in my practice when I was heir to all the lower castes and troublesome chronics. It was tempting to dismiss these people or get rid of them the quickest way possible. They were odd, malodorous, abandoned shipwrecks, but I had to remind myself that they were no less worthy than any other patient. Given different circumstances, any of us might be sleeping on a park bench and scrounging for scraps in a dumpster.

Emma carried her shopping bags wherever she went, and together with her coat, they contained the sum of her earthly possessions. Carolyn and Daphne had tried various tactics, determined to sneak a look into her bags.

"Emma, we need a urine specimen," said Carolyn on a previous visit. "Here's the washroom. I'll watch your stuff while you go."

Emma fixed her with an unwavering eye. "I'll take them with me," and crammed all her gear into the tiny washroom.

Carolyn had tried the direct approach, "Emma, can you show me what you have in your bags?"

"None of your damn business," she snapped, and pulled the bags tightly around her legs.

"I just want to see if there's anything we can get for you."

"Got everything I need," Emma had said. The bags remained a mystery and a continuing quest for the office staff. It must be a female thing – I hadn't the slightest interest in knowing the contents – I had seen the inside of my wife's purse.

"Hello, Emma," I say as I open the door. "The nurse tells me you have pain and a rash."

"Yeah," says Emma. "There." She points to her backside.

"Ok, we might as well get to the bottom of this. Let's have a look." I pull back the curtain. "Take off your clothes and put on this gown. You can hang your clothes over there behind the table."

"Don't need no gown." She unceremoniously sheds her coat and her bags in a jumbled heap on the floor, drops her drawers, and bends over the examining table. I warily approach her exposed anatomy when a breaker hits me – my eyes water, and my nose hairs begin to curl. I decide then and there we need to invest in biohazard gear.

Emma needs intensive care – a bath, even a carwash would be a start. I take a deep breath and crouch down to have a look. I decide against laying on of hands, except to do a quick swab for bacteria. There is a perianal rash and excoriation from scratching – she has long, dirty fingernails – but the main problem is a ripe purple plum protruding from her anus.

I back out of range. "There's a rash alright," I say. "But the major problem is a thrombosed hemorrhoid."

"What?"

"It's a blood clot in an external hemorrhoid, so it gets inflamed and painful." Emma pulls up her bloomers, and begins gathering her bags. "Hold on, Emma. We need to fix that. I'll put a little freezing in there, cut open the hemorrhoid, and remove the clot, and then…"

"No, you're not! No freezing. No cutting."

"Listen, Emma. Those things are very painful, and it will heal faster if I take out the blood ..."

"Not on your life. I'm getting out of here."

"Okay, okay," I shrug. "No cutting. You need to soak your bottom several times a day in warm water, and after a bowel movement, and then dry the area well. Can you do that? Maybe we can get the nurse to give you some instructions."

She gives me a scornful look. "I haven't lost my marbles. I can look after myself."

"Emma, where are you staying?"

"On the street... sometimes."

"Are you staying in that old rooming house down by the skating rink? That's a terrible place."

She seems startled at being found out. "Yeah," she replies, gathering her bags. "I did a few nights. Now I'm on the street or sometimes stay with a friend. I don't want people snooping around, so I sleep in the park."

"We should find you something better, maybe the nursing home? Have you talked to the welfare people – perhaps they can help you?"

"I'm fine! Don't need any help." Her jaw is set, and her eyes blaze.

Previous attempts had been made to find her decent housing, but she would have none of it. She is fiercely independent, and has no truck with meddling do-gooders. I give her a few more suggestions about hygiene, not certain that she either cares or can find the necessary amenities, like hot water and a bathtub. I hand her a tube of ointment from our sample cupboard. "Here, apply this crème to the rash twice a day after washing. It will relieve the itching and pain, but that will take a while. You should have a checkup, Emma. Sometimes diabetes causes fungal..."

"No checkup."

PETE & TILLIE: A REAL LIFE NOVEL

"Okay, okay." I raise my hand in surrender. "Come back in four or five days if it's no better."

"The bags are back," says Carolyn the next afternoon. "Emma told Daphne she needed to see you right away. The offices are all full. Should I tell her to wait?"

"No, no. Might as well show her into the treatment room and I'll talk to her," I reply.

Carolyn motions to a stool. Emma shuffles into the room, sits down, and sets her bags around her feet.

"Hi Emma, your backside isn't any better yet?"

"It's no better. Itches like hell, and hurts."

"Well, we should take out the clot."

"No cutting. You gonna look at my ass?"

"Well, we're very busy and the rooms are all full. It won't have changed from yesterday."

"You're not gonna help me?"

"You don't want to do what I recommend, so you'll have to give the treatment a little more time, Emma. Are you doing the sitz baths? No? Well, come see me again in a couple of days if it's no better. Okay?" She gets up, grabs her bags and leaves.

I walk down the hall to see the next patient. I can hear Emma complaining to Daphne within earshot of the crowded waiting room, "That Dr. Giesbrecht is no damn good. He won't even look at my ass."

Emma is back in several months. The rash is gone. This time she has a painful mouth from a dental abscess around one of her molars. "You should see a dentist and get that fixed."

"Don't need a dentist. I don't have money. Just give me penicillin."

"I'll get you some antibiotics, but you should still see a dentist. That tooth is going to give you more problems. I'll phone one of the dentists in town and get him … "

"I said no dentist."

"Emma," I persist, "I'll talk to him. It won't cost you any..."

"No dentist! Just give me penicillin." Her jaw is set, and she lifts her chin in defiance.

"Alright, alright. I'll give you Cloxacillin. That's a better antibiotic for an abscessed tooth. Just a minute, I think we have some samples."

As I walk back into the room, I notice Emma had a mild tremor of her right hand. She immediately clasps her hands and the shaking stops.

"How long have you had that shaking in your hand?" I ask. "Here, let me have a look." I take her hands and stretch out her arms in front of her.

"I'm fine." She pulls back, and hides her hands in her coat.

"Just let me have a look, Emma. Rest your arms on your lap." After a minute or so, the tremor is back in her right arm. It's slight, but unmistakable, the involuntary 'pill-rolling' tremor of Parkinson's.

"Have you had any trouble walking?"

"No, there's nothing wrong with me."

There are no other obvious signs, and I decide not to push my luck. If she is still functioning well, it's probably better to wait for further testing. The diagnosis could not be made simply based on the tremor. There's no point antagonizing her. In any case, she'll be noncompliant unless she develops serious problems. I wasn't used to patients who defied me at every turn. This was still the 80's – a physician was rarely challenged. Patients were not always compliant, but that was usually because of lack of money for drugs, ignorance, or careless disregard, not out-and-out defiance. Emma was somewhat of an anomaly – an independent soul who wouldn't take my advice.

"Why don't you come back to see me in two or three months, and we'll see how things are going." I say.

Emma is a challenge, not the least of which is her constant eristic behavior. The practice of medicine can be a great pleasure when people are clean and cooperative, and hang on every word that emanates from my lips – I've known one or two mentally challenged patients like that. Emma repeatedly tested my resolve to treat her with respect, no matter the radiation level, lice, or lack of compliance.

The next time I saw Emma was in ER. She had been brought in by a passerby who witnessed her fall on the sidewalk.

"I think she has a dislocated shoulder," says Cathy. "But she is more concerned about her belongings than her injury."

"Hello Emma. We meet again. What happened?"

"I had a fall. It hurts like hell," she says, brusquely. "Don't touch it."

"Well, I have to look at it. I'll be very careful, okay? We'll have to get some of your clothing off first."

Cathy helps Emma remove her coat and sweater amid colorful prose. I can see the shallow depression where the humeral head should be. I gently palpated the shoulder – the normal smooth roundness of the deltoid muscle over the joint is gone.

"The shoulder is dislocated. We'll have to get an x-ray, and then put it back in place."

"No operation," Emma protests. "I don't want no operation."

"This is not an operation. I'll put some freezing in the joint and give you something for pain intravenously."

"No IV. You're not going to poison me." I roll my eyes and look at Cathy.

"Emma, we're not going to poison you. All I'm going to do is put some freezing into the joint, and give you something to make you a little drowsy. You won't go to sleep completely. I promise you, no one will look into your bags or take your things."

The x-ray shows the head of the humerus sitting anteriorly and inferiorly (in front and below the joint). Pain causes muscle tightness and will not allow us to put the humerus back in place. I inject xylocaine into the area, and push four mg. of midazolam into her IV. Emma's eyelids begin to droop and her arms relax. "Okay, let's do this quickly while she's out. Cathy, hold the shoulder while I pull." I grab the forearm bent at the elbow, and pull with all my strength rotating the arm outward, and then bring the elbow back across the chest, Cathy providing counter traction. There is a gratifying thunk as the head settles back into its socket.

Emma murmurs, "Is it fixed?"

"Yes, it's fixed," I reply. "Cathy will put your arm in a sling. But you can't manage on your own – you won't be able to use your arm for a while. It will be painful when the freezing comes out. We'll have to phone home care to find you a place, or admit you to hospital for a while."

"No hospital," she spits. "You're not going to get me in there."

"You know what, Emma," I say. "Listen! It's time for us to make these decisions. You're not a young chick any more. Now you have a bad shoulder. We can't just let you go back to the street. There's no way."

For several minutes Emma says nothing. You could see the battle going on in her mind. She looks at Cathy, then back to me. Her face softens and the defiance in her eye slowly melts, like a furious gale that finally blows itself out.

"Okay," she sighs. "Give me my bags." She points to a ragged handbag. She rummages through the contents with her good hand and produces a small scrap of paper. "Here, phone my sister Isabel. She'll come pick me up."

"You have a sister?" I ask incredulously. "Emma! You always told me you had no family. Where is your sister?"

"She lives in Winnipeg with her husband."

"Really? So why are you on the street? Wouldn't your sister help you?

"I used to live with her after my husband died. We had a huge fight years ago. She begged me to come back, but I told her to go to hell. I haven't seen her for years."

Cathy phones Emma's sister. An hour later Isabel arrives and takes Emma with her. She promises to take her to see her own doctor in Winnipeg. Emma seems almost happy, now that she's dropped the pretense and the battle is over.

I drive home with Emma's story on my mind. Had it all been an act, a means of survival? Defiance that took on a life of its own? Now she was vulnerable and cooperative. I couldn't decide which was the real Emma.

Clare Bially is a contrast – pleasant, cooperative, and compliant, but like Emma, challenging and intimidating. She is a new patient – a twenty-year-old woman, recently married, with long burgundy hair, deep coffee eyes, and an infectious smile. She asks for a complete physical. "I want to make sure I'm in good shape to have kids," she says sweetly.

"Are you pregnant?" I ask.

"No, but we're trying to make it happen." She smiles coyly.

"Anything you're concerned about? Any past health problems? Any surgery?"

"No, everything is fine. I just want a physical and Pap test."

"Okay, take your things off and put on the gown. I'll be back in a few minutes."

I come into the room and pull back the curtain. There is not a stitch of fabric to be seen except for the patient gown hanging on a hook on the wall. Clare is nonchalant, sitting cross-legged on the edge of the table. She has an uncommonly perky, Playboy figure, at least from what I've been told.

"Maybe you should wear the gown." I say, hastily drawing the curtain again.

"Dr. Giesbrecht, don't tell me you're embarrassed?" she taunts. "Don't you like the view?" I like the view – what's not to like? But I'm uncomfortable – gorgeous women can be intimidating, particularly naked ones. Most nudists are people you wouldn't want to see naked, but Clare… Disease and deformity I could handle, perfection not so much.

I weigh the right words. "Oh, the view is... great," I say. "And no, I'm not really embarrassed. Uh... it's just more appropriate if we expose one small section of your anatomy at a time. I'll get the nurse to come in."

"Okay, you don't need to do that. I'll use the gown."

That settled, I'm about to examine her heart and lungs. Clare says, "Oh, there is something I should mention – I did have an operation – breast augmentation several years ago."

"Oh," I say, "that would explain the... scars. No problems with the surgery?"

"No, everything went well."

This was the early 80's, long before breast augmentation became a trendy procedure. It was the era when *Mash* ended and Cabbage Patch kids began.

I complete the examination. "Everything's fine, Clare," I say. "You're cleared for take-off."

Two months later Clare is back in my office. I'm surprised to see her back so soon. I begin with some small talk, but she's in no mood. "I want you to look at this," she says. She unceremoniously pulls her sweater over her head and removes her bra. The right breast is as perky as ever, but the left is as limp as a leftover party balloon.

"That's really weird." I frown. "How did that happen?" I wonder fleetingly what sort of activity might have deflated the left side.

"You tell me," she says dejectedly, "Look at my stomach and my left leg."

Her lower left leg and ankle are swollen and lumpy, but there is only slight tenderness. Her abdomen also has several odd bumps that squish under my fingers like a lump of cookie dough.

Clare is no longer very intimidating.

"Would you look at that," I exclaim. "I've never seen anything like it. You know what has happened, don't you?"

"Yeah," she says, "My left boob is exploring the rest of my body. I never should have had that surgery. It's a disaster. What do we do now?"

The implant was obviously defective; the capsule has ruptured, and the silicone has slowly seeped down through her tissues to enhance her ankle. I referred Clare to a plastic surgeon to repair the damage, but she elects to have the implants, including the one around her ankle, removed.

"I get a fever for a few days, and then it goes away," Clare says one day. It is some twelve years and several children since the meandering mammary. She looks pallid and worn beyond her thirty-two years. "I thought it was the flu, I'd feel better for a while, and then the fever was back. My joints get sore, and after a day or two they get better again. Right now my hands and knees are painful."

"This has happened a few times?" I ask. "Always several joints at the same time?"

"Usually the fingers, wrists, and knees. Sometimes the elbows."

"Have you had any chest pain or shortness of breath? Any skin rashes?"

"Some patches on my face, arms and chest, but it goes away in a couple of days."

"Okay, Clare. Let's have a look." Her finger joints, wrists, and elbows are slightly tender and swollen. She has trouble clenching her hand and there is stiffness in many other joints as well. Up close, I can see a faint erythema over the nose and cheeks in a butterfly pattern. Her heart sounds are normal and the lungs are clear. "Any numbness anywhere, muscle weakness, double vision, loss of balance – anything like that?"

"No, not really. I feel quite tired when I have a fever, and maybe a little dizzy at times. So what is going on?"

"I'm not certain. We'll have to run a few tests, and have you come back in a week."

"But you must have some ideas," she persists. "I'd like to know."

"Well, okay," I say. "I'm not sure, but the history, the joint pains, the rash – it sounds very much like lupus."

"Oh," she says. Her face falls and there's a hint of fear in her eyes. "That's not good, is it?"

"Well, it can be serious, but often the disease is mild, and may go away for months or years at a time. We'll have to do some tests, and get you to see a rheumatologist."

I give her a moment to digest the information.

"So what is lupus, anyway?"

"Lupus is an autoimmune disease. A person's own immune system gets side-tracked and attacks various organs or cells in the body." Lupus is often called the great imposter – it can affect many different tissues or organs and mimic many other diseases. The symptoms and health problems will depend on which areas are affected.

I give her a requisition for the lab work, chest x-ray, and urinalysis. In several days, the results start arriving on my desk. Urinalysis shows some protein, and many red cells, both of which should not be there – they are signs of renal involvement. Her ESR, a nonspecific test, elevated in many inflammatory illnesses, is 50, much higher than normal. The antinuclear antibody test (ANA) is positive as in ninety percent of lupus cases. A blood smear reveals the characteristic large white blood cell (LE or lupus erythematosus) under the microscope. (This test has now been obsolete for some years – a more accurate test, antinuclear (DNA) test is used now.) Clare's hemoglobin (blood count) is 105, moderate anemia, accounting at least in part for her fatigue and pallor.

When Clare returns in a week, she is worse. Her customary joie de vivre is clearly taking a beating. Her shoulders sag and her face shows the fatigue. "I've got some shortness of breath, and my chest hurts. I've got some sores in my mouth, too."

"Does it hurt when you cough or take a deep breath?" I ask.

"Yes, it hurts to breathe."

Her oral cavity has a few ulcers, like canker sores. I put the stethoscope to her chest wall, and there is a characteristic sound, like coarse sandpaper on wood. "You must have pleurisy – the lining that covers your lungs is inflamed, so it hurts to breathe when the two surfaces rub over one another." Her urine shows a few more red cells and a lot of protein.

"I'm sorry, Clare. The tests all show that you have lupus. Your kidneys, lungs, and joints are all involved to some extent. The nervous system and your heart seem fine so far. You should start using some ibuprofen for pain and to relieve the inflammation. We'll have to keep watching for kidney damage. Stay out of the sun – that can often cause flare-ups, or use a good sunscreen. We'll get you started on some steroids to get this under control. I'll call Dr. Samuels – he's a rheumatologist, we'll get his advice. With any luck, he can see you soon."

"Here's a prescription for the prednisone – start at fifty mg a day, and then taper down to ten mg. Hopefully, by that time you'll be able to see the specialist, and he'll advise you further. I'll talk to him today, and call you if he suggests anything else."

Some patients have an aggressive form of the disease and die within the first few years. However, the vast majority of people with lupus live full active lives, and suffer only minor symptoms, with intermittent relapses and long periods of remission. The prognosis also depends on concomitant problems like anemia, hypertension, high cholesterol, and kidney disease. Most deaths from lupus occur because of renal disease or infection.

Clare fared well once the lupus was under control. She had a long remission, followed by mild symptoms – some joint pain and fatigue. She was fortunate – she didn't suffer kidney failure, heart attacks, or strokes that may develop with severe cases of lupus. She was able to avoid the use of chemotherapy and further steroids. She did, however, require repeated use of an antimalarial, hydroxychloroquin, which eliminated most of the flares of LE and controlled her fatigue and joint pains.

In the years following Clare's initial diagnosis, I looked after another pregnancy, her children's chicken pox, ear infections, routine physicals, and her husband's diabetes. She matured into a wonderful wife and mother. Aging and the lupus did, of course, take its toll on her body, but it was peculiar how, in a reversal of the usual course of events, Clare had most of her serious health issues early in her adult life.

Clare and her family moved to northern Manitoba, but the last I heard, they were still thriving. Looking after their health needs was family practice at its best – involvement with the whole family as they matured and family circumstances evolved.

## Chapter 10

# SERPENTS

"Why don't you and Rose come to the Kinsmen social on Friday?" asks Dan Morgan, a colleague from the early years in Steinbach. It's the early 80's and we have both been in practice for some 15 years. We both have our interests and social networks, but they don't intersect a great deal. "There'll be music, dancing, and lots of food. You'll get to meet some of the guys from the club."

"Friday. Let me think." I find a Coke in the small refrigerator in the staff room and sit down on one of the ancient chrome and bile-green vinyl couches. Hmm... music, dancing, and beer flowing like the Amazon. My ancestors would turn over in their graves. "Oh, I remember... we're busy Friday. But thanks for the invitation."

"Church again?" Dan fills his cup from the coffeemaker and sits down. "You spend your whole life in church."

"As a matter of fact, Friday has nothing to do with church. We have theater tickets."

"Okay, then I'll give you lots of advance warning for the next one. We'll be getting together again four weeks from Friday for a regular business meeting. You can see what it's all about then."

"Dan," I say, "I have to be honest with you. I don't know if Kinsmen is exactly my cup of tea – we're not really into drinking and dancing. Besides, we're busy and can't really add another thing to our schedule."

"C'mon. You need to break out of your mold," declares Dan. "You'll have fun. And we have some great community service projects."

"I know your community work is very worthwhile. We have fun, too, you know. You guys have this bizarre idea that if we're church-goers, we can't possibly be having any joy in life."

"You take religion way too seriously," argues Dan. "You don't actually believe all that Bible stuff, do you?"

The animated chatter in the room suddenly dies away. I become aware of a rapt audience.

"I go to church too," Dan continues. "But our minister explained that the Bible was not meant to be taken seriously – it's mostly fables. It's no different from any other book about religion."

Carolyn and Daphne look at me expectantly, like ringside spectators at a WWF match waiting for a decisive hold. I take another sip of my Coke. Dan has thrown down the gauntlet.

"You have some warped ideas about the Bible," I counter. "The Bible is historically accurate and can be verified by archeology, parallel historical records, and many other disciplines. So if it's accurate, why would the message not be accurate? It's true there are many allegories; Christ himself uses them in his teachings. You can't take everything literally, but the Bible still speaks the truth about the human condition. It's a worldview and ultimately a matter of faith. Faith is not the same thing as religion, you know. A relationship with God is not something you add to your life; it's supposed to *be* your life. Most people know the twenty-third Psalm, but don't know the shepherd."

I surprised even myself. A concise one-minute sermon. Pastor Keller would have been impressed. Carolyn and Daphne are grinning in anticipation of the next salvo.

"There are too many thou-shalt-nots," says Dan. "You have to loosen up. You're being held hostage by your religion."

"It's not about the negative. Faith is about joy and hope. It's about the positive things you can do through the power of God. Why do I have to loosen up? My life is interesting and fulfilling. You think I'm a Victorian prude, but my lifestyle is a bit different from yours, that's all. Christian faith isn't about prohibitions – it's about the positives."

"All that hell and damnation – how can you take that week after week?"

I roll my eyes and glance at Carolyn, who is struggling to keep out of the fray. "You really have no idea, do you?" I retort. "Have you ever been to a Mennonite church, or any evangelical church for that matter?" Dan shakes his head. "I didn't think so… Tell you what, I'll come to a Kinsmen meeting if you come to one of our church services." Carolyn eagerly nods approval – score one for Dr. G.

"Nah," says Dan, "I don't think so."

"Why not? Seems like a fair deal to me."

"Yeah." Carolyn jumps in. "I agree with Dr. Giesbrecht. Seems fair. If you don't want to go to his church, you can come to ours. You're welcome any time. Is that okay, Dr. Giesbrecht?"

"Absolutely," I say, "it doesn't have to be our church."

"Your churches are too holier-than-thou for me to ..."

"How do you know if you won't come and check it out?" demands Carolyn impatiently.

"Now who's being closed-minded?" I add. "Surely you're not afraid of what your friends will say? Anyway, you've talked about this before. Why is this so important to you – do you have some repressed guilt or a secret fear we may be on the right track?"

"Nah, that kind of religion is just too serious for me. Anyway, I've got to get back to work." With that, Dan empties his cup in the sink and disappears around the corner.

"Well," says Carolyn, "I think you won that round."

"Yeah, maybe. I'm not concerned about winning or losing. Arguing about religion is never very productive, I guess. It's just that people like Dan are forever accusing us of being narrow-minded and ignorant. We don't have the corner on the truth, but isn't his attitude just as intolerant? Anyway, I have to get back to work, too."

Next day I meet George Jamieson in the treatment room of the clinic. "How about we go to Winnipeg after office hours tonight for that seminar on heart disease," he says. He seems unusually eager. "Dan wants to go too. We can get a bite to eat at a restaurant before the lecture."

"Okay," I say, "I hadn't heard about that. Where is it – the medical college?"

"Uh, yeah."

"Sounds good. I'll phone Rose and tell her I won't be home for supper. Who's the speaker?"

"Oh…uh, Jeff Hughes."

"Great. He's always good."

It should be an informative evening. Dr. Hughes is a well-respected cardiologist. Downright nice of them to invite me – a good way to bridge the social barrier, perhaps. The invitation is a bit of a surprise. Though we had already worked together for years, outside of work, the spring barbecue, and Christmas staff party, we didn't see each other socially.

George offers to drive – he wants to show off his new Mercedes. As we pull into Winnipeg, Dan suggests we stop at the Nisswa hotel for supper. I had never been there before – its reputation was on the greasy side of respectability. No matter, it was their invitation, and I could slum with the best of them.

"We have plenty of time," says George. "Why don't we stop for a drink before supper?" Okay, more surprises. We make our way to the bar. It's like a dark tribal cave, with a caustic miasma of male body heat and cigarette smoke so thick you can hardly see into the corners. George orders a martini, and Dan has a beer. I order a Bloody Mary – I'd heard of that before and it sounds hip. Coke is totally uncool and I know nothing about beer. You'd think I'd have learned some of these things in university – drinking was an essential element of training for medical students, though not on the official program of studies. Dan lights a cigarette, and George pulls out a stogie, which he favors for special occasions.

There were, of course, no bars in Steinbach. For that matter, there were very few restaurants of any kind – people ate at home where they belonged. An occasional meal or coffee break might be forgiven, but eating out was costly and frivolous. In the 60's, there were only three eateries in town: Pete's Inn, the only restaurant with any style or decorum; Fred's Lunch, a small dingy café; and Johnny's Grill, another nondescript eatery, all on Main Street. We were a dry town, and no alcohol could be served publicly. The fact that we repeatedly voted no in liquor referendums, but drove to Winnipeg or St. Anne in convoys to purchase alcohol was something we couldn't always explain.

Herb Siemens, a patient of mine, had a ready excuse for imbibing. He stoutly maintained to his very conservative wife and fellow church brethren that beer in sufficient quantities was the only effective way of flushing out his kidney stones. He did have a remarkable number of stones from what he confided to me.

Belonging to a church wasn't a prerequisite to living in Steinbach, although some might have liked it that way. In fact, the majority of people were churchgoers. Movies had gained a grudging acceptance, although the small musty Main street theater was poorly attended. Dancing was a definite no-no... sort of.

Our interpretation of the Bible sometimes made us look silly in the eyes of outsiders – every liquor referendum or controversy over high school dances had the media salivating. People were frugal and hardworking and were rewarded with prosperity, but financial rewards sometimes engendered greed and marginal business practices. The pursuit of material prosperity occasionally blurred our Christian morality, and a visitor to Steinbach might wonder who was in charge – God or Mammon.

Sometimes we forgot that loving our neighbor was just as important as saving him from eternal damnation. We didn't always get it right, but the teachings of the Bible were the foundation for most. We believed in the centrality of God and the power of prayer in our lives.

"Cigarette?" Dan asks, as we sip our drinks.

"No, thanks," I answer. Being cool has its limits, and doesn't extend to inhaling carcinogens. I look at my watch – six thirty. "What time did you say the lecture started?"

"Eight o'clock," says George, "Relax, we've got lots of time."

Suddenly, a tiny floodlit stage appears out of the haze. A blast of bone-rattling music explodes from a set of tinny amps. "Gentleman," a male voice booms, "Welcome to the Nisswa. It's show time. Tonight, we have some exciting entertainment for you. Let's welcome the beautiful, exotic Rena, direct from the bright lights of Las Vegas, Nevada."

The music rumbles like a quake deep in the bowels of the earth. My skull starts pounding and I'm beginning to sweat from the stifling air. This is okay – I'm an educated, mature adult, an MD in fact. I've worked in the inner city emergency department of the Health Sciences Centre where life is raw and naked. I've seen it all. I can handle this.

A woman in a satiny red gown and stiletto heels undulates onto the stage clutching a sizeable snake. Rena begins writhing savagely to the beat. 'Dancing' applies to a wide spectrum of contortions – Rena has the grace of a decapitated chicken. I appraise her with a clinical eye – she was high mileage, her plastic face glistening with thick make-up like a fresh coat of latex which fails to hide the sags and wrinkles. She was zaftig, but could use the services of a structural engineer to shore up her hanging gardens – an over-zealous bump-and-grind and she'll hand herself a concussion. The snake, on the other hand, is a prime specimen, lithe, well-muscled, and firm. I glance at George and Dan, and shout above the din, "Do you think we should get something to eat? We'll miss the lecture."

"Relax," Dan yells back. "Have another drink. Aren't you enjoying this?"

"The snake is kinda cute," I say. I'm wondering how her attire can stay in place with all her contortions, but soon realize it's not supposed to. She begins tossing portions of her costume into the crowd. Now we are truly enjoying life – alcohol, tobacco, a serpent, and a woman about to bare her soul to a roomful of degenerates. There are hoots and catcalls. When Rena has finished molting, she wears nothing except the twelve-foot serpent draped strategically across her body.

Amid the testosterone-fueled hooting and catcalls from the floor, there came sudden enlightenment – my little grey cells had finally put the pieces together – *there is no lecture* – this was George and Dan's selfless contribution to broadening my views. They are both grinning like Cheshire cats – enjoying what they think will set me back twenty years in my quest for sainthood.

"Thank you so much for the educational evening," I say, when the music has faded into the gloom. "If you're trying to make a point, I guess you've made it. Now can we eat? I'm starved."

The next morning the news of our escapade had spread quickly through the office staff thanks to George, and I endured a lot of good-natured ribbing about my choice of leisure pursuits.

# Chapter 11
# DAISIES

Aconsiderable portion of my practice consisted of drug pushing, mainly in the form of anesthesia, beginning in the first years of my career. The drugs were strictly legal of course. I have framed documents from the University and the Government of Manitoba that attest to that fact. There was a time when I displayed my credentials proudly on my office walls, but they don't seem that important anymore. I have, of course, the blessing of the health care system and a signed consent from the patient.

I enjoy most the anesthesia component of my drug practice. I am in total control – a carefully scripted power trip. Noncompliance is never an issue, and patients don't grumble about their bunions, hemorrhoids, or husbands. If they do, I can discreetly turn up the pump and cut them off in mid-gripe. They may be talkative, anxious, and reluctant to be there, but soon after I arrive, they are serene and well-behaved. Most people are apprehensive about being put to sleep, and are exceedingly annoyed if they don't wake up. That generates a lot of bad press. Of course, I do take the responsibility of the lives in my care very seriously. And, except for some high-risk patients, I find anesthesia less stressful than listening to patient woes for hours at a time in the office. An anesthesiologist, someone told me, is a doctor who delays the pain until you get the surgeon's bill. In our benevolent system, the government pays both my bill and the surgeon's, so patients have little fiscal pain, except perhaps at tax time.

To do anesthesia well, you must have confidence that you are always in control no matter what the complication – a drop in blood pressure, an abnormal heart rhythm, or a frail elderly patient.

Anesthesia was simpler in the '60s and '70s. The only monitors we had were our eyes and ears, a stethoscope, and a blood pressure machine. Pentothal was used for induction (initiate sleep). Halothane, an inhalational drug, had replaced ether and chloroform. Ether was a primitive anesthetic agent, which sometimes caused serious explosions, even a few lungs. Chloroform was another agent with nasty side effects like potentially fatal cardiac arrhythmias. Halothane was much safer and more effective, but could also have rare toxic side effects, like respiratory or cardiac arrest and liver damage.

In those days, there was minimal ventilation in the operating room, and nobody worried about the effect of drugs on operating room personnel. When the patients were done with the halothane, they breathed it into the room air, where I could enjoy it second-hand. This may explain some of my mental aberrations. Fortunately, by this time, the early '90s, OR ventilation had improved and scavenging devices were introduced.

The first case of the day is a wizened old gentleman, Herman Kehler, who requires an amputation for a gangrenous foot. His health is precarious. I had seen him a day prior to assess his fitness for anesthesia and I'm aware of his fragile condition and the risks involved. He has a common medical condition – PPP, (piss-poor protoplasm - another of those crude medical acronyms), the consequence of aging and multi-organ failure.

The family is having a hard time with the proposed surgery. David Kroeker, the family physician, had talked to the family at length. "Your dad is not doing very well, as you can tell. He has some kidney failure, but at the moment his diabetes is stable and his heart is okay. The nursing staff is concerned about your dad's pain. His care is difficult – cleansing the foot and applying the dressings causes severe pain. There is little blood supply to that limb and it probably will never heal."

"But dad isn't going to live very long anyway, is he?" asks Helena, one of his daughters. "Why put him through the surgery?"

"Well, he may not live very long, but we don't know that. We do know he is suffering. With the surgery, he will be much more comfortable whatever time he has left. Why don't you talk it over with the rest of your family and let me know."

"We'll try a spinal," I say to Candace. She has the spinal tray ready.

"Yes, I know," she says. "I saw your note in the chart."

"You mean someone actually reads that stuff?" I feign surprise. "I'm impressed. I'll have to be careful what goes into the chart." Spinals were often used in high-risk patients, particularly in those with compromised cardiac or respiratory systems.

Mr. Kehler lies quietly on the operating room table with his eyes closed, mouth open, his face pallid and gaunt. I bend down to his ear. "Good morning, Mr. Kehler." He opens his eyes slightly, but they are unseeing. Age and dementia have claimed his mind.

We gingerly turn Mr. Kehler on his side – he seems as brittle as a delicate Ming vase. "This is not going to be easy," I mutter to no one in particular, as I feel the spine for a space large enough to insert the four-inch spinal needle. I draw up 1.2 cc of marcaine and 10 mcg of fentanyl in the syringe. I feel for the spinous process of the vertebra and angle the needle slightly. Just as I feared, the needle hits bone – with arthritis and calcification, the spaces between the vertebrae have disappeared. I check the landmarks and change the angle of the needle. Bone again. Fortunately, Mr. Kehler is oblivious. "Candace, can you pull his knees up a bit more, but don't break anything." That maneuver usually helps to open up the spaces between the vertebrae. I probe once more, and after another stab, I feel the needle pop through the ligament protecting the spinal cord. The clear spinal fluid drips slowly onto the drape. I attach the syringe and push in the marcaine.

We all hate amputations. Removing a diseased gallbladder or appendix is a normal, rational thing to do, but an amputation is different. It seems barbaric and violent, as if we are in an abattoir. The rasp of the saw on human bone is always grating, but the moment when the leg is handed to the circulating nurse is especially inspiring. The leg is wrapped and placed in a large container to be sent to the pathologist for examination. With time and experience, we develop some degree of immunity to the brutal and mutilating parts of medicine.

With the spinal and a little sedation, Mr. Kehler does well. The dementia is actually a blessing – he has little awareness of the assault to his body. Mr. Kehler lives only another ten months, but his pain and infection have been minimized.

The next case is a hemorrhoidectomy – not the stuff of Grey's Anatomy. "They may be piles to you," Jim Sanderson is fond of saying, "but they're bread and butter to me."

Max Sandler is on the receiving end of the surgery. "So you guys are amputating my grapes of wrath?"

"Yes we are," Jim says as he walks in the door. "No more grapes and no more wrath."

I'm about to fire up the anesthesia pump. "Here comes the happy juice, Max."

"Happy juice? You mean Jack Daniels?" Max asks. "By the way, no harvesting of organs while I'm asleep. I keep a complete inventory, so I'll know if something is missing."

"Oh, c'mon," Jim replies. "You wouldn't miss a kidney, would you? You'd still have one – people get along perfectly well with only one kidney."

"Well, okay, but I expect a good deal – maybe a new BMW or something like that."

"Not to worry," Jim says. "We'll give you a good cut."

Max groans. "Good cut! That's terrible."

"Okay Max," I interject. "Starting to see double and feel single?"

He is too far gone to reply. Candace and Michelle begin the surgical prep. They hoist Max's legs into the stirrups and burst into laughter. "Dr. G, you have to see this," says Candace. I put Max on autopilot and walk around to have a look. Peeking coyly from between his buttocks is a small white daisy.

The next case in the OR is an add-on. Kyle, 22 months, had fallen and suffered a large laceration of the tongue.

"Are you okay putting him to sleep for suturing?" Jim Sanderson asks. "Mom gave him half a cup of water an hour ago."

"Just water?" Jim nods. "He'll be fine. It's a short procedure. I'll intubate and watch him closely to avoid aspiration."

Kyle has other plans. No amount of mothering from Candace can stop his sobbing. He thrashes and sputters bloody saliva in every direction. Lois, another operating room nurse, is trying to apply the monitor pasties and get a blood pressure, but it's impossible with arms and legs flailing wildly. It's like trying to put a halter on a wild stallion.

"Dr. Giesbrecht," says Candace. "You'll have to use your charm on him." I turn on the oxygen and halothane, and place the mask over Kyle's face.

"At this age, there's no way we can reason with him," I say. It takes three of us to gain control. I turn the Halothane up to five percent, and in a few breaths, Kyle stops struggling. "Okay, let's start the IV. Hold the mask." I turned the anesthetic down to two percent. In short order, Kyle is fully anesthetized and the monitors are in place.

"Look at how well-behaved he is," I say to Candace. "You just have to know how to handle kids. And no, you can't take any of this stuff home. Dr. Spock would frown on a parenting technique like that."

The surgery is done and the patient delivered safely to the recovery room, I complete the anesthetic record and turn to leave when the ward clerk comes around the corner. "Dr. Giesbrecht, they need you on main floor right away. One of your patients crashed."

I grab my stethoscope and head for the stairs, just as the message comes over the PA: "Nine-nine, room 103, Medical Floor, nine-nine, room 103." There goes coffee break. My pulse quickens. Someone's life is hanging in the balance, and we're expected to tip the scales in the right direction, playing God, or stalling for time until He makes up his mind. I quickly put the apprehension out of my mind – just another job to do.

I walk into Room103 already swarming with people. It's a scene of fevered activity with the aura of death. Herb Froese is on a cardiac board, a rigid wooden panel, to facilitate resuscitation. Laura has a mask on his face, periodically squeezing the bag to push oxygen into his lungs, while another nurse, one knee on the bed, is doing chest compressions to keep as much blood as possible flowing to his vital organs.

"What's the story?"

"We heard a clatter," says Laura, without looking up, "and found him on the floor, unconscious. He had been walking to the bathroom, I guess. We're just getting the monitors hooked up." Alice, the ward clerk is recording, and several LPN's are running for equipment and drugs.

"I was going to intubate," says Dan Morgan, the ER physician for the day. "Maybe you should do it."

"Okay, let's have a look." I grasp the laryngoscope and insert it under the tongue to the base of the epiglottis, then angle upward to flip it out of the line of sight. I could just get a glimpse of the glistening white vocal cords. "Laura, a little cricoid pressure, please." She pushes down on the trachea cartilage to bring the larynx into better view. I slide the tube into the trachea. With ventilation, Herb's color improved immediately.

Herb is a fifty-four year-old farmer who had arrived in hospital two days earlier with chest pain. He had experienced minor warnings before arriving at our door – shortness of breath and mild central chest pressure while wrestling with hay bales or directing cattle traffic. He had dismissed the symptoms as indigestion or fatigue. This time it had been much worse – a severe crushing pain with sweating and nausea. So his wife brought him to hospital. His cardiac enzymes and ECG had been normal, so there was no tissue injury (muscle damage from a heart attack). I had started him on metoprolol, a beta-blocker, to reduce the work of his heart and slow the rate, and nitroglycerin to dilate his coronary blood vessels and increase the blood flow. I had ordered anticoagulants to prevent blood clots and possibly a major heart attack. Herb had been stable and pain-free with therapy. Angiograms to outline the blood vessels supplying the heart had been planned whenever Winnipeg could accommodate him.

But now the crash cart with emergency equipment, ECG monitor, and defibrillator is there. Jim Sanderson makes his way down when he hears the page. The ECG – the tracing of the heart's electrical conduction system looks indecipherable, like the hieroglyphics of a lost Mayan civilization.

"There's too much interference, stop the resuscitation for a moment," says Dan. The tracing stabilizes, and we can see the coarse, disordered squiggles of ventricular fibrillation – random uncoordinated spasms of the heart muscle, fatal if left untreated.

"Okay, keep the resuscitation going," I say. "We have to defibrillate. Set it for 100 joules." Dan places the paddles on Herb's chest, one just left of the sternum and the other on the side of the chest, so the current will flow directly through the heart.

"All clear!" Dan barks. Everyone steps away from the bed. Herb's body heaves from the charge. We watch the monitor. "Keep up the resuscitation."

There is a straight line, one or two normal beats, then a few more until the spikes from the heart's own pacemaker become a regular rhythm. That doesn't necessarily mean good muscle activity, but it is a hopeful sign.

"Right," I nod. "We've got sinus rhythm. Keep on ventilating. Do we have a blood pressure? What's the timeline?"

"It's 70/40," Laura says.

"Ten minutes," replies Alice. She's keeping a minute-by-minute log of the resuscitation effort.

I place the stethoscope over the heart – there are normal sounds as the valves of the heart rhythmically open and close. "Sounds good. Keep ventilating." A perceptible wave of relief sweeps over the room.

It is short-lived. Almost immediately, the monitor reverts to the chaotic pattern.

"Drat! There he goes again," Dan groans. He glances at me, and I know what is going through his mind: we have to do this, but it isn't going to work. "Shock him once more – 200 joules. One mg of epinephrine."

"One mg. of epi," repeats Laura. She draws up the contents of the vial and pushes it into the IV line.

Cardiopulmonary resuscitation was another of those concepts that had come into prominence since my graduation from medicine. The first guidelines were published in 1966, but it took a few years for CPR to become common practice even among physicians. We had rehearsed mouth-to-mouth ventilation and chest compression on 'Resusci Annie', (and also heard the apocryphal story that Annie's face was modeled after a physician's daughter who had drowned in the Seine river). Cardiac monitors, defibrillators, and crash carts were soon purchased and put into general use.

Resuscitation on Herb continues. Six more defibrillations. I stay at my post ventilating the lungs, while several nurses take turns doing chest compressions.

"Has anyone called the fam..."

"We're losing him," Laura interrupts. "The blood pressure is going down. I can just barely hear something at 60."

"Another mg. of epi," says Jim. "Add some bicarbonate to the IV."

We give several more doses of epinephrine to give the heart a nudge and bicarbonate to correct the metabolic imbalance that takes place with cardiac arrest. With each successive shock, the normal rhythm lasts a few minutes, then only a few beats, until finally repeated defibrillations don't change the confused pattern.

"No blood pressure," says Laura.

I shine a flashlight into Herb's eyes. The pupils are wide and don't constrict with the light. Probable irreversible brain injury from too little oxygen.

"His pupils are fixed and dilated," I say dejectedly. "How long since we started?"

"Fifty minutes."

No one speaks. Everyone knows the moment has come. The room is eerily quiet.

"I think we should call it," I say finally. "There's obviously no viable myocardium left. Jim, what do you think?" He nods in agreement. "Dan?"

"I agree," he says. "Too much damage, and we've been at it almost an hour."

"Okay, that's it," I say.

For a few seconds no one moves. It always happens that way – a sense of betrayal in a battle we wanted so desperately to win – a feeling of bewilderment that someone with so much living left to do could be snuffed out in a fragile moment. We should have been able to fix this. He should have been given another chance.

"He was really looking forward to his second grandchild," Alice says. "He told me this morning that he was going to Shopper's Drug Mart to load up his half-ton with diapers." We laugh ruefully.

"Has his family arrived?" I ask.

"Yes," Laura replies. "They're waiting in the hall."

Most of the team slowly drifts back to their duties elsewhere in the hospital. The staff from the ward begin removing the monitors and tubes to clear away evidence of the indignities Herb's body had suffered.

I dread the next task. What do you tell a distraught family, who an hour ago believed their husband and father would be okay. Certainly, he would've needed more investigation and probable surgery, but in the end, he would have returned to the family circle. I walk resolutely into the hall. Sara, his wife, is there surrounded by her family. Her eldest daughter, Emily, holds her in her arms as they sob quietly.

"I'm so sorry," I say to Sara. She grasps my hand in hers. "He had a major heart attack. We did everything we could, but there was just too much damage."

"Thank you." She bites her lower lip and blinks through her tears. "I know you all did your best."

"He seemed fine yesterday," says Emily. "He was in such good spirits. He just wanted to go to Winnipeg and get this over with."

"Well, he was ready to go," Sara says between sobs. "He always said he talked to God every day, so He wouldn't be surprised if he suddenly landed on his doorstep."

"Do you want to go in to see him now?" I ask gently. Sara nods. "Just one thing before you go in. I'm sorry I have to ask this, but in a sudden death, we are required to get an autopsy. If the family is absolutely opposed to it, I would have to talk to the coroner's office. Talk it over with your family, and let Laura know what you decide."

I walk slowly down the hall and up the stairs to the operating room. I hate these things. There was no other way, I suppose – sometimes resuscitation works, but in the majority of cases, it doesn't. In any case, we had to play through the drama. Herb Froese had been doing well, his cardiac condition stable – we reasonably expected him to be safe for a few days until the system could fit him in. I review our resuscitation efforts in my mind. He was discovered on the floor almost immediately, and resuscitation started within minutes. Protocol was followed. We had done everything possible.

But we had failed.

A death like this is emotionally draining. There is the frenetic urgency of the effort, and a poignant reminder of our own mortality. Most people witness death only once or twice in their lifetime; we are there repeatedly.

We always tell ourselves that death is inevitable, that we all have to go sometime, that sudden death is welcome in an elderly person whose body is slowly disintegrating from cancer or diabetes, but that doesn't make it any easier. We don't get to choose, but why Herb? The health care system doesn't always work the way it's supposed to. Someone with acute coronary syndrome should have angiograms and angioplasty or surgery within twenty-four hours. It's in emergencies where the crunch is the worst. It's always the same – no beds in the tertiary care hospitals, so we add another name to the list. The system never gets fixed. Or maybe it shouldn't be fixed – we have come to expect a second chance for those whose deaths were accepted just a few decades back. Medicine progresses relentlessly. We have more technology, innovative surgery, and miracle drugs, so our expectations rise. In rural hospitals, we do the best we can with fewer resources and less technology. We wonder whether we are being taken seriously when we call for help.

The defenses I have learned slowly take hold. The emotional assault is over. We have more work to do. The day is far from over. You can't let emotions get in the way of objectivity, or you won't do anyone any good.

# Chapter 12
# DOCTORS HAVE PAIN TOO

C olds are caused by viruses – nasty little bits of protein and DNA looking for a friendly host to put them up for a few days and allow them to procreate. In return for our hospitality, they make us miserable and ill-tempered. Viruses cause colds, pneumonias, polio, influenza, and many other forms of human suffering. We have no treatment for viruses (preventative vaccines, yes) – at least no effective, inexpensive treatment. Modern medicine now has anti-viral drugs that are useful in some conditions, but of no real benefit for colds.

It is often difficult to tell the serious from the innocuous condition that will disappear in a few days. A high fever, a productive cough, a painful ear – these may require checking for bacterial infections that take advantage of our body's weakened defenses after a viral assault. An adult averages two colds per year. Southeastern Manitoba has approximately thirty thousand people, so that adds up to a lot of snot and sniveling. Fortunately, only a small fraction of these people show up at my office. If everyone who had a cold came to the see the doctor, we would have no time for anything else. According to a recent study, the common cold costs Canadians about four billion dollars per year from work absence, complications such as sinusitis and pneumonia, visits to the doctor and medications. That works out to around one hundred ten dollars per person per year. In reality, the physician can do little except confirm that it isn't a serious bacterial illness, and offer common-sense advice that grandma knew without the medical training.

I haven't found the common cold that objectionable – I have paid for a good chunk of my mortgage and the Jeep Cherokee as a result of all this wretchedness. (Incidentally, I have also found the 'useless' appendix very useful financially.) Viruses are very helpful for a good medical practice – when we can't make a diagnosis, we can always tell the patient it's a virus.

Maggie Jenson looks as bleak and bedraggled as a five-day autumn rain. She clutches a package of Kleenex in one hand, and winces with each raspy cough.

"Hi, Mrs. Jenson," I smile. "Not feeling so great?"

"No, I'm not," she whimpers. "I've had this now for three days. I could hardly get out of bed this morning."

"Any fever?"

"I felt hot, so I took my temperature, but it was normal."

I can pretty much predict what I will find. Her throat has only a hint of redness, her lungs are clear, and there are no swollen neck glands. The thermometer says 36.8. I take a throat swab for strep, suggest some lozenges and decongestants, and give her the standard advice about fluids and rest.

"I think I need some antibiotics," Maggie says, with a convincing honk.

"I'm sure you have a virus," I say kindly, "so antibiotics won't help. Why don't we see how you feel in a day or two? The throat swab results will be back by then, and if it's positive, I'll get you some antibiotics. I know it's tough, but chances are you'll feel better in a day or two."

She hesitates, plotting her next course of action. Advice without a prescription is no advice at all. She doesn't need a doctor to tell her to take decongestants and fluids. She pulls out a tissue, covers her nose, and delivers a productive blast. It is impressive, but doesn't change my mind. "Well, okay," she snivels. "I guess I'll have to wait and see."

The next day after the last patient has left I tackle my list of messages. "Mrs. Jensen? I called to see how you were doing."

"I'm feeling much better today," she says.

"That's great. It just needed a little time. I wanted to let you know the throat swab was negative."

"Oh," she says, brightly. "I went to the ER yesterday evening. Dr. Morgan was there. He knew right away what was wrong with me. He said my throat looked terrible and gave me some Amoxil."

"Okay... that's wonderful, Mrs. Jensen," I said, as graciously as possible between clenched teeth. *Dr. Morgan knew right away what was wrong?* But I did not inveigh. "As long as you're feeling better."

What could I say? Antibiotics would not have helped unless she developed a complication, like sinus infection or bacterial pneumonia. In any case, it would take twenty-four to forty-eight hours for the Amoxil to make any difference. Her body's defensive artillery had done its job, and I was a birdbrain.

I didn't blame my colleague. This was Mrs. Jensen's second visit that day, and when there are a dozen people waiting in ER, it's much easier if you give in to a demanding patient. It's not very satisfying, but there is much less physician wear and tear. One has to judge the patient – some are okay with calling their malady 'just a virus.' Others need a specific diagnosis – don't say you don't know – call it galloping dandruff or whatever, but have an answer. A time-honored tactic is to ask the patient what their diagnosis is and then agree with them.

Mrs. Jensen, like many people, expected the medical establishment to be at her beck and call. She appeared at the clinic or the hospital ER regularly with life-threatening hemorrhoids or blood blisters. Medicare has even brought a nervous breakdown within the reach of everyone. But then, her life *might* be very difficult, and she deserved good medical care even if she abused the system from time to time.

Every six months or so, I make a new resolve not to cave in to requests for antibiotics, and to patiently explain that viruses are the cause of colds. I emphasized the rising menace of antibiotic resistant bacteria from overuse. Bacteria of different strains, in a form of kinky sex, exchange DNA; in other words, they mutate and may develop resistance. We also have trillions of bacteria in our bodies that are essential to our health, and antibiotics often wipe those out. People think they should be treated anyway – their suffering is unlike anything humankind has experienced before, and one more case of antibiotic use will not make any difference to the resistance problem. Twenty-five years earlier, when I started my practice, antibiotic resistance was not yet a problem. There were only a few main antibiotics, so prescribing was much simpler.

The *science* of medicine is not usually the most important thing to a patient. It took me a while to learn more of the *art* of medicine – listening, getting to know the patient, and giving them hope and compassion. Sometimes it *is* better to prescribe an antibiotic for a viral illness, or visit a patient at home, even if you are certain little can be done there. It's easier to acquire a mountain of information than the judgment needed to apply it wisely.

One group of researchers reported that the use of cough and cold kits, loaded with over-the-counter cold remedies, provided relief from symptoms and reduced the use of antibiotics. Kits included Tylenol, Sudafed, Robitussin DM, throat lozenges, teabags, and educational pamphlets. Even Jewish penicillin (chicken soup) was measurably helpful.

We have fostered a mindset that says everything can be cured with a pill, and no one should have to suffer. This is a change from my early days in practice. At that time, we could not treat many conditions very effectively, like schizophrenia or coronary heart disease. The only antibiotics we had early on were penicillin, tetracycline, and sulfa drugs. The more "wonder drugs" we have, the more people believe we can cure everything. Now we have pills to help us urinate, eliminate, coagulate, and copulate. So when there is little else to offer, capitulate and prescribe another pill. People love pills. Doctors feel pressure to prescribe; patients are demanding and we must send them away happy. Half the modern drugs could be thrown out the window, except that the birds might eat them.

Over the years, doctors have frequently been accused, mostly by ivory-tower academics who have, of course, never treated a patient, of over-prescribing and treating only illnesses, and having no interest in promoting preventative medicine and healthier lifestyles. I recall the thousands of hours talking to patients about their well-being – ninety percent of it could be distilled into one dictum: Stop smoking, lose weight, exercise more, and follow a proper diet.

Enough pontification. Back to my story.

Daphne comes down the hallway from the receptionist's desk. "Dr. Giesbrecht, your wife is on line two."

I pick up the phone on my desk. "Hi, honey, what's up?"

"Could you bring the otoscope home after you're done?" Rose says. "Scott came home from school with a bit of fever and a painful ear."

"Sure," I say. "I'll have a look when I get home."

The last patient of the day, John Martens, is a routine physical. One of the more pleasant aspects of my practice was doing pilot physicals. Most of these people were private recreational or crop-spraying pilots. They were typically healthy individuals who required little medical sleuthing. I was not a pilot, so DOT (Department of Transport) physicals indulged my interest in flying. Pilots love to share stories about their Cessna or Glasair. The majority of the pilots are men, invariably leaving their renewals until the last minute, when it becomes a matter of great urgency. Letting their license lapse is worse to a pilot than losing their nuggets.

John is requesting a pilot's license renewal. He's a long-time pilot and a prominent businessman and politician. After the vision tests, I place my stethoscope on his chest – good air entry on every lobe, heart sounds normal. Wait... I listen again... four or five regular, then an early beat. I keep the stethoscope on his chest for several minutes – there are frequent extra beats. There's also a soft murmur during systole, the muscle contraction part of the cycle. That murmur has not been there before.

"John," I say, "Everything else is fine, but your heart is not behaving. The rhythm is out of kilter – there are many extra beats. In other words, the heart's internal pacemaker is not functioning properly. It's only been a year since your last cardiogram, but we need to do another one. I'll give you a requisition and you can get it done this afternoon. Anyway, the bad news is that you can't fly until this is sorted out."

"What do you mean, I can't fly? Of course I can fly. I have to fly – I promised a couple of guys we were going fishing up north, and I'm the pilot."

"I'm sorry, but your heart has some irregularities that weren't there before. The rhythm problem could be a sign of something more serious. I can't let you fly until we find out what is going on. You'll need an ECG, possibly a stress test, and maybe a consultation with a cardiologist."

"Hey, doc, I'm fine. I've never had any problems."

"Well, you have now," I shrug. "Sorry, John, I just can't let ...

"Just sign the damn thing," he explodes, gesturing at the form, the color rising in his face. "We can figure out what the problem is later. I'm sure there is nothing wrong with my heart."

"I'm sorry," I repeat. I take a deep breath and exhale slowly. I'm weighing my words carefully. "I simply can't do that. If something should happen to you while you're flying, it could be very dangerous. That's the most important consideration." I make my way to the door, hoping to end the confrontation. "I'm responsible to see that pilots are in good health, so I'm legally liable as well, and you can't fly until this is investigated. Those are the rules."

"You arrogant SOB," he sputters. The veins stand out from his neck, and he shakes his fist in my face. "You forget who I am. I'll see that you never do another pilot's physical." I back away as he storms out of the office.

Well! As they say in Latin: *vescare bracis meis* (eat my shorts). Who does he think he is? I knew I was right, but it was disconcerting to be treated like that. I can't flout regulations, or even common sense, for that matter, to meet his agenda. He'll just have to find out he can't always push people around.

"I was simply trying to do my job," I tell Rose when I get home that evening. "There are good reasons why pilots must be in good health."

"Well, that's John Martens. You know him; he's got money, and he's used to having things his way."

"That's no reason for him to be such a jerk. I guess faith doesn't extend into everyday life for some people. If it involves making money or furthering their agenda, flaunting the law or swearing is okay. Where are his principles?"

"I know," Rose agrees. "He thinks the world revolves around him because he has a few bucks. Do you think he'll cause trouble?"

"I don't know. I checked the DOT manual before I left the office, and I followed regulations."

"Don't worry about it," Rose says gently. "I'm sure it will blow over. Don't let it spoil your evening. Can you check Scott now?"

I check his ears. The drums are a little dull, but no bulging or redness. His throat looked fine. "He'll be okay. Nothing serious."

"Doctor, are you sure he doesn't need antibiotics?" Rose asks with a gleam in her eye. "Maybe I should take him to ER to get a second opinion."

"Mrs. Giesbrecht, the vast majority of these things are viral congestion. They don't need antibiotics – the recommended treatment is watchful waiting and analgesics as necessary."

"Thank you, doctor, for your fabulous advice. Can you check my sons' ear again tomorrow?"

"Certainly, Mrs. Giesbrecht, I'll be glad to do that. I'll even make a house call."

"Oh, doctor, you have such a wonderful bedside manner."

"You guys are sick," says Scott, rolling his eyes and feigning nausea. "Do I have to go to school tomorrow?"

"We'll see how you feel in the morning," I reply. "I think you'll be okay."

"Scott," says Rose. "You know your dad. If you're warm and have a pulse, you're going to school."

"Okay," says Scott. "But if they have to call a hearse to take me home, you'll be sorry."

A doctor's family endures more than most. Everyone assumes a doctor will immediately spot serious trouble in members of his own family. Alas, he is so busy bringing health and healing to the masses, he wouldn't even notice appendages falling off or impending rigor mortis. His family suffers not unlike the shoemaker's barefoot kids

A few days later I take a call from the regional Department of Transport officer, Dr. Browning, "I got a call from Mr. John Martens," he says. "I've heard of him. He is really fuming about his pilot's license. I promised I would look into it. Oh, and I'm supposed to fire you."

"Yeah," I reply. "He's a local businessman. He doesn't like being told what he can or cannot do."

"He's been a pilot for many years," says Dr. Browning. "Is there really something seriously wrong with his heart? He says he's fine and has never had any problems."

"Well, he has been well until recently. Now he has a lot of extrasystoles and his cardiogram shows some early ischemia (lack of blood flow to the heart muscle). These are new findings, so I thought this should be checked out before he flew again."

"If that's the case, I agree. I'll back you up, but he's making a lot of noise."

The case hangs over me like the Sword of Damocles. A month later, I'm in Regina at a Department of Transport in-service, a regular requirement for licensing physicians. I'm chatting with the head of the DOT medical division in Ottawa, Dr. Sigurdson.

"So where are you from?" he asks. "Are there many pilots in your area?'

"I have a practice in Steinbach. I do about a hundred DOT physicals a year."

"Ah, Manitoba. Say, do you know a Mr. John Martens – he's from Steinbach, right?

"Yes, I know him very well," I say. I frown, trying to make the connection. "How would you know him? Oh, let me guess – he phoned you."

"Yes, as a matter of fact, he did," he answers, "He was incensed about your denying him his license. He demanded that I reinstate him, but I told him I would have to wait until I heard from Dr. Browning in Winnipeg."

I explain the situation once more, and Dr. Sigurdson agrees that John's condition should be investigated and he will have to go through the regular channels.

I'm not surprised that John Martens had contacted Ottawa. Nor would I have been surprised to get a call from the Minister of Transport, perhaps even Brian Mulroney, but it never comes. I'm thankful my superiors have backed me up – I'm off the hook for now. It's schadenfreude – guiltily enjoying John Marten's misfortune. I don't wish him anything dire, but he needs to learn the world doesn't revolve around him.

Several months later, I scan the list of patients for the afternoon clinic – there's John Marten's name. I'm in for another session of name-calling and accusations. Being a peaceable guy, I intensely dislike confrontation, but I do have righteousness and the Department of Transport on my side.

My flight-or-fight response had already kicked into high gear. My chest tightens as I walk into the examining room. John Martens is smiling, and stands up to shake my hand. "How are you, doc?" he says. "Nice to see you again."

Okay… this is not in the script. Is he trying to disarm me with a change in tactics? The stick hasn't worked, so perhaps the carrot? I sense this is a different man. John has lost weight, and looks haggard, as if he has spent several months in a concentration camp. The commanding arrogance has vanished. I'm anxious to learn what has brought about the transmogrification.

"How are you, John?" I ask warily. "I must say I'm surprised to see you here. Please sit down."

"Yes, I knew you'd be surprised. First, I want to apologize. I'm truly sorry about my behaviour last time. I hope you will forgive me."

I lean back in my chair and feel the tension drain away. "Yes, of course I forgive you. I'm glad you came back to talk to me – not many people do that." It's also easier to forgive when you were right in the first place – there is no pillow as soft as a clear conscience.

"I used some awful language," he says. "That was inexcusable. I was a real jerk."

"Well… I know you were upset, but I was just trying to do my job. So what has happened? I haven't heard anything more from DOT – do they still want you to get some more tests?"

"Actually, I guess I won't be flying for a while, maybe never – I don't know. I have a little story to tell you. Several weeks after I was here, I was driving in Winnipeg with my wife, when I suddenly got this terrible pain like someone had my chest in a vise. It cut off my air and I almost passed out. I thought I was dying, so I pulled over, and my wife drove me to St. Boniface hospital – we were only a few blocks away. Anyway, they got me into emergency, and the doctors said I was having a heart attack. They gave me some morphine and nitroglycerin, and finally the pain eased up. By the time I woke up next morning, I was recovering from a triple bypass."

"Wow!" I answer. "Isn't that something? So, everything is going well?"

"Yeah, pretty well. Dr. Corning said I'm doing fine. I'm still weak, my stitches hurt a bit, but I'm alive. I can't drive; my family has to take me everywhere. You were absolutely right. Thank God, you were right! I could have been up there in my plane with my family, and we probably would have crashed. Thank you for what you did. The Lord was looking after me even though I behaved like a jackass."

"He *was* looking after you. That's an amazing story."

"Yeah, isn't it, though? By the way, Dr. Corning wants me to have a stress test and wondered if you could do it in Steinbach."

"Sure, let's talk to Carolyn. She'll give you a date."

There is a firm energy in my step as I emerge from the room. Sweet vindication. "Yes!" I exclaim as John Martens disappears through the lobby.

This evening is our clinic barbecue – physicians, staff, and spouses. The party is at our house, so I leave the clinic early to make sure the yard is tidy and all the supplies are ready.

Jim Sanderson had suggested we have a lobster feast. He had some contacts in the Maritimes, so he had arranged for a hundred pounds of lobster to be shipped live to Manitoba. Air

Canada had assured him the lobster would arrive this afternoon. Jim has gone to Winnipeg to meet the plane, due to land at 4 PM.

Jim phones from the airport, "Dennis, Flight 292 arrived on time, but no lobster. Air Canada says the shipment will be on the five-thirty flight, so I'll wait here."

"Okay, everybody is supposed to arrive at six-thirty, so we should be okay. We'll get everything else ready, and have the pots boiling by the time you get here. Think you'll be here by seven?"

"I sure hope so. See you later."

There is great anticipation as people started arriving. Many have never eaten lobster, certainly not an eat-all-you-want lobster fest. We start with raspberry punch and a few appetizers. The baked potatoes and salads will wait until the lobster arrives.

"Dennis," Rose calls from the house, "Jim is on the phone again. We have a problem."

"Hi, Jim," I say. "You're still at the airport? Don't tell me there's no lobster? Everyone is waiting."

"There won't be any lobster," he replies. "Apparently, they are sitting in a warehouse in Toronto. They won't be arriving until tomorrow morning. That's Air Canada for you."

"You're kidding," I groan. "Oh, man. What are we going to do now? We don't have anything else to barbecue."

"I don't know," says Jim. "But it's not going to be lobster."

"Well, I guess we'll have to go to Penner Foods and see what we can find."

Steaks would have been a reasonable substitute, but the supermarket only has a few that are ready. It will be impossible to rustle up enough beef in time for supper. Our lobster fest morphs into wieners and farmer sausage.

"This has been an amazing day," I say to Rose after everyone has left, and we have cleaned up.

"We had a nice party, even without lobster," she says.

"Yes we did, and we still have the lobster to look forward to. Anyway, you know what happened this afternoon at the office? John Martens came back to see me."

"Same arrogant jerk?"

"No," I say. "Not at all. That's the amazing thing." I tell her the story.

"I never would have believed it. It kind of restores your faith in people, doesn't it?"

The crustaceans arrive the next day, none the worse for the sleepover in a Toronto. Jim and I divide the lobster and load our freezers. For the next several months, we entertain in a sort of crustacean carnival of boiled lobster, lobster Newburg, lobster salad, and lobster bisque.

## Chapter 13
# SCURVY AND SCHIZOPHRENIA

July has been suffocatingly hot and dry. Even the nights give little reprieve. I get up early one morning to do yard work before the heat of the day. I don a pair of shorts and tee shirt and wander into the garden. It's hard to keep up with the yard work. Without constant watering the lawn rapidly scorches and the flowers look like a two-week-old corsage. The air is cool and faintly fragrant from the last of the Littleleaf lilacs. Tiny points of light glisten from the dew. I listen to the sounds of the new day awakening. A red-eyed vireo sits high in the cascading arms of the willow to the south, trilling through a remarkable reper-toire – apparently using music to defend his territory, though it sounds more like pure joy. I turn on the sprinkler, and a robin appears, hopping under the spray, cocking her head, looking for a worm. A crow sits on the ridge of the roof, cawing raucously, then flies off to the back yard. I go to check. He's sitting on a rock in the fishpond, hungrily eyeing the goldfish swimming lazily in the water, but takes off at the sight of me.

Wait… what is that black blob in the water? There's an unmistakable white stripe down the center of a furry back. The skunk looks exhausted, its fur waterlogged, and the poor animal is struggling to gain a purchase on the overhanging ledge. It turns its head and looks pleadingly at me. What to do? I could let it drown, or get my 22 and end its misery. But I can't bring myself to do that. Besides, I would still have to dispose of the body – I'd have to phone the RCMP and the coroner, ask the family for an autopsy...

I get the pool net and a short plank, which I lay across from the edge of the pond to a large tub of water lilies. I use the net to help the skunk crawl onto the plank. It lies there for a moment, looks at me with its beady little eyes as if to say thank you, and slowly makes its way to safety into the tall grass at the edge of the property. Another life saved, and I haven't even left the house yet.

I finish the edging and go into the house to get ready for work. It's peaceful as I drive the short distance to work, though the cares of the day will soon come crowding in. I wonder fleetingly what I'll encounter. No surgery this morning – the day will start with rounds, a few outpatient procedures, and end with the usual clinic marathon.

Oscar Hayworth is one of the highlights of the office slate. He's a large, unwieldy man, grubby and unkempt, fifty-eight years of age, but with the facial furrows and grey hair of a seventy-year-old. He always wears the same threadbare clothes that probably haven't seen the inside of a washing machine for months. They are stretched over his frame with patches of pink flesh bulging between the buttons of his olive green shirt. He wears faded jeans that hang loosely from a leather belt. He grimaces and chews non-stop.

"Hi, Oscar, how are you doing?" I say, as I sit down at my desk.

"Not too bad." A man of few words, he speaks in a breathy halting voice as if each word is an enormous effort.

"Good," I say. "Before we check anything else, let's get your weight." Three hundred pounds. "Oscar, every time you come

in, you've gained three more pounds. You can't keep doing that."
Oscar is diabetic and hypertensive, and has been spectacularly
unsuccessful in controlling his burgeoning profile in spite of
mounting health problems. Some people are born to fatness,
but Oscar has worked at it all his life.

"Yeah, I know," Oscar replies, avoiding my eyes. "But I
don't eat much." An astonishing phenomenon encountered
with virtually every obese patient – eating very little and yet
able to defy the laws of thermodynamics.

"What exactly do you eat, Oscar?"

"For breakfast I have bacon and eggs. For lunch I have
cereal, and for supper, I have macaroni. I eat lots of bread, too."

"Every day? No vegetables or fruit?"

"Yeah, every day. I don't like vegetables. Fruit is too expensive – and it gives me gas."

"Oscar, that's not a healthy diet. You should eat some fruit
and vegetables every day. And how about some other protein
– maybe chicken or fish. Do you go out to eat once in a while?"

Oscar scowls and scrunches his eyes tightly. "I don't like to
go out. People talk about me."

"What do you mean, people talk about you? Are you
hearing voices?"

"People say all kinds of stuff. Somebody wants to kill me."

"Nobody is trying to kill you, Oscar. Why would they want
to kill you? Did you stop taking your pills again?"

The demons were back in legions. Oscar was a schizophrenic and had been on anti-psychotic medications for thirty
years. When the assassins emerged from the shadows, I knew
he had quit his medications. That's a recurring thread among
schizophrenics – medication takes away the voices and paranoia,
and since they're feeling better, they stop taking their drugs.

Oscar had been born in Saskatchewan, and had spent
many years in a mental hospital until the 60's and 70's when the
first generation of anti-psychotic drugs like chlorpromazine and

trifluoperazine became available, and many schizophrenics were able to leave hospital or mental institutions. A more enlightened attitude put these people back into the community, sometimes in foster homes, sometimes on their own with support from local health services. Some did well with this approach; some did not.

Oscar had been more or less abandoned by society. He had one living relative, a sister Beatrice who lived in Alberta. I asked Oscar about her – perhaps she might be a resource, an anchor for his rudderless existence, but he had little contact and had last seen her many years before. From time to time Oscar volunteered that he would be visiting Beatrice, but it was always six months in advance, because "she's too busy right now." When the time came and he called to make arrangements, she had heart trouble, or a new husband, or she had to work overtime. I felt sorry for Oscar, but it was hard to tell if it bothered him. He had learned through a lifetime of being ignored or shunted about, not to expect much. He seemed to have lost the capacity to feel failure or disillusionment. Typical of the snarled cerebral circuits of schizophrenia and years of potent drugs, Oscar was emotionally flat and unmotivated. If only there were some way, like a computer programmer getting in there and rewiring the motherboard.

It wasn't hard to relate to Oscar, though. He was amiable and cuddly like a huge teddy bear, except for the repulsive smell of sweat and cooking fat.

Albeit somewhat tarnished, Oscar, too, shone as the image of God, and deserved respect and good health care. Madness is just another facet of being human – for some of us it might only be a scrambled snippet of DNA or a crushing life circumstance away. Sanity is sometimes more ephemeral that we think it is. It was easy just to give Oscar a powerful drug to take away his delusions, and not deal with the whole person. Fortunately, he had Jake, a single pensioner who put his charity into action, and made it his business to befriend Oscar, take him to appointments, and invite him to church functions. Jake and another friend cleaned up Oscar's place once or twice a year when the refuse threatened to take over the last vestige of usable space.

I knew Oscar had a fondness for the demon rum, though he assured me that he was on the wagon. His paranoia would have to be treated aggressively. "Oscar, you have to take the pills. I'll give you a new prescription to take for a couple of weeks, and the voices will go away. When that medication is done, you start taking your chlorpromazine again. Okay? Don't stop taking your pills!"

"Okay, doc," he replies, "Thank you."

Oscar is usually cooperative, although his memory loss and an innate obstinacy make compliance unreliable. I give him three weeks' supply of haloperidol, another anti-psychotic, which in previous delusional periods had worked well to banish the fiends. I phone Gwen, his home care nurse, to check on him and make sure he takes his medications. If necessary, we could resort to a monthly injectable anti-psychotic.

Oscar is back in a month. "It looks as if you've lost some weight this time," I say as I walk into the examining room. The scale reads two hundred, ninety-five pounds. "That's great, Oscar, that's five pounds less. How did you do that?" This is a surprise – I don't need my homily this time. Either he has made a supreme effort or he's ill.

"I can't eat, doc. I'm so weak."

"Just not hungry? No stomach trouble?" He shakes his head.

"Are the voices still there?"

"No."

"Good. Make sure you keep taking your medications."

I look him over. His face is pasty white, and his skin dry and scaly. He has the typical facial tics and masticatory movements of a schizophrenic on chlorpromazine for many years,

161

behavior known as tardive dyskinesia, a fine tremor of his head and the 'pill-rolling' movement of his hands, parkinsonian signs, a common side effect of antipsychotic drugs.

I have Oscar lie down – his generous abdomen spreads out across the table like a huge pizza dough. Even through his bulky abdominal wall, I think I can feel an enlarged liver. There are islands of raised, red spots on the skin of his arms, and legs. He has nasty bruises and a bit of swelling of his legs. There's some disease process at work here other than the diabetes and obesity, but what is it – cirrhosis, a nutritional deficiency, maybe a malignancy?

"There are a few things we need to check," I say slowly, still puzzled. "We'll do some blood tests and a chest x-ray to begin with. Here's the requisition. Take it to the lab at the hospital. I want you to come back to the clinic in two weeks."

"Okay, doc," he says as he shuffles out of the room. "I'll try."

The lab results start to trickle in over the next few days. The hemoglobin is a bit low at 12, nothing startling. The BUN (blood urea nitrogen, a measure of kidney function) and creatinine are high, but again not far off the mark. The blood sugar is high at 10, but normal for Oscar. The chest x-ray is unremarkable. Liver function tests are slightly abnormal in keeping with early cirrhosis, but nothing that would explain the weight loss and skin problems. The white cell count, platelet count and prothrombin time (measure of blood clotting) are also normal. Oscar's bruises are not likely a result of a coagulation problem.

I leave the office and head home, mulling over Oscar's case.

"Hi, sweetie," says Rose as I walk in the house. "Time for a break?" We saunter to the patio and sink into the patio chairs on the deck.

There are no houses, cars, or people to be seen, just hundreds of virid shades. The air was still and hot, almost oppressive, like a steam bath. The sky is clear, but there is a bank of blue-black clouds gathering behind the poplars on the golf course. "It looks like a thunderstorm on the way."

"Well, rain would be nice," says Rose. "As long as we don't get the wind again." We had had a formidable late June storm; its fury had taken the top of our tallest cottonwood and hammered hundreds of unripe apples from our prize tree into the ground. Since then there has been no rain, and the soil is cracked and parched. "Anything interesting at the clinic?"

"Well, actually, I have an interesting case. Remember my telling you about Oscar Hayworth?"

"Oh, you mean the big guy with schizophrenia?"

"Yeah, that's him. He's sick and has a drinking problem. He gets paranoid, mostly when he stops his medication, and thinks people are trying to kill him. But now there's something else going on with him." I go on to describe his new symptoms and the lab results.

"Maybe he has cancer." Rose gets up to pick a few spent blossoms from the pots and check the soil for moisture – ingrained habits only a gardener would understand. She sits down again. "Or maybe he has a nutritional thing, like scurvy or something…" Rose sometimes surprised me – it might appear she wasn't paying attention, but at the cellular level she was really quite busy.

"Wait a minute – scurvy? Hey, smart woman! I hadn't thought of that… it's possible in a guy like Oscar – he abuses alcohol, and his diet is dismal to say the least."

I'd never seen a case of scurvy. That sort of thing rarely happens in Canada anymore. You check for the common stuff first. "Don't look for a nightingale if you've got a sparrow in your hand," a professor used to say. It was always nice to get the diagnosis right before the pathologist figured it out at autopsy.

"So did you admit him to hospital?"

"No, not yet. He's coming to the clinic in a couple of days, and I'll see how he's doing."

"Is he still hearing voices?"

"Well, we're making progress – he still hears the demons, but they've agreed not to kill him … No, I'm kidding, he is much better. Haldol to the rescue."

"Anything you need to do before supper? We have to eat a little early – Jodi has baseball today at seven, if it doesn't get rained out."

"Oh, right. I was hoping to work on the yard this evening. I guess I'd better be a good dad and take in the game."

Later we walk out to survey the yard as we often do after the chores of the day. Twilight and the soft evening air, still warm, settle around us like a cloak. Overhead, a nighthawk's shrill cry pierces the evening air. A few mosquitoes are making reconnaissance flights looking for the blood bank. In the neighbor's undisciplined meadow of bromegrass and clover are thousands of fireflies. We walk to the edge of the field – there are countless pulsating points of light dancing and swirling over the tall plumes of grass. We stand mesmerized until Rose breaks the spell, "Do you realize they're all hunting for sex, like one massive singles' bar?"

I thought no more about Oscar – he would be coming back to the clinic in a few days, and we'd have another go at his problem. He was an intriguing problem, rather more interesting than bunions or brothel sprouts (genital warts). A week after his last visit, a memo lying on my desk at the end of the day read, "Call Oscar Hayworth" and his phone number. I return the call after the last patient has left that afternoon.

"Oscar, its Dr. Giesbrecht. You called?"

"Yeah, Doc. I'm very sick." His voice is distant and breathy, and I could hardly make out his words.

"What's the problem?"

"I'm so weak, and I can't eat. I have the runs."

"Okay, can you come to the emergency department? I'll meet you there."

"I don't think I can make it by myself."

"Should I send the ambulance to pick you up?"

"No, no. I don't want to go to the hospital."

"Well, you might have to, Oscar. Okay, I'll come by to have a look."

Oscar lives in a tiny, ramshackle house near the middle of town. There is a dimly lit entry with the door ajar. The small windows on each wall are covered with dirt and cobwebs, several panes are cracked or missing. I knock on the door.

A feeble voice calls, "Come in."

I stop in the doorway. The scene of devastation startles me for a moment. It's as if a corner of Steinbach's landfill had been dumped into Oscar's house. The orangutans at the zoo had better accommodations. The house has one room roughly twelve by fourteen, but there are only a few square feet of useable floor space. A narrow path leads to the bed and to a filthy toilet, then to a semicircle around the potbellied stove and the bed. The room reeks of stale food and urine. Bags of garbage line the walls. The rest of the floor is covered with stacks of firewood and newspapers, small mounds of underwear and outerwear in varying shades of grey and brown, a few chairs and a table under more trash. There's a small cabinet with a sink near the door covered with dirty dishes, a frying pan, and a few grease-covered pots. The stove has a metal stovepipe leading horizontally to a hole in the wall. Jake and his friend have evidently not been here for some time.

The sheets on the bed are grey with a patina that could only have come from human skin and sebum accumulated over an unknown period. I make my way to Oscar's bed. My shoes make a ripping-Velcro sound with each footstep. It's fortunate I have a cast-iron stomach and not easily deterred.

"Hello, doc. I feel awful."

"Hi, Oscar, not doing so well? Let's have a look at you." He's pale, the skin on his hands is dry and cracking, and the bruising is worse. I look in his mouth – his tongue is dry and coated, likely due to dehydration. He is weak and breathing as if he had run the half marathon. But what caught my eye are the raw, bleeding gums.

Scurvy.

Scurvy played a significant role in the history of exploration. It was a disease associated with sailors with limited diets on long voyages. Many died during the Age of Sail until the British discovered that eating limes or other citrus fruit was a cure, hence the sailor's nickname, 'limey.' It is estimated that several million sailors died of scurvy worldwide, more than died in shipwrecks, combat, or other causes combined. Scurvy also figured in the early history of North America with the deaths of many settlers until the native Indians showed them that drinking a tea made from boiled pine bark would reverse the effects of their poor diet. Scurvy was also a factor in the Irish potato famine, the American Civil War and the Crimean War.

"We have to get you to the hospital, Oscar, and see if we can get you up and running again. I'll call the ambulance to come pick you up."

With Oscar in hospital, I order the routine blood tests again – something might have changed. I phone Brad, the lab director, "Do you do blood levels of ascorbic acid here? I've never ordered it before that I can recall."

"What have you got?" he asks. "I don't think we've ever done that. We would probably have to send something like that to Winnipeg."

"Okay, let's do it. I think this patient has scurvy – that's a first for me."

Vitamin C or ascorbic acid is required for normal body tissue health to produce the enzymes that make collagen, the mucilage of life, which binds cells and tissues together. If the collagen breaks down, bones, teeth, and cartilage start to come apart. There is blood loss because the walls of the blood vessels disintegrate, so bleeding gums are a common sign.

While we're waiting for the results, we get Oscar degrimed and sanitized. The dietician starts him on a balanced diet. He is given tablets of Vitamin C 250 milligrams three times daily. He improves rapidly – his gums heal and the bruises disappear. The diarrhea stops, his appetite and energy level improve. Meanwhile, the ascorbic acid blood level comes back at 0.12 milligrams per deciliter, well below the normal threshold.

"Honey, remember Oscar?" I say at supper soon after. "You were right – he has scurvy," Rose has a barely perceptible smirk evident only in times of personal triumph like finding the perfect handbag.

"Oh, really," she says smugly. "That's twice this year."

"What's twice this year?"

"That's the second time this year that I was right – I'm getting better."

"Okay… when was the first time?"

"A month ago when you were convinced that plant in the north flower bed was a weed, and I said it was a perennial, Russian sage."

"You remembered that? Wow, it must have been a momentous occasion for you."

"Oh, I don't forget things like that. It doesn't happen that often. Anyway, how's Oscar doing?"

"He's a lot better with good old vitamin C. He'll be going home in a few days."

"What's scurvy?" asks Scott.

"Well, it's a lack of vitamin C in the diet. It's needed for healthy tissues in the body. Sailors used to die from it because they had such a poor diet on the ship. And that's why you have to eat your vegetables." I was never one to pass on an opportunity for an object lesson.

Oscar was sent home a week after his admission. "We found out what was causing your problem, Oscar, but you have to keep taking the tablets. And you have to start eating better. No more booze."

"I'll try, Doc," he says, unconvincingly. There's still that vacuous look on his face.

"We'll get you hooked up with AA. Is that okay? You could use some help – it's also time to get you into a nursing home, don't you think? You'll be much better off with someone else providing your meals and living quarters. By the way, Oscar, are they still trying to do you in?" That shouldn't be the case – we had switched him to an injectable anti-psychotic in addition to his oral medication.

"No, Doc," he says. "No more voices."

Oscar's name slowly inched up the long waiting list for nursing home placement. With round-the-clock supervision and good nursing care, the demons were banished and Oscar's health improved remarkably.

## Chapter 14
# DEMENTIA

"*Dokta Giesbrecht, Eck jleewe eck sie en dee teit.* I think I'm in that time (pregnant)."

It had been some time since I'd last seen Sarah Reimer – an elderly woman beginning to fray around the edges. She is spidery and frail with a thin, sad face. Her grey, wispy hair is kept from straying by a pale green *Düak* (kerchief) tied firmly under her chin. Her eyes dart about the room from the floor to ceiling to the body chart on the wall and back, the movements magnified by thick glasses perched precariously on her nose. She won't look me in the eye, except for fleeting, furtive glances while she's talking, as if to establish that we are, in fact, communicating. She seems more ill at ease than usual, fidgeting with her hands, winding and rewinding a small embroidered handkerchief around her knobby fingers.

Sarah speaks Low German – she knows virtually no English. She fidgets and waits for me to respond. The tempo of her eyes quickens with her anxiety. I shift in my chair, thinking. I can't just dismiss her; this is obviously not a frivolous concern. "Whatever makes you think you are pregnant?" I ask finally.

"*Doa weelt irjentwaut unja e'room.* Something is wallowing around down there. *Eck jleewe daut ess en Bäbe.* I think it's a baby."

"Mrs. Reimer, you are too old to be pregnant – you're seventy-four. And…ah… you're a widow. How could you be pregnant?"

"*Yo, eck weit.* Yes, I know. *Oba doa mott irjentwaut senne.* But there has to be something."

"What you are feeling is probably bowel spasms – just gas," I reply. There is a marvelous medical term for the rumblings of fluid and gas in the intestines – they're called borborygmi. Feel free to use the word at your next dinner party. Sarah likely has borborygmi. In any case, no examination or treatment is needed for her borborygmi, just lots of reassurance.

"*Best dü sejcha?* Are you sure?"

"Yes, Mrs. Reimer," I say earnestly, taking her wrinkled hand. "I'm very sure. At your age, pregnancy isn't possible. Why don't we just wait for a bit – those rumblings will go away. In any case they are nothing to worry about." Sarah nods her head, but hesitates. She slowly gets up and trundles down the hall.

Carolyn is waiting for me, her eyes bright with curiosity. "She seemed quite upset, but she wouldn't tell me her problem."

"She thought she was pregnant." I respond. "At seventy-four! Talk about miracles. She felt some commotion in her abdomen, and was positive it was a baby. I tried to assure her that wasn't possible, but I'm not sure she's convinced."

"What?" Carolyn shakes her head. "That's what she was worried about? Mrs. Reimer always was a little strange, but this takes the cake. Is she losing it?"

"I'm not sure. She's rational most of the time, but things are starting to unravel a bit. I guess she didn't think far enough to realize pregnancy wasn't possible."

"You want a Coke before I finish getting supper?" Rose asks when I get home from the office. That was our ritual provided we both made it home in regulation time. It was a useful time of communication, although it was more like a debriefing after an espionage assignment. Rose had a great interest in my work – she was an RN and inordinately curious. "Oh, nothing much," was not an appropriate response to "So what happened at work today?" Not to describe my day in exquisite detail meant we weren't sharing and our marriage was doomed. In any case, medical information was confidential and would never leave the walls of our home.

"Okay, I'll get the Coke," I say.

"Good. I'll just put the potatoes on to cook and I'll join you."

I pour the Coke, Roses' Diet, and my Classic, and take them to the sunroom. Rose comes from the kitchen. We sit in silence, enjoying the solitude.

"It's so peaceful out here," she remarks.

"Yeah, it certainly is. So how was your day?" I ask, trying to be sensitive and ask first.

"Pretty good, mostly. It just seems there are more meetings and more meetings – I hardly get to see my clients anymore. Endless paperwork and bureaucracy. That Lasalle family is driving me nuts. I received a letter today asking for another ministerial review."

"Ministerial? You mean the Steinbach Ministerial? I knew they would catch up to you eventually – you've gone over your allotment of indulgences again." Rose smacks my shoulder.

"Minister of Health, wisenheimer. He got a complaint from one of my families. Agnes Lasalle has MS, so we put in home care. We were providing some meals and basic house cleaning. Her husband claimed he had a bad back and couldn't work, and wouldn't do a thing to help. They protested that we weren't supplying enough care, so Susan and I went for a home visit to check things out. Mrs. Lasalle said they needed someone to clean the basement and move some furniture. I told her that's beyond our mandate."

"Aren't there some family members who can help?" I ask.

"Exactly. There was a seventeen-year-old daughter lying on the sofa watching TV, so I asked if she couldn't help around the house. She said, "Pay me." I looked out of the window and there's Herb Lasalle with his bad back jumping off his half-ton unloading an ATV. So I pulled the homecare, and they sent a formal complaint to the Minister of Health."

"I've seen a few people like that on Compensation," I remark. "So now you have to justify removing the homecare."

"Yeah. I know I'm right, but it's always a huge hassle and a ton of paperwork. There are more and more problems with abuse of the system from unreasonable families. Anyway, that's far too depressing. Let's talk about something else."

We watch a flycatcher dart from his perch in the green ash by the fishpond to nab an insect on the wing. Overhead the contrails of a jet slowly congeal into tiny puffs of cloud.

"It's your turn," Rose says. "How was your day?"

"Interesting. Sarah was in the clinic today."

Rose's brow furrows. "Who's Sarah?"

"Remember Sarah, the lady of Old Testament fame, whose biological clock had been ticking for ninety years, and she was barren? Anyway, I had Sarah *Reimer* come to see me – she is seventy-four and thinks she is pregnant."

"You've got to be kidding! Is she senile, or just strange?"

"Well…" I reply. "Probably a little of both. Anyway, she felt some movement in her abdomen and was convinced she was pregnant."

"Yeah, that is weird. I remember Sarah in the Bible," Rose says. "She was old and lived in shame because she had no children. She had given up on Abraham getting her pregnant – have you ever wondered why?"

"Maybe Abraham's testosterone was down a pint or two, and his aging boys couldn't get the job done. Abraham was supposed to populate the earth like the stars of heaven. In the

PETE & TILLIE: A REAL LIFE NOVEL

meantime, Sarah told Abraham to get her maid pregnant. You don't hear that from too many wives these days."

"That would make for some interesting family dynamics. Sarah finally did get pregnant – God intervened and Abraham was able to father His chosen people. I wonder how God did that, anyway?"

"Perhaps he had to untwist Sarah's fallopian tubes."

"I know," says Rose, "Abraham took a bottle of Wonder Oil." Wonder Oil was the nostrum for every ailment the past generation had suffered.

We laugh and laugh. After a stressful day, it doesn't take much to get us going.

"Mrs. Reimer thinks she's pregnant," I say, wiping my eyes with a sleeve. "But she's a widow. At least Sarah of the Bible had Abraham to help her with the job. Maybe Mrs. Reimer is God's second attempt at a chosen people."

"Well, there's already tons of Mennonites," Rose retorts, "And besides, they wouldn't qualify as an obedient nation. The French maybe, but the Mennonites?"

"The French? Yeah, right!" I snort. "You know the French are near the bottom of the list."

"Listen, buddy," Rose jabs her index finger in my direction. "You better watch your step. I'll get the priest to stop selling me indulgences, and then look where you'll be."

"You used up all your credit marrying a Mennonite."

We laugh again. The tension and stress of the day has melted away. These inane conversations happened from time to time – probably a subconscious means of relieving stress. We get up to go – Rose continues with supper, and I change to get some gardening done before dark.

I'm surprised when Mrs. Reimer is back three weeks later, still convinced there is a bun in the oven. An occasional delusion is harmless as long as it doesn't involve garroting or other violent recreation, but her fantasy has persisted much longer than I would have predicted. Mrs. Reimer isn't as agitated as she was at her first visit, as if she has already accepted the responsibilities that motherhood would bring.

"Okay, Mrs. Reimer," I say. "We'll have to do a pelvic exam. Then we'll know for sure. Let's check your tummy and your pelvis. Why don't you go behind the curtain, take off your clothes, and put on this gown." I'm hoping an examination will convince the dear soul of her ungravidness.

Sarah starts to extricate herself from layers of material, like an astronaut after a space mission. I had forgotten the extent of her wardrobe – it has been some time since her last physical. A mound of fabric slowly grows beside the table. This could be a long afternoon, all that stuff would have to go back on again. I go next door to see another patient. I walk back to see Mrs. Reimer, but she's still disrobing. Rivers flow into the ocean, and the leaves on the elm outside the clinic window turn from green to yellow. Finally, I can wait no longer – I pull back the curtain. She is sitting there in the most peculiar garb I have ever seen. She's wearing a hand-made bra – an eight-inch band of heavy fabric, something I recognize from my farm days as unbleached flour bag. The band has two round holes, into which she had stitched twin peaks. She looks like an aging Xena, warrior princess. The bottom half of her unmentionables are bloomers, also home made, as voluminous as a back-up parachute.

"You'll have to take off a little more, your bottoms. I'll get the nurse to help you."

There is, of course, no evidence of a pregnancy. "Mrs. Reimer, you are not pregnant. There is no baby."

She gives an audible sigh, her eyes stop darting for a moment, and her shoulders wilt in relief. "That's good. I didn't want a baby. How could I ever raise a child at my age?"

"That's right," I say, equally relieved. I smile benevolently. "That would be very difficult for you. Is there anything else I can do for you?"

Sarah has no other health concerns. I send Carolyn into the room as wardrobe assistant.

The story should have ended there, but it didn't. Mrs. Reimer returns a month later. "Dr. Giesbrecht, you were wrong. I *was* pregnant. Yesterday, I had a cramp sitting on the toilet, and I passed something. I'm sure it was the baby."

"That wasn't a fetus, Mrs. Reimer," I say impatiently. This is getting ridiculous. "Probably just some tissue from the vagina. Did you bring it?"

"Yes, I did." She looks me directly in the eyes and triumphantly pulls a Kraft jam jar from her purse. A small blob of amorphous tissue is floating in the water. I put it on a glass slide and examine it under a low-power microscope. There is no recognizable tissue, merely bloodstained mucus.

No amount of explanation could convince her that this had not been a fetus. But she assured me now that God had willed her unborn child's life to end, she could get on with hers.

I saw Sarah Reimer during the next several years for other age-related problems: arthritis, poor eyesight, and constipation. It also became more obvious with each visit that her dementia was progressing. This happened in the mid 80's, before the first useful drugs for dementia were available. It wasn't long before she was admitted to a local nursing home. Her admission history read: 'Alzheimer's dementia, failure to cope.'

There are the jokes about hiding your own Easter eggs or constantly making new friends, but Alzheimer's can be a devastating diagnosis for the patient and family, particularly when the individuals are in their forties or fifties. It's difficult to diagnose Alzheimer's in the early stages – frequently the family first notices the changes: loss of memory, difficulty doing ordinary things like following a recipe, keeping track of car keys, or writing a cheque. Inability to program a cell phone doesn't count. The memory loss goes beyond the usual lapses that we all experience.

There are no definitive tests to confirm Alzheimer's dementia. Tests of memory, cognition, and simple arithmetic skills like those in a Mini-Mental exam often give an indication, but may not pick up subtle early changes. A CT scan will sometimes show atrophy, or shrinkage of the brain, but that is nonspecific and may appear only in the late stages of the disease. It is often at autopsy that the neural tangles and senile plaques of Alzheimer's are discovered.

Yet there are some brains examined at autopsy that have a high degree of these tangles and plaques known as amyloid beta-peptide, but in life, the patient had not displayed lack of cognitive function. The lessons learned from these people are that they seem to be able to override the decline with larger brains (more brain reserve) and possibly higher-level brain functioning or more education. I advised people to go back to school – a PhD at seventy-five has been done. Read, write, do crossword puzzles, interact with people. Bigger brains? We'll have to wait for evolution to do that for us.

Recently, a vaccine was developed that was effective in clearing the amyloid plaque and in some patients slowing the progression of Alzheimer's symptoms. However, many of these people suffered severe allergic symptoms and the trials were abandoned. Work is still progressing on a better vaccine or a more effective drug.

When I was in training back in the Dark Ages, we had hardly heard of Alzheimer's disease. We called it dementia, progressive mental deterioration, or senility. You get old and your brain turns to mush. There were many other illnesses emerging, like carpal tunnel syndrome, misdiagnosed and poorly treated for decades, until a precise understanding of the disease developed and a successful treatment by a small incision to free the median nerve in the wrist became common practice. There was osteoarthritis, rheumatoid arthritis, and gout – now there are over 100 known causes or subtypes of arthritis. All these changes required constant study – journals, seminars and lectures. Doctors have had to double or triple their medical knowledge – new research, new diagnostic tools, and new drugs. I'm counting on the fact that all this CME (continuing medical education) will delay the onset of my dementia.

Nobody wants to get old, but aging is the only available way to a long life. Losing your hair, virility, teeth, eyesight, or hearing is not something to be welcomed, but it is part of the human experience, just like birth, finding an occupation, and getting married. The difference is, of course, you can choose your occupation and usually your marriage partner. You can do precious little about aging. Old age is like being increasingly penalized for a crime you didn't commit.

Getting a good education, building wealth, having a loving, stable family and following all the rules for good physical health have been shown to add a few years to our lives, but they don't stop the aging process. Aging is built into our genetic framework. Our body cells, all ten trillion of them, are programmed to age and die. With each division of our body cells to replace worn-out and dying cells, a part of the gene sequence called a telomere becomes shorter, and when the chain is gone, the cell stops replicating itself and dies.

We accept old age with a certain amount of equanimity, but it is remarkable to note the things we fear. We fear sharks, poisonous snakes, and airplane crashes. Yet more people are killed by coconuts each year than by sharks and more by donkeys than by plane crashes. More people are killed by champagne corks than by poisonous snakes. This isn't going anywhere, except to say our fears are not always rational. We are terrified by a SARS outbreak, but many thousands more die from causes that are preventable by a change in lifestyle.

Later in my practice during the 90's, I looked after Anna Bartel, another patient with dementia. She was eighty-five and had been active and involved all her life, but during the previous year there was an obvious slowing; she had lost her ability to read and couldn't seem to manage her knitting. What most concerned her daughter was her loss of interest in the family, which had always been the focus of her life.

Mrs. Bartel's devoted daughter accompanies her to the clinic for all her appointments.

"So how are things going, Mrs. Bartel?" I ask on one of her routine visits.

I would get more information from her daughter, but I speak directly to Mrs. Bartel which takes a deliberate effort. I learned that in medical training from Dr. Maclaren. "Don't talk down to elderly people," he had said. "It's demeaning. People with dementia deserve the same respect as anyone else."

"Good," Mrs. Bartel says cheerily. "You want to see my knitting?"

"Sure," I say, "Did you make me some socks?"

"No, I didn't." She peers at me over the rim of her glasses and jabs the air with her knitting needle. "You wouldn't wear them anyway."

I fumble for a reply. Mrs. Bartel's daughter laughs. "She's doing good," she adds quickly, coming to my rescue. "She's reading again, and making some meals."

"That's great." I reply.

"I beat her in rummy yesterday," says Mrs. Bartel with a triumphant smile and a nod toward her daughter.

"Maybe we'll play cards next time you come." I say.

"You wouldn't have time. I'll play with my family."

"You're still pretty sharp, Mrs. Bartel. You really are doing better. I guess we should continue with the Aricept. I'm glad you have such a good family – that's more important than any drugs. Come and see me again in three months."

Our current drugs for Alzheimer's don't always help, but in Anna Bartel's case, they made a real difference. She had had the MMSE (Mini Mental State Exam), which tests cognitive function in areas such as orientation, attention, calculation, recall, and language. She had scored in the mental deficit range at 20, but on Aricept improved to 24. The real bonus was that she had become an integral part of her family again.

Researchers have also found promising help from statins, the drugs used for cholesterol control. It seems that in a roundabout way statins inhibit the production of the amyloid or some of its precursors. There is no cure yet for Alzheimer's, but I'm trying to hang on until it arrives.

*The advantage of a bad memory is that one enjoys several times the same good things for the first time.* Friedrich Nietzsche

## Chapter 15
# FIRE IN THE FURNACE

Summer has matured into sultry August heat and a palette of gold and crimson sunsets. The incessant chirping of crickets begins on early twilights. The headlong growth of summer has slowed. Green berries on the elder are turning red and the branches on the apple tree hang low with burgeoning fruit. Everywhere fields of ripening grain spread out like vast golden carpets.

The urgency of summer chores is waning, leaving a little more time for golf, barbeques, and long drinks on the patio. I'm fortunate that Brent enjoys golf and doesn't mind playing with his masochistic father who sticks with the game no matter how appallingly it treats him. Yet, the golf course is relaxing – a brilliant sun in a blue sky, the grass green and luxuriant, and a pair of king birds scolding noisily in a tree overhead – until I swing my club and invariably have to retrieve my ball from a sand trap on an adjacent fairway. Hope springs eternal, and begins with the next shot, the next hole, or the next game. I long to hear those encouraging words, "Good shot, dad!", but they are rare. I tried to calculate the percentage of decent shots it takes to keep me in the game – it's probably around twenty, which just proves it doesn't take much to make me happy. I enjoy golf more as I grow older and take pleasure in the company of Brent and later, Scott, and several sons-in-law. Their scores improve even as mine hover above the three-figure range. If ever by great good fortune or creative score keeping I break 100, I'll think I'm in a new universe. I need ideal conditions, not too hot, not too cold – even then my game is an endless series of tragedies, punctuated by an occasional moment of sheer brilliance. Someone has said that in primitive cultures, when native tribes beat the ground with clubs and yelled, it was called witchcraft. Today, in civilized society, it's called golf.

I had passed my midlife crisis some time back without too many serious injuries. I could have used it as an all-purpose excuse for buying a Corvette or climbing Mt. Kilimanjaro, but my wife and a flattened bank account kept me in check, and I settled for new golf clubs.

Sunday arrives with morning church as usual. Rose and I are standing in the foyer after the service exchanging pleasantries with friends Randy and Sheila, who suggest we go out for lunch. I ask Rose if that's okay.

"Are you kidding?" she says. "Is the sky blue? You know I'll never refuse eating out. The kids are all coming over for supper, though, so we can't stay too long. I'll ask Scott and Jodi if they want to join us."

Not surprisingly, the kids aren't interested in dining with their elders, so we drop them off at home. Just as well, our conversation would be hampered by their young ears. Going out for lunch seems to have replaced the fine old tradition of roast-beef dinner at home with family after church, dissecting the Sunday sermon and the preacher.

The restaurant is noisy with the after-church crowd. Steinbach had changed. In the '60s and '70s, it was impossible to find a restaurant open on Sunday. Everybody went to church. Well, almost everybody – those who didn't stayed under cover. There were no gas stations or convenience stores operating, either. There was no hockey, baseball, or other sports. The only traffic consisted of good folks driving to church morning (and possibly, evening, too) or visiting relatives.

"We've only seen Pastor Keller behind the pulpit a couple of times so far," I comment after we are seated. "What do you think of him?"

"I think he's very good, and I hear he works hard," says Sheila.

"But his prayers are way too long. Good thing he wasn't hired to preach every Sunday."

"Well," Randy says thoughtfully, "there are always plenty of things to pray for, so maybe that's okay."

"Not in public," replies Sheila. "If he wants to pray for half an hour, he can do that at home. And you know what? Private stuff like Gloria's D & C doesn't need to come from the pulpit. Gloria can share that with anybody she likes, but don't announce it to the congregation. That's stupid. If I miss a period, is the pastor going to pray about that in church?"

"If you miss a period," counters Randy, "I hope the whole congregation prays."

"Yeah, I guess you're right," says Sheila amid the laughter.

"I agree," adds Rose. "There are some things that are private. I know we are supposed to support one another, and share our burdens, but not when its hemorrhoids or my kids have lice."

The waitress appears with two coffee pots. "Regular of decaf? Is everyone ready to order?"

"Brenda is the pastor's wife, right?" Sheila continues after we've ordered. "She seems nice, but do preacher's wives think that frumpy is more pious? She ought to get a decent hairdo and maybe new glasses."

"Well," says Rose. "Maybe she's not that attractive, but she's very pleasant. Just think what people would say if she dressed like Cher. Then we'd all complain she was a floozy– you know, not spiritual enough."

"Just a minute." Randy puts down his coffee cup. "Shouldn't we be more concerned about her contribution to the life of the church and her walk with God? So she's not a fashion plate – maybe that's just not important to her. I agree with Rose – you don't want someone like that looking like a bimbo, either."

"Sure," replies Sheila, "but she could still make herself a little more attractive. I still think preacher's wives, or missionaries for that matter, should make a little effort to keep up with clothing and hair styles."

"Well, we haven't analyzed the other pastors yet," says Randy, as our orders arrive. "But I guess we can pick another one for next Sunday."

We went on to compare families, movies, and shopping. One-thirty, and we all head for home.

It's August 12. "There's a meteor shower tonight," I report at supper. "Do you guys want to go out and watch?"

"Sure," exclaims Jodi. "So we can stay up late, right?"

At midnight, we shut off all the lights, go out on the front lawn and lie on our backs watching the sky. It is a beautiful moonless night, the air warm and still. Somewhere in the distance, we hear the mournful howl of a coyote.

"The August meteor shower is called the Perseids," I say. "Watch the zenith of the sky, straight over our heads."

"Where do these things come from?" asks Jodi.

I treasure this moment of wonder with the kids. It's not often one can connect with them – friends, blood-curdling music, and surges of independence are often impenetrable barriers to communication. "Perseids just refers to the constellation Perseus where we see the meteors. The meteors are little bits of dust from the orbit of the comet Swift-Tuttle. When the earth passes through the orbit, the tiny particles burn up in the atmosphere."

"What are those bright stars right overhead?"

"Those three bright stars? That's called the summer triangle – Deneb, Altair and Vega. Deneb is the one there to the north. If you look at the other stars around it, you can see the shape of a cross, called Cygnus, the swan."

"Oh, look, there's one!" exclaims Scott, as a small blaze of light streaks off to the north.

"There's one," says Jodi. "Wow, there's another one."

Every minute or so a tiny blaze sprints across the sky. We lie there for twenty minutes, transfixed. Jodi breaks the silence, "Scott, move over, you keep jabbing me with your elbow."

"*You* move over," Scott retorts, giving her a shove. "You don't have to lie so close."

The spell is broken. "Okay, kids," I say, "the show is over. Time for bed." The weekend is gone and Monday rears its ugly head once more. The morning's surgical slate proceeds as scheduled and I'm able to get to the office to see the first patient on time. This is somewhat of a rarity, but welcome. I like an orderly day where I can indulge the perception of being in control. When late, I would spend the whole afternoon racing to catch up. Patients were annoyed and I was stressed.

Armand Gudreau was never upset at having to wait. Clinic visits were part of his social scene and he happily plied his peculiar brand of small talk on waiting-room patients.

"Hello, Mr. Gudreau," I say. "Pretty hot out there today?"

"Yeah, Doc, too 'ot. I 'ave trouble to breathe when it's so 'ot."

"You're not doing so well?"

"Not so good," he says. "My 'eart is going funny."

Armand Gudreau is eighty-four with a corroding chassis and burning a little oil. But as he told me on every visit, "Dere's snow on de roof, but dere's fire in de furnace." He has a perpetual mischievous grin on his face and a twinkle in his eye. He wears several days' worth of stubble – he's convinced this adds to his charm. His jokes, of which there are many, are banal, even crude. Despite his age, he thinks it his duty to flirt with every woman he meets. A vintage Casanova. There are none so old as those who have outlived enthusiasm, and by that standard, I admired his irrepressible spirit. He has a long history of hypertension and gout controlled with medication.

"What do you mean, funny?" I inquire. "Is your heart going too fast, or skipping beats?"

"Yeah, it's missing. I need new spark plug. An' I got no air."

"You're short of breath? How long has this been going on?"

"Coupla day."

I pull out my stethoscope and place it on his bony chest. His heart is irregular and sputters like a badly tuned racecar. The normal pacemaker is no longer in control, and his heart is beating erratically due to atrial fibrillation, which at his age meant underlying heart disease. Averaging 130 beats per minute, his exhausted pump is inefficient and fluid is pooling in his lungs. The shortness of breath comes from too little oxygen and carbon dioxide exchange as the alveoli, or tiny air sacs, are being flooded. He has gained two kilograms, likely due to the extra fluid. Mr. Gudreau is in the early stages of congestive heart failure.

"You've got heart problems, Mr. Gudreau," I say. "The pacemaker isn't working. We'll have to try to fix that. We'll have you come to the hospital and do a little shock treatment to put your heart right. And we'll get rid of the fluid in your lungs so you don't feel like you're drowning."

"Jes give some pill to take 'ome? I 'ate de 'ospital."

"Well, no, your heart is too irregular, it's like an engine that's missing and has no power. We need to fix that. We won't keep you in hospital for long – just a few hours, okay?"

He throws up his hands in a helpless gesture. "Ok, Doc, you de boss."

Cardioversion attempts to bring the electrical activity of the heart to a complete standstill, turning off the ignition, so the normal pacing center, called the sinus, resets. If possible, cardioversion should be done early in the game, as it is more likely to be successful. Waiting several weeks may also allow blood clots to form in the atria because of stagnant blood. The clots can dislodge and cause a stroke.

None of this was available when I was in medical school. Cardioversion, CPR, and defibrillation with cardiac arrest were new techniques that had been developed more recently. We had only heard about ultrasound and CT scans. A host of new drugs like beta blockers and powerful new antibiotics were being marketed.

Armand shows up next morning as arranged. His condition has changed little, although his heart rate is a little slower. When I arrive, Myrna, the ER nurse, has already started an intravenous line and hooked up the cardiac monitor.

"Hi, Mr. Gudreau," I says, cheerfully. "Your heart is still not firing on all cylinders. We're going to give it the shock treatment. I'll give you some intravenous medicine, some homebrew, to make you sleepy."

"Okay, doc. Jus' don' kill me. The old lady still want me, eh?" He grins and nudges me with his elbow.

"You'll be fine, Mr. Gudreau. This fix doesn't always work, but we'll give it a try."

I slowly push five milligrams of midazolam, a drug used for conscious sedation, into his vein. Mr. Gudreau mumbles for a minute, then begins snoring.

"Okay," I tell Myrna, "set the energy at fifty joules."

I apply the two paddles to his chest so the current will flow across the heart.

"Everyone clear?" The nurses step back and I press the red buttons. Mr. Gudreau's muscles contract and his body lurches. He grimaces and moans softly. I watch the monitor. A straight line. An agonizing four or five seconds while you wonder if you've fried the heart. Everyone is silent, waiting. The doors clatter in the entrance as the ambulance crew brings another patient. Then the first few blips appear – signaling the heart is recovering from the assault.

"It's still atrial fib," I say. "We'll give it another shot. Increase to a hundred joules."

I give Mr. Gudreau another two milligrams of midazolam. Another cardiac standstill from the jolt… one beat, then two, picking up speed until there is normal sinus rhythm.

"Good. Let's hope it holds. Leave the monitor on until he's fully awake."

I come back to see Mr. Gudreau in half an hour. He's alert and talking. His own pacemaker is still in the driver's seat.

"Much better, doc. Didn' feel a ting."

"Good. You'll have to take digoxin pills to keep your pacemaker steady, and give your heart a boost, sort of like high-octane gas. And you'll have to take a water pill to get rid of the extra fluid in your body, and a potassium supplement. Here are the prescriptions. Come back to the clinic in a week and we'll see how you're doing. But I have to tell you, your heart is sick and you may have more problems."

"C'est la vie. I come back in a week." His crooked grin is still there.

The medication kept Armand out of trouble for nine or ten months, but it was only a matter of time. One day he arrived in ER in a panic.

"Doc, I need 'elp." He's gulping for air, and he looks exhausted. "I tot it was jus a cold in the 'ead, but now it's my ches." I thump his ribs with my fingers – it's dull, like knocking on a watermelon. I place my stethoscope and listen for the telltale sound of fluid. There's little air entering the base of the lungs, and what there is sounds like bursting bubbles. I can see the distended jugular vein in his neck and a visible pulse above his clavicle, signs of backpressure from a heart that is not keeping up with his body's demands. His liver is enlarged, and there's edema of his legs. Armand is supporting his torso with his hands on the table in a typical unconscious attempt to increase his lung capacity.

"Mr. Gudreau, it's your heart again – it's running out of steam. Your lungs are filling up with fluid. Your heart isn't keeping up. We'll have to get you a hospital bed and get rid of the fluid. We need to do some blood tests and a chest x-ray. You'll have to be in hospital at least for a few days so we can see how the medications work. The nurses will take you to the ward and I'll check on you in a couple of hours."

Thirty minutes later Laura calls from the medical floor. "Mr. Gudreau looks pretty bad. I think we're going to lose him. You better come and have a look."

I bolt out of the office. "Carolyn, Mr. Gudreau is crashing. I don't know how long I'll be – I'll let you know. Don't cancel anyone just yet."

Mr. Gudreau's face is dark and mottled, the color of eggplant. His eyes are closed and he's fighting for air. With the hypoxia (low blood oxygen), he has become comatose. I place the stethoscope on his chest. Silence. In spite of straining chest muscles and diaphragm, there's little air movement. We may be too late – heart failure can sometimes cascade like a set of falling dominoes, and nothing you do will reverse the sequence. I have the feeling of inevitability, but we have to attempt a rescue. Laura already has an oxygen mask on Mr. Gudreau's face and an IV running.

"Let's give him furosemide 80 mg IV stat, and get me some digoxin." I turn to his wife, who has just arrived, "It doesn't look good, but we'll do what we can." I draw up .25 mg of the digitalis in a 3 cc syringe, and pushed it slowly into the IV tubing. I insert a Foley catheter through the enlarged prostate into his bladder with no protest. I wait anxiously for fifteen minutes and give him more furosemide and digitalis. We hover around his bed, watching as he struggles for breath. I call Daphne to cancel some of the afternoon's appointments.

"We'll just have to wait, but I'll stick around for a while," I tell Laura. "Can we make rounds while I'm here? I didn't have time this morning."

As it happened, that was one of the last times a nurse made rounds with me. The next morning Laura says, "Dr. Giesbrecht, sorry, but we're not supposed to be making rounds with the doctors anymore. We've been told our time is too valuable, and the doctors are to make rounds on their own from now on."

"What? Where did that hare-brained idea come from? Isn't it better if the doctor and RN see the patients together?"

"I'm sorry. You'll have ask the Director of Nursing about that."

She turns on her heel and makes a quick getaway. More bureaucratic interference. Doctor's rounds and looking after patients aren't important? But there is more charting to be done, forms to complete, and manuals to write.

There was hot debate and vehement objections at the next Medical Staff meeting to no avail. Doctors could not be allowed to thwart progress.

Thirty minutes has gone by. Mr. Gudreau remains unresponsive. I put my stethoscope back on his chest and check all quadrants. "He's beginning to diurese," I say. "There's a little more air entry."

Laura bends over Mr. Gudreau to listen. "You're right," she says. "His color's a bit better, too."

"Good, I'll be back in a couple of hours to see how he's doing."

When I come back after the office, Mr. Gudreau is very weak, but his color has changed from purple to dusky red and there's a noticeable improvement in lung aeration. "Mr.

Gudreau." I shake him gently by the shoulder. "How are you doing?" His eyes open briefly, but he only grunts in reply. "Start the oral meds in the morning, and get a chest x-ray," I tell Darlene, who had started her shift several hours before. "He should be okay for the night." A bit of bravado – I go home fully expecting to be called back. It's a quiet evening. I call the hospital – Armand is holding his own. After mulling over the day's events, I fall into a restless sleep.

"Hello, Mr. Gudreau," I say in amazement next morning. "Look at you! You're a lot better." He's grinning and scarfing scrambled eggs and cold toast.

"Amen, for sure," he says, "Mush better. Tanks, doc. What you pump in dere do de trick." He points to the intravenous bag.

I put my stethoscope to his lungs. "Take some deep breaths, Mr. Gudreau." There's the rush of air in and out of his bronchial passages, but a dull, airless band at the base of both lungs – pleural effusions, an accumulation of fluid between the lung sac and the ribs, which would take a few more days to disappear.

"He's made quite a recovery," Laura says, back at the nursing station, "but he's such a dirty old man. It doesn't matter how careful I am taking his blood pressure, he always manages to brush my boob with his hand. Yesterday he was knocking on the pearly gates, and today he's back to his old tricks."

"I know," I say, "He does that to Carolyn at the office."

"Mr. Gudreau," Carolyn had said on more than one occasion. "Please keep your hands where they belong." He was unfazed, his grin broader than ever. "Oh, sorry," he would say innocently, smirking. "Sorry, jus' accident."

Armand continues to improve and is discharged home in five days.

"Your lungs are clear now," I say on his follow-up at the clinic.

"Tha's good," he says, "You damn good doc. I almos' die, an you save my life. I feel good now. I got some action…you know, las' night." The patented grin as always.

"Oh, really." I blinked in disbelief, wondering what that might do to a severely beleaguered heart.

"Yeah," he says, "Da prune juice kick in." He chortles until he almost chokes.

Total compliance with doctor's instructions was rare, but not in Armand Gudreau's case. "What you say, dat's what I do," he would say. His devotion knew no bounds – he followed every bit of advice to the letter. He did well for five or six months. The statistics for heart failure were dismal, and Armand's age was against him. It was only a matter of time before he would turn in his time card. There were several times when I advised him, (in more subtle language), not to buy green bananas, but he always rallied. This was before the days of medications like ACE inhibitors, widely used angioplasty, and bypass surgery. Implantable defibrillators and other therapies had not yet been developed.

Then one morning at 4 AM, I was called to the hospital. Armand Gudreau had been brought in by the ambulance after a call from his family. He was DDD (definitely done dancing), as one of the RNs was fond of saying. We did not attempt any resuscitation. He had died peacefully in his sleep.

## Chapter 16

# A TOUCH OF PREGNANCY

I was called to ER to see a young couple who had been brought in by the RCMP.

"There are a couple of kids here who were in a motor vehicle accident," explains Dora Kingston, the nursing supervisor. Dora was a portly matron, single, a career nurse, efficient and no-nonsense, her kindness and compassion hidden under a gruff exterior – the sergeant-major of Florence Nightingales.

"Teenagers shouldn't be allowed to drive – they're too irresponsible." Dora sprays the examining table with Dettol disinfectant as she speaks, and carefully wipes every inch. "They're into drugs and alcohol, and who knows what else. I guess they're too old to spank, but Lord knows they need it." Dora isn't a wellspring of medical wisdom, but she does know that microbes were the cause of much illness, and she would do her part to keep them at bay by sterilizing everything within reach of her spray bottle, which she carried like a sheriff's revolver. She was compulsive when it came to properly made beds, and ensuring that all flowers and potted plants were put in the hallway for night so they would not rob the patients of oxygen while they slept. No one could persuade her that this had no scientific basis and was quite unnecessary.

"I'll get the kids into a room," she says gruffly.

I approach the officer. "Hi, I'm Dr. Giesbrecht. What's the story?"

"Hi. These kids were driving just outside of town and rolled the car," he says. "I brought them in to get checked."

"How did that happen?"

"The driver lost control on a gravel road. Going too fast or not paying attention – I'm not sure. This kid just got his license a couple of months ago."

I watch the teenagers as Dora ushers them into the examining room. Two scared kids, standing in the hall holding hands, nervously eyeing us. "Okay. They seem fine, but I'll check them out."

"Yeah, they're probably okay," says the officer. "But we like to be sure. We can't say they're okay until you say they're okay. I'll phone their parents once you've seen them."

I glance at the ER form. Brian is 16, Sheila 15. They look flushed and shaken, otherwise none the worse for their experience. I examine Brian and discover nothing more than a few bruises on his chest and arms. He has a small goose egg on his forehead, but no headache, memory loss, or neurological evidence of concussion.

When it's Sheila's turn to be examined, Brian pulls me aside, as if to share some shameful family history.

"I'm kinda worried about her," he says in a fatherly tone.

"I'll check her over," I reply, "but she's probably fine."

"Yeah, but I'd like you to make sure…uh… she could be pregnant," Brian says, a hint of pride in his voice.

"Oh, really?" I raise my eyebrows in surprise. "She might be pregnant? Has she seen a doctor? How far along is she?"

Brian looks at his watch. "Oh, about an hour or so."

"Uh… an hour?" I turn my head and cough vigorously while I regain my composure.

"Sorry – bit of a cold I picked up. You know, Brian, if she were pregnant, no damage would occur at this stage. It will be two or three weeks before we can even do a pregnancy test. I really don't think there is anything to worry about."

Sheila has no visible injuries. Brian and Sheila leave with the officer. I double up with laughter. "Dora, did you hear that?"

"I don't know what this world is coming to," Dora fumes. "That's disgusting! These kids shouldn't even be dating. When I was fifteen, I wasn't even allowed to look at boys."

Obviously. She still isn't looking. She hasn't discovered a sense of humor, either.

"Don't you wonder exactly how the accident happened?" I chuckle again. "I'd like to be a fly on the wall when these kids try to explain this to their parents."

Dora tut-tuts indignantly. "They should be taken over the knee and spanked."

"Well, teenagers are a walking hormone bank. They know what to do, but have no idea why or why not, though they probably wouldn't listen anyway." There's nothing wrong with teenagers that reasoning with them won't aggravate.

Some women do not want to become pregnant, others desperately do. Gerda Meier was a quiet, intense woman of forty, married for many years but childless, which, in her eyes, was a fate worse than death – like Sarah from the Old Testament who was scorned even by her own maid because she was barren. Gerda had come to see me – she had missed a period two weeks before – wondering if she might be with child.

"I would be so happy to be pregnant. We wanted for years a baby. We are married sixteen years already. My sister and brothers all have children. I have no children."

"Mrs. Meier," I say, "you have just barely missed your period, so a pregnancy test will likely not tell us anything yet. It's a bit early to do a pelvic exam, too. Why don't you come back in a month? We'll do a complete physical at that time."

Gerda agrees, and promises to be back in four weeks. It would be a wonderful thing for her, a miracle after all those years, but at her age, a higher risk of a complicated pregnancy or congenital abnormalities. When she appears again in a month, Gerda is quiet, but she's beaming. She's pregnant and the curse of sixteen years is about to end.

"So how are you doing, Mrs. Meier? No period since last time?"

"No," she exults, "No period. Isn't that wonderful?"

"Yes," I say. Her joy is contagious. "That is wonderful. Let's get you on the examining table. We'll do a physical and a pelvic exam."

Her general examination is normal. There does not seem to be any enlargement of the uterus, but she carries a few extra pounds that make it difficult to be certain. The cervix is normal, and the Brevindex (pregnancy test) is negative.

"I can't feel the uterus very well, so I'm not sure," I say. "The pregnancy test is negative, but it's still early. Everything else is fine, so why don't you come back again in a month."

"When will my baby move?" she asks.

I was tempted to answer, "With any luck, right after he finishes high school," but she would not likely appreciate the wisecrack. "Probably not until about sixteen or eighteen weeks."

"I'm waiting so much for that," she says.

"No period," Gerda says at the following visit. "I'm bringing up – what you call it morning sickness? I'm so happy. My family happy. Now we all have children." Not too many of my patients are ecstatic at having nausea and retching.

"You're well, other than the nausea? I see from your chart, you have gained a few pounds. Let's do the pelvic exam once more."

I examine her pelvis, but still can't be sure. The abdominal wall is too thick to feel the uterus with certainty, like trying to feel a pea through a mattress. The pregnancy test is still negative.

I'm troubled. Something is amiss, but she has all the symptoms, so I'm willing to give her the benefit of the doubt. This was before the advent of ultrasound to examine pregnancies. Occasionally, if an abnormality was suspected, an x-ray could be done, but we tried to limit radiation as much as possible during pregnancy.

The following month, Mrs. Meier is wearing maternity clothes. She had been buying baby clothes, she says. She still looks radiant – the mysterious glow that anoints an expectant mother. Her belly is beginning to swell below her navel and her breasts are mildly engorged. It's three months now, but there is no pregnant uterus. This time I'm certain. The pregnancy test is negative for the third time.

"Mrs. Meier," I begin slowly. "I don't know how to tell you this, but you are not pregnant. Your urine test is still negative." Her eyes register shock and disbelief. "I know how very much you would like to be pregnant, but there is nothing …

"What do you mean, not pregnant. Of course I'm pregnant." She stands up. Her hands are trembling and the glow had been replaced by her blazing eyes.

"I'm really sorry," I say gently. "I know how much you want a child. Sometimes a woman's desire to have a baby is so intense that it can trick the body into these symptoms and signs. Sometimes it can be due to hormone changes. But there is no baby."

"Dr. Giesbrecht, you don't know what you talking about. I go and see different doctor." Gerda storms to the door in a rage of tears.

"I'm so sorry," I say humbly. "Please do see another doctor."

I was certain I would not see her again, but I was wrong. She came back several weeks later. The nausea and breast tenderness were gone. Her enlarged abdomen was gone, the maternity clothes were gone. Gerda's glow and exhilaration had disappeared, too. She was, in a word, deflated.

"I was foolish," she says. "I wanted so much a baby. Please, Dr. Giesbrecht, if you could maybe help us, we would be so thankful."

"You mean help you get pregnant?" A woman had never before asked me to get her pregnant. Not even my wife.

"Yes, if you can, please."

"Well, there are some things we can do. The first thing is to have your husband bring in a sperm sample. I'll explain that to you. That's probably the easiest thing to check. Very often with infertility, it's because the husband has a low sperm count. The other thing we can do is a salpingogram – an x-ray where we inject dye into the cervix to see if the tubes are open. We should refer you to a gynecologist for a consultation." She listens attentively – this is her last hope. "But you know, Mrs. Meier, I have to warn you – you are forty, and the specialist will tell you that at your age pregnancy is more risky. But I'll certainly get you an appointment if you wish."

She said she would think about it, but I did not hear from her again.

The medical term for Mrs. Meier's baffling condition is pseudocyesis, or phantom pregnancy, where a woman exhibits physiological symptoms of pregnancy, but is not pregnant. It may not be entirely wishful thinking – nutrition and hormonal factors may play a part. Pseudocyesis may last for the full nine months and even end with false labor pains. The condition has been observed since antiquity – Hippocrates gave the first written account of cases around 300 BC. The most famous case in history involved Mary Tudor, Queen of England (1516 – 1558), who thought on several occasions that she was pregnant when she was not. She was motivated in that direction, no doubt, when she recalled her father, Henry the VIII's second wife, Anne Boleyn, who lost her head for not producing a male heir.

Pseudocyesis is becoming increasingly rare, what with modern, reliable pregnancy tests, ultrasound, and more patient health knowledge.

I had not quite finished the afternoon's list of patients when I was called for an emergency Caesarean section. I told Carolyn to rebook the remaining patients. Susan Hoeppner was in labor with her first baby. She had progressed very slowly, and was in painful distress. David Kroeker decided that a section was needed.

"Please, please, Dr. Giesbrecht," Susan pleads between groans. "Do something. I can't take it anymore."

"Yes, I will as soon as I can. At this stage, it'll mean some narcotics. I understand you don't want anything like that."

"I don't care what you do, just stop the pain." She moans with another contraction. Her tone changes from pleading to screaming, "Just get that baby out of there!"

I quickly explain what I'm about to do – the intravenous and the spinal. She nods assent between groans.

The spinal takes only a few minutes to do. She has one painful contraction while the medication floods her spinal cord, then relief.

"Thank you, thank you." She sighs and takes my hand. "You're my hero."

"Oh, good," I say. "It's been a while since I've been one."

Jim Sanderson is there by this time, gowned and gloved. "Hi, Susan," he says. "We're going to start the section very soon. I'm going to test you first. Can you feel anything?" He takes forceps to pinch the skin of her lower abdomen. "Feel anything sharp?"

"No," she says, "Nothing."

"Right answer," says Jim. "Okay, we'll go ahead."

The OR is calm and Susan closes her eyes with fatigue. The nurse quietly hands me a three-page typewritten document, a sort of magnum opus of obstetrical care, which Susan had assembled from her own research during the pregnancy. "She gave us this when she came in." I shake my head in disbelief as I read. There are patients who think the best time for an epidural is right after they find out they're pregnant. This is the extreme opposite.

*PROCEDURES FOR MY HOSPITAL STAY*
*No one is to enter my room without permission, other than my husband and the head nurse*
*I shall be allowed to vocalize as I wish*
*I shall be allowed any light foods or beverages*
*No students or residents allowed, but my doula may be present. I reserve the right to ask anyone to leave my room at any time*
*No bright lights or loud voices*
*My husband shall be allowed in my room at any time*
*My husband shall be allowed to stimulate my nipples*
*No artificial induction of labor*
*No painkiller is to be administered without my permission. I am to be given no narcotics of any sort, except in an emergency. Then morphine may be given, but no Demerol*
*No episiotomy under any circumstances*
*Immediate skin-to-skin contact and breast-feeding allowed after the birth*
*Etc…*

Susan has abandoned her carefully planned delivery with amazing alacrity once hard labor set in. The nurses were all experienced, caring professionals, and several of them had been through childbirth themselves. They were there to help Susan deliver a healthy baby with as little trauma as possible. Susan's document was a mite insulting, as if the staff were all incompetent amateurs, not to be trusted to provide good care. In the end, their baby was delivered safely, and she and her husband were delighted.

But times were changing and I might as well get with the program. Susan had been aware of her rights as a patient and had adopted the consumerist attitudes emerging everywhere. No longer was the doctor's word the truth, the whole truth, and nothing but the truth. Like every other physician, I had to adapt – give more information and treatment options. The time when husbands were persona non grata in the delivery room was long gone. During my early years in practice, I might never meet the husband during the entire pregnancy and delivery. Now, however, they were expected to participate in birthing classes and the blessed event itself. As a doctor, this took a bit of getting used to – some husbands were more squeamish than their wives and required attention themselves when they fainted or felt nauseous. However, they could be a great support to their wives and begin bonding with the new arrival.

Husbands were also allowed in the operating room with Caesarean sections. It was disconcerting to have a non-professional watching my every move, invading my territory. It turned out most men couldn't care less what I did, as long as things were going well.

I thought back to the time our youngest, Jodi, was born. I had been at the hospital for emergency surgery at that time, too. When I walked into the house around seven-thirty in the evening, Brent was waiting in the hallway. Rose was on the phone trying to reach me. A small suitcase stood on the staircase.

"Thank goodness you're home," she exclaimed, as she dropped the phone. "The pains started about an hour ago and are coming every five minutes. We had better go."

I took one look at her face. "Yes, I guess we should," I said. "You've got everything?" I grabbed the suitcase.

"Yes, I'm ready. Brent, you okay with Scott? We'll let you know what's going on as soon as we can."

We were headed to St. Anne, a small hospital where my wife would avoid being delivered by a colleague of mine. "You doing okay?" I said as we started out of town down the highway.

"Yeah, I think so. The contractions are a little stronger now."

The trip was quick – I was not about to deliver my own son or daughter in the car. We arrived at the hospital and the nurses quickly got Rose settled in bed. She was in good labor. "Hey, it will soon be over – won't that be great?" I said.

This was a role reversal. I was used to being the obstetrician – efficient and professional. Now someone else was in charge, and it was *my* wife in labor. I was just a dumb husband. So what was it I'm supposed to be doing? I know – forget the professional stuff, just be supportive and comforting.

"Do you want something for pain, honey?" I said. I jumped up to call the nurse.

"No, no, I'll be okay. I don't think it will be very long."

"Okay. How often are the pains coming?"

"Every three minutes. Help me sit up."

I leaned over, grabbed her by the shoulders, and heaved.

"Ouch, that hurts. You doctors don't know much, do you? Just give me your arm so I can hoist myself up."

"Sorry." I know – just talk to her – that'll get her mind off her pain. "Honey, remember a few year's back when Scott was born?" Every mother thinks their newborn is gorgeous. "I remember seeing Scott in the hospital – he was so red and wrinkled – he was kinda ugly, wasn't he?"

Rose shot me a withering look. "Of course," I said quickly, "he's such a handsome boy now." I thought for a moment and tried again. "I was reading about these fascinating Australian birds in International Wildlife magazine. The male Mallee fowl builds a Taj Mahal of a nest. He gathers a huge pile of sand and green vegetation, and the female lays her eggs in a little hollow in the middle. When the female has finished laying the eggs, the male covers them with more leaves and grass. The eggs are kept at the proper incubation temperature of 92 degrees by the heat given off by the fermentation of the vegetation. Isn't that something? I thought that was so amazing. The male bird can sense if the temperature is too high, and uncovers the eggs to cool them off, or if the temperature is too low, he will cover the eggs with more stuff. Is that a good father or what? That's what you call a sensitive male."

Rose turned to me with a look somewhere between nausea and homicide. "Have you lost your marbles? Will you stop about that stupid bird already? Can't you think of anything better to talk about?" She rolled on her side trying to find a comfortable spot.

She seemed genuinely upset. I think she meant: If you don't shut up, I'm going to wrap the umbilical cord around your neck!

"Okay, sorry," I murmured. "I was just trying to get your mind off your pain. Is it better if I just shut up?"

"Yes, it is. Just sit next to me and hold my hand."

I took her sweaty palm and tried to look compassionate. She moaned softly every few minutes.

"You better call Ann," Rose said suddenly. "I think the baby's coming."

Ann was a seasoned professional. She took one look at Rose and wheeled her off to the delivery room. I went to the doctor's change room to put on some greens. Dr. Bergeron arrived just as I was about to go into the delivery room.

"Hi, Ray," I said, "How are you?"

"Oh, pretty good," he said. "So, another addition to the family?"

"Yeah, but I think this will be it. Six kids now. You're as busy as ever?'

"It's been a long week," Ray said. "I had a College meeting two nights ago, and last night I was on call for ER. I think I was called every hour until four. One case was a bad MVA, and I had to send a guy in with closed head injury – I don't think he's going to make it."

"Have you done any golfing?" I asked. Ray was hunting through the shelves for a cap and mask.

"I was trying to get in a couple of games. Spring is well on its way, and I've only been out once."

"Yeah, I know how it goes," I said. "I usually don't get out 'till I've done a month of yard work. Have you tried out that new course at Oakhills? It's supposed to be very nice."

"No, I haven't, but I intend to once things slow ..."

There was a loud knock at the door. It was a nurse aide. "Dr. Bergeron?" she said. "Ann says to get out there – the baby is coming."

We hurried to the delivery room across the hall. It was too late. Ann had just delivered the baby. Ray quickly grabbed a pair of gloves and took over. After the delivery of the placenta, he examined the baby.

"She's perfect," he said. "Apgar 10."

There was my beautiful little daughter, loudly voicing her displeasure at being wrenched from her warm spa to meet her lame father. My wife, bless her heart, was too relieved and happy to comment. If she had known we missed the delivery because of golf talk...

This was the end of the line for us, kid-wise – I had done my part in populating the earth, and hopefully a few of the other Biblical imperatives as well. Any more children and I'd be paying for diapers with my pension cheques.

Scott, who was now four, was enamored of his baby sister. "Mom," he said to Rose while playing with Jodi one day, "We should have another baby."

"You would like a baby sister or brother?"

"Yeah, a sister."

"Well, you have a baby sister, and there are the older kids. Your dad doesn't want any more kids."

"Why not?"

"Well, Rose replied, "He has six kids now, and he thinks that's enough."

Scott thought about that for a moment. "You can get another baby, Mom. Dad isn't the only doctor in town, you know."

## Chapter 17
# PETE AND TILLIE

M arion MacDonald was been another long-time patient, dating back to my salad days as a physician. She was militantly cheerful, her visits like a January chinook after a month of 30-below weather. Many patients enjoyed their illnesses; Marion was reluctant to complain as if it reflected badly on her character.

Marion lived in the wilds of southeastern Manitoba in a settlement called Sandridge, a metropolis of nine or ten houses, and a gas station/hotel-pub/convenience store/post office. "It's a one-horse town," Marion said, "but the horse died." That corner of the planet was flat with rocky, marginal soil. It grew aspen, poplar, some birch, several species of evergreen, eccentric hermits, and a few grow-ops. In Plautdietsch, we call this topography *Struck* (bush). If you came from the *Struck*, you couldn't really cling to any pretensions.

The bush provided few ways of making a living other than wood cutting and raising cattle. Blueberries, saskatoons, and peat moss were the only other natural resources. Marion was married to Bill, a contractor, who had a crew of seven or eight, cutting and transporting pulpwood. In doing so, they had managed to double the economic impact of the region and make a decent living for themselves.

"We're okay," she said, "We're making a living. And we don't mind the isolation."

"So, what do you do for excitement out there?" I asked.

"Oh, there's bingo and cards. If we get tired of that, we start rumors. On Saturday, we go out and hit the pub. Once in a while we have a murder so people don't forget about us entirely." They did in fact have a homicide some years back, which had cemented their image in the minds of Manitobans as an uncivilized backwater.

Marion was conscientious and sensible about her health. She came to my office every two years like clockwork for a physical, a Pap test, and a mammogram.

"Make sure you check the begonias – they're a great blessing to my husband. This one we call Pete," pointing to her right breast, "and the other one is Tillie. Tillie is his favorite. After a trip to Wyoming, he called them the Grand Tetons. Bill says big boobs are good because they pull the wrinkles out of my face." She laughed heartily, as she always did at the slightest provocation.

Marion had mild hypertension, controlled with a small dose of diuretic and a beta-blocker. She was moderately overweight from "all the rich living we do out there."

Some time later Marion arrives at the office as a walk-in one day on a particularly crazy afternoon – I'm an hour behind schedule. It's the middle of July and several colleagues are on holidays. Daphne asks would I see her, or should she send her to ER? No, I'll see her. It's probably important – Marion wouldn't show up without an appointment unless it was something a more critical than a cold.

She walks haltingly into the examining room, her husband Bill steadying her on his arm. Her face is flushed with exertion and she winces as Bill helps her to a chair. I frown – this is not the feisty woman I had known all these years.

"Marion," I say in astonishment. "What's going on? This isn't like you."

"You tell me," she says, wearily. "Strange things are happening. It's like I'm drunk without a party." She forces a laugh. "My legs started to get numb and tingle the day before yesterday. I've been getting weaker by the hour, and now I can hardly walk."

"This does look very odd," I say, puzzled. "Two days ago you were fine? Do you have tingling or weakness in your arms or face, too?"

"Yeah, two days ago I was okay. I have a bit of numbness and weakness of both arms, mostly the left, and my face feels funny, too. This morning my speech was slurred and I was dizzy, but that part is better now."

"Have you had any chest colds or flu recently?"

"She had stomach flu two weeks ago," Bill offers.

I take Marion's arm and help her to the examining table. "I want to check a few things." "First, we'll do a quick physical." I examine her head and neck, lungs, heart and abdomen – everything is textbook. I grab her hand. "Let's check your muscle strength – pull toward yourself." It takes little effort on my part to straighten her arm. There is definite weakness in her legs as well. I tap the knees and ankles – virtually no reflexes. She has some facial weakness raising her eyebrows or showing her upper teeth. Her pulse rate is rapid and she looks flushed. I go through a quick differential diagnosis in my mind. Stroke? The symptoms are too varied and there are deficiencies on both sides of the body – rare with strokes. Plus, she's fully alert. Multiple sclerosis? Unlikely – the progression of symptoms is much too rapid. Brain tumor? Again, too rapid and her symptoms are bilateral.

Guillain-Barre! That would fit – substantial disability within a couple of days, multiple symptoms, and onset after a viral illness.

"Marion, I'm not quite sure what is going on, but this sounds like something called Guillain-Barre."

She grimaces. "I've never heard of that."

"It's a nerve disorder, thought to be an auto-immune problem, where the body's immune system gets confused and attacks its own tissues. There may be inflammation and destruction of the myelin sheath, the insulating tissue around the peripheral (outside the brain) nerves. We'll have to get you in hospital for observation, and do a few tests."

I see Marion the next morning. She's cheerful, but the weakness has progressed – she is unable to walk, and has more facial paralysis. I perform a lumbar puncture to obtain some spinal fluid for analysis. There are no blood cells, which would suggest infection, like meningitis or abscess, or a bleeding abnormality of some kind. However, there is increased protein in the fluid, part of the picture of Guillain-Barre.

"Guillain-Barre can progress rapidly to respiratory failure," I comment to Laura after rounds. "She may require intensive care and a respirator. She worries me – this is really more than we can handle here. I'm going to contact Dr. Middleton in Winnipeg. She should be transferred before we run into trouble."

I manage to track Jeff Middleton down at Health Sciences Centre, and tell him Marion's story. He's sympathetic, but Marion isn't in respiratory failure, in other words, not an emergency, and their intensive care beds are occupied. I agree to continue observation in our hospital. I would have liked Marion in a larger center with all the facilities needed if a crisis should arise. We didn't have a respirator or an intensive care unit at Bethesda hospital.

I leave orders to monitor her breathing and blood pressure. We put her on a cardiac monitor and oximeter to check the oxygen saturation in her blood. I leave the hospital with a feeling of unease that won't go away. But Marion holds her own, and after several days, she has partially recovered. Her facial and arm weakness has improved slightly, and she is able to walk the halls with another person by her side.

The next afternoon clinic was routine and I managed to get home by six o'clock. No one else was home that day. I had planned to golf, but it was too late to find anyone to join me. Besides, it was a blisteringly hot day, and golf was cruel enough in pleasant weather. I scrounge in the fridge hoping to discover something delectable, but settle for some leftover chicken and rice. I check the vegetable drawer, but there are only a few carrots and celery from the Diefenbaker era. I toss them in the garbage. I nuke the chicken hoping for a miracle of rejuvenation – perhaps some Botox would help. I grab a glass of ice water and sit under the patio umbrella. A moment of peace, patients briefly forgotten.

It's a claustrophobic airless heat. The air buzzes with honeybees around the potted flowers on the deck, and an occasional dragonfly passes by, its transparent wings whirring softly. A slight breeze springs up and I listen to the wind talking in the tall poplars. There's a hint of dark billows on the far western horizon – perhaps the makings of a thunderstorm.

Overhead the high-pitched whine of an airplane catches my attention, distant, yet familiar. There are many private single-engine planes that fly overhead; our property is in a direct line with the runway of the local airport, a half-mile to the north-west. I recognize the drone immediately – the sky diving plane, circling for altitude to drop its cargo of human bombs. The aircraft is barely visible in the hazy cloud to the west. I run for my binoculars. There's a drop in pitch of the engine's whine as the pilot cuts the power and the first tiny speck falls from the plane. As the pilot circles for the next drop, I hear a snap like the pop of a balloon as the first chute opens and brings the plummeting figure up short. I follow several of the colorful sails drifting lazily to earth behind the trees.

I finish my leftovers and go into the house to change into my summer grubbies. Scott has mowed the lawn, but I will do the finishing touches like edging and trimming. Back to nature, like primitive man, now a bit more technical with gas-powered tools, chemicals, and plant hybrids, and a chance to exercise some of the farming skills I had learned as a boy. Even in the stifling heat of mid-summer, I find gardening to be a healing touch, a creative endeavor, picking and choosing from the bounty of nature, and shaping it to our needs. I like the molecular biology part, too – the combinations of DNA that orders one blob of plant tissue to become a patch of inconspicuous moss on a rock in the pond, and another, a towering cottonwood on the north side of the yard. How is it possible for these infinitesimal spirals of protein to direct the petals of a cranesbill to grow to a five-point velvety star of white with blue edging? My botany lectures come to mind: the mechanism that makes a water lily close for night, and open to welcome the sun, called heliotropism, a system that triggers motor cells by the movement of potassium in and out of cells. Or gravitropism that uses a plant hormone called auxin to make roots grow down and stems grow up in response to gravity. I'm fascinated by the fact that you can make hydrangea bloom bluer with acidic soil and pink with alkaline soil.

The universe is marvelously complex. Is it possible that evolution could have brought all this about without the guiding hand of a Creator? Functionally, evolution makes sense, but why a gorgeous sunset, a sky sparkling with stars, or the endless colors of plants, birds and even fish, the abundance of which seems to serve little purpose other than beauty itself. I have spent years reading natural history and science – the more information I glean, the less certain I am about the process. I have been through the spectrum from six-day creation to

Darwinian evolution, but do not yet know the truth, not that it really matters.

I like the search. I'm not concerned about the answer. I understand the adage, "walk with those who seek the truth, shun those who have found it." The Creator must have a good laugh now and then at our relentless, divisive, and often futile attempts at explanation.

After the edging, I bring out the chainsaw. I hate to bring down any tree. It's a remarkable thing to watch it grow, provide pleasure to the eye, and shelter for many creatures. However, several apple and linden trees have succumbed to a harsh winter. And there's nothing quite like a chainsaw burning fossil fuel to get rid of pent-up aggression and bring male instincts to the fore.

A chainsaw and a truck. One couldn't really claim masculinity without owning a half-ton, even if it's a 1968 GMC with extras like through-the-floor ventilation, and tires as smooth as a bowling ball. It once had a beautiful blue exterior, now leprous with rust.

My pager interrupts my thoughts as I work. I go indoors to phone the hospital. "Mrs. Macdonald is not doing so well," Laura says. "She's having trouble breathing, and she seems a little confused. Her oxygen saturation has dropped to 88 percent." Normal is 95 to 100.

I clean up and race to the hospital. I head straight to her room. "Hi, Marion, how are you doing?"

My question is answered straightaway – Marion is flushed, and her lips have a ghastly bluish tinge. She doesn't have the labored breathing of most other respiratory conditions because her chest muscles are quitting on her, signals from her respiratory center are not getting through. She rouses only when I shake her gently, and she partially opens her eyes. "Hi, Bill," she says. "I can't breathe." She's becoming confused from the anoxia (low blood oxygen). I listen to her lungs – little air entry anywhere.

"Okay," I tell Laura, "we have to transfer her. Get the ambulance crew here. Do we have the emergency equipment for the ambulance? I'll have to intubate her before we go."

"While we're getting things ready, can you see if you can get Dr. Middleton on the phone?" I ask Jenna, the ward clerk.

I find the laryngoscope, and a number 7 endotracheal tube. I give Marion 120 mg of succinyl choline to paralyze her vocal cords, and insert the tube. Mona connects this to the oxygen outlet on the wall, and to an ambubag, a balloon-like apparatus that is compressed at regular intervals to breathe for the patient.

The team is ready in 30 minutes, and begins transferring Marion to the waiting ambulance. Arlene, another RN, will accompany us to the city. She will handle the ambubag for respiratory assist. Meanwhile, Dr. Middleton was nowhere to be found. I ask for the resident from the intensive care unit.

"Sorry, no beds," he says. "Try St Boniface hospital."

I talk to the intensive care resident at St. Boniface. He's sympathetic, but the answer is the same, "Sorry, we're jammed – no beds." I can feel my anger and frustration mounting – always the same run-around.

"You know, doctor," I protest, "the patient is in the ambulance. She is not doing well. She is intubated and needs an intensive care unit. If I phone another hospital, I'll get the same answer. That's just a waste of time – I'm taking her to your ER."

"Well, okay," he says, "I guess I can't stop you."

I hang up. "Okay, let's go, St. Boniface." When Marion lands in ER, they will have to deal with her. I have no other choice. The system often fails, and sometimes we have to disregard niceties and protocol, and do whatever is necessary.

Things do work when they are compelled to – Marion Macdonald is admitted to the intensive care unit. She has a stormy course in hospital and requires several months of convalescence. With rigorous physiotherapy, she makes a virtually complete recovery. Her illness happened before the modern treatment of plasmapheresis, where the patient's blood is removed in stages, the serum separated, and the blood reinfused so the body builds a new complement of antibodies.

After that illness I hadn't seen Marion for several years. She had continued follow-up with her physicians in Winnipeg. I had forgotten her – patients don't always come to mind until they show up one day and you realize you haven't seen them for some time.

Marion had come for an office appointment. I hardly recognized her – she had lost weight, and her face was drawn and pallid. There were lines and furrows I hadn't seen before. Her hair didn't look right somehow, and I realized she was wearing a wig.

"Tillie got it," she says matter-of-factly after the initial exchange of greetings. "I think they made her into soap. Pete is so lonely." Marion's laugh seems forced and weary.

"What?" I say, "Tillie? What are you talking about?" Then I remember – the blessed twins, Pete and Tillie. I chuckle, at the same time aware that it seems inappropriate. "What happened to Tillie?"

"Well, I had my last mammogram in Winnipeg. The doctors found a spot on the x-ray which turned out to be cancer, so I was referred to a surgeon."

"Oh, wow, I'm so sorry to hear that. So you had a mastectomy? How are you doing?"

"Well, I'm okay so far. I had the surgery, and I've just finished radiation."

"What was the operation? Probably modified radical mastectomy with axillary dissection."

That was the gold standard for breast cancer – mastectomy with removal of as many lymph nodes as possible from the armpit. The nodes are examined for tumor spread – necessary for staging – determining what radiation or chemotherapy should be used.

215

"Yeah, that's the one. That's not the boob job I had in mind. A lift, maybe – I couldn't cross my legs anymore without getting them caught." Another rueful laugh. "Anyway, I'm almost finished the radiation, and the specialist at the cancer clinic said I should go back to you for follow-up care and my blood pressure. So here I am, what's left of me."

"Are you okay? You've lost weight."

She sags momentarily, then brightens as if lifting her spirits by her own bootstraps. "I'll be okay now that the treatments are done. I have to get back to a normal life. I know I look pretty sad. I think I'll go to the beauty salon for an estimate. Too bad they can't bring Tillie back. You know this nonsense about beauty being only skin-deep? That's deep enough for me – what do I want, an adorable liver?"

I laugh. Some of the old gumption is back – she wills it to be back. "You could have reconstructive surgery done," I say.

"No," she sighs, "that's like new paint on an Edsel– it's not that important any more."

With the weight loss Marion's blood pressure is normal and we stop all her medications except the tamoxifen. That was the accepted cancer drug to prevent tumor recurrence. I contact her surgeon for a report on her mastectomy. The operation had been uneventful, but the cancer was aggressive with spread to her lymph nodes – Stage III, which meant a 50% chance of surviving 5 years.

Marion does well for the next nine or ten months. She puts on some weight, and her hair grows back. Then at one of her monthly checkups, I sense immediately something is wrong – the energy and sparkle have vanished again. "I've got pain in my chest, and I'm tired again," she says, rubbing her left arm.

"Any cough or fever? Are you short of breath?"

"No, not really. Maybe a little short of breath with vacuuming or heavy work like that."

I examine her chest wall and axilla (armpit where the dissection of lymph nodes was done). There are no enlarged glands, but there is some diffuse rib tenderness. I have that sinking sensation – her cancer had been an aggressive one, but this is still awfully soon for a recurrence. "We'll have to get a chest x-ray and some blood tests and check this out," I say. I try to keep my tone matter-of-fact and cheerful, despite what I know will not be good news.

"I knew it! The cancer is back, isn't it?" For the first time in her life she looks exhausted – not the fatigue of physical exertion, but the comprehension that it's over.

"Well, I don't know yet. Hopefully it's something else, but I'd be lying if I didn't tell you it looks like a recurrence. Go over to the hospital and get the x-ray done. You should probably make an appointment with me for next week."

The next morning, I go to look at the chest x-ray. There are several lucent spots on her ribs.

"These are metastases, right?" I ask Mel Levitt.

"Yeah, doesn't look so good," he says. "There are some metastatic lesions in the ribs, and the mediastinum is widened and irregular."

The mediastinum is the central structure in the chest containing the esophagus, trachea (windpipe), and the aorta, the large vessel taking blood from the heart to the rest of the body. The mediastinum also contains many lymph nodes that may enlarge with infections or tumor spread.

Marion returns in a few days with Bill. I tell them the verdict. "I phoned the oncologist, and you have an appointment with him for Friday."

"There isn't much they can do, is there? I mean, it's only ten months since I finished the chemotherapy."

"Well, I don't honestly know. I guess the best we can hope for is to shrink the tumors with some more radiation or chemotherapy. Dr. Elwood will tell you what the chances are. I'm sorry, Marion. That's really awful news."

"I've had a good run," she replies. "God has been very good to me, and I can't expect much more. I guess I can see Dr. Elwood, but he probably can't do a whole lot."

God? I'm almost startled. I lean forward. "Well…you're right, there may not be much they can do, but there is always a chance. You seem to have a very good attitude. I'm a bit surprised. I've never heard you mention God before."

"You know, Dr. Giesbrecht, after I almost died from Guillain-Barre, my neighbor Gwen came to see me. She and her husband run the little church in our area. She had called me before, but I thought she was a Bible-thumper who just wanted to add another scalp to her belt, so I had told her to get lost. Anyway, she asked if she could come over. I thought why not – at this stage what do I have to lose. Anyway, we got to be friends, and she turned out to be such a wonderful caring person. She never once preached to me, until one day I asked her what she knew about death, you know, what would happen when she passed away. She told me about her abused childhood, and the terrible pain and rejection she suffered, and how she slowly overcame her past with God's help."

"So you go to her church?"

"Sometimes. Sometimes Gwen, a few other women, and I have our own sessions. We read the Bible or other books; sometimes we just talk. At first I thought there must be some loopholes around this dying thing, but I couldn't find any. Anyway, God has opened up a whole new world to me. There are so many people who are hurting out there, and we're trying to help them. So I'm doing whatever I can until the time comes."

"So what are you doing?"

"Well, there is an elderly couple who need some help – they are both frail, so I go there a couple of times a week and make meals or clean. And I volunteer if the health nurse has a young mom who needs some help. Anyway, if I live a little longer, that's good – I'll do more, and if I can't, that's okay too."

"That's an amazing story," I say. I lower my head. "I should have talked to you a long time ago."

"No, I would have told you to go to hell, and I would never have come back."

The oncologist started Marion on radiation, but it brought on waves of nausea, and more lethargy. She decided to stop all her treatments except for pain medication. With metastases to her ribs, spine and liver, she required large doses of morphine and fentanyl patches to control the pain. She died in hospital several months later, her indomitable spirit and faith intact to the end. She had not run an orphanage in Calcutta or won an Olympic medal, but she was a champion nevertheless – from a one-horse town in the *Struck*.

## Chapter 18
# TRUTH SERUM

The morning slate listed a diagnostic laparoscopy, hernia repair, and cholecystectomy (removal of gallbladder), a typical surgical day. But you never know what interesting twists may develop. Like snowflakes, no two people are exactly alike, not even identical twins, and people sometimes respond to therapy and drugs in curious ways. Standard doses work for most people, but may still have unusual effects.

Jennifer, twenty-something, long on shape, but a little short on intellect, headlined the day. She needed a diagnostic laparotomy for intermittent abdominal pain during the previous year. Her health history was otherwise unremarkable except for mild seasonal asthma.

"Good morning Jennifer," I say, tying my mask as I walk in. "I'm Dr. Giesbrecht, the sleep doctor. We met at the clinic the other day, remember? How are you?" I quietly begin filling syringes with my favorite potions.

"Hi," she says. "What is all that stuff? That scares me."

"You'll be just fine. We'll take good care of you. Did Nora give you the Ventolin before you came?"

"The what? Oh, you mean the mask? Yeah. Are you sure I'll be okay? I'm afraid of needles."

"Trypanophobia." She looks at me quizzically. "Fear of needles, medical procedures. You have an IV running – no more needles," I reassure her. "You're in good health and this is a short procedure. It's not a big deal with keyhole surgery. Everything will be fine," I say in my best operating room tableside manner. "I'm starting the happy juice now." I turn on the electronic pump and the propofol begins flowing smoothly into her vein.

Surgery and anesthesia had changed considerably by the early '90s. Many surgical procedures were now done with laparoscopic equipment to view the abdomen and remove an appendix or gallbladder. The abdominal anatomy is viewed in enlarged detail on the monitor screen. We had also begun using other anesthesia techniques, particularly the intravenous agent propofol.

"What's that white stuff?" Jennifer asks. She is apprehensive, eyeing the 60 ml syringe in the pump.

"This? It's called propofol – it's the sleep medicine. It'll be lights out in a minute or two."

"Have a good sleep," says Eleanor, the circulating nurse that day. "When you wake up, you'll be back in recovery room on your stretcher." As the drug starts to percolate through Jennifer's cerebral cortex, she changes from nail-biter to Chatty Kathy. There is only twenty or thirty seconds between trepidation and out for the count, but often it's long enough for a bit of unplanned exposé.

"Ohhh… this is so fun," she slurs. "It's feels like I'm floating in an airplane." She smiles dreamily. "My boyfriend and I went for an airplane ride last week – you know, the Mile-High Club?" I put the pump into overdrive and her words trailed off. "That was so cool… we want to…"

This was more medical history than we needed to know.

"What's the heck is the Mile-High Club?" queries Eleanor after the initial flurry of activity had settled and the surgery begins.

"Never heard of the Mile-High-Club?" I grin behind my mask.

"No, I have no idea what she was talking about."

"Really? Well, you may want to look into that. It's a very exclusive club. An enterprising pilot takes you up in his private plane. There's a cot in the back, and when they reach an altitude of one mile, he draws a curtain behind the cockpit and the couple, ah, you know... "

"What?" Eleanor bursts out laughing. "Really? Oh, for goodness sake! No wonder she was so enthusiastic." She waggles her finger at me. "Don't you ever give me any of that stuff."

"Got some deep secrets?" I inquire. "I won't tell anyone. I've heard that people sometimes become card-carrying members on regular airline flights, too."

Eleanor giggles, "Dr. Giesbrecht! How do you know about that?"

"Oh, I read about it... in a magazine, MD Review, as a matter of fact."

"Yeah, right! That's a likely story."

"It's true," I protest. I glance at the patient monitor – O2 sat, blood pressure, heart rate normal. "That's where I heard about it. People will do anything for a thrill. Some climb Everest, some sail around the world, and some... well, do this. If anyone has ever done it on Mt. Everest I can't say."

Jennifer had no serious pathology. There were some small areas of endometriosis, tissue from the lining of the uterus on the ligaments, ovaries, or fallopian tubes, sometimes even the intestines. With the hormonal changes of a woman's cycle, these trouble spots can swell and cause pain. These were cauterized and the normal appendix removed.

The next patient, Juan, needs a hernia repair. He looks a little shop-worn for 22 – pock-marked skin, unkempt dirty hair, and brown teeth. He's Mennonite with a few Mexican genes added for flavor. He had recently arrived in Canada. He has been tight-lipped about his health history and the reason for leaving Mexico. He knows some English, but is more comfortable in Spanish and Low German.

I don't like surprises, so I pursue his medical history again when he arrives in the OR. I can't help thinking there's an unsavory past. "Juan, any health problems? Any previous surgery? Are you taking any medications?"

"No operations," he assures me, "No pills. Everything good."

"Okay," I say. "Everything good. Siesta time, Juan."

I start the propofol, and Juan begins talking. "I take cocaine, but no more when I get out of jail. The doctor give pills for depresh, uh, nerves…"

"Depression?" I say. I glance at Eleanor. "I thought you weren't on any drugs, Juan. Which doctor was that?"

"The jail….doc…. I don't …" Too late, his frontal lobe has been immobilized like a shot from a taser.

I added a note to the chart about his history. "Interesting what the truth serum will reveal," I say to Brad. "I wonder what else there is to the story."

Brad, a medical resident in Steinbach for several months, has already scrubbed in as assistant, waiting for Jim Sanderson to arrive. "Hey, do you think I could have some of that stuff? Some of our parties are pretty dull."

"Well… that's kinda illegal," I reply, "I don't think Health Canada will approve it as a party drug. However, in return for immunity, I might bring some if I'm invited. Actually, most people don't get talkative with the drug – they just drift off. By the way, Eleanor, have you called Dr. Sanderson?"

"We've called him twice. He'll be here shortly. He's just seeing someone in ER."

"I'd start the operation myself," says Brad. "But the nurse won't give me that sharp pokey thing."

As fate would have it, I see Juan a number of times after that operating room encounter. He comes to ER on a Saturday morning during my shift. He is agitated and looks like a casualty from a back-alley brawl. I'm not that surprised after the revelations during his anesthetic.

"Hello, Juan," I say. "We meet again. You look like you're in trouble."

"Yeah, I think I had stroke. My arm hurts. It's like dead." He lifts his left arm and tries to straighten his wrist.

"This just happened overnight? What about these bruises on your face?"

"Yeah, this morning I wake up, no feeling on my hand. I can't use it proper."

"And your face?"

"Oh… I fall." Acute gravity attack.

Right, and my grandmother was Anastasia, the last surviving member of the Romanovs. I'm beginning to see some flaws in Juan's business plan.

"Let's have a look," I say. Juan has a wrist drop – when he pronates (palm down) his arm, the hand droops and he can't straighten the fingers. With gentle pricks from a 25-gauge needle and the touch of a Kleenex, there's loss of sensation of the back of the hand and along the thumb and index finger. His right arm is fine except for Rothman's sign (tobacco staining of fingers).

"Juan, let's cut the bull. Where exactly were you last night? Were you stoned, or had too much to drink?"

He looks sheepishly at the floor. "Too much beer, I pass out."

"Ah, brown bottle flu. Drugs, too? Let me guess – you fell asleep on a chair or bench, and probably had your arm slung over the back." Juan says nothing, but his face tells me I'm warm. "Well, you have radial neuropathy. It comes from hours of pressure on the nerve here in your arm." The radial nerve is stunned, and some of the fibers can be beyond recovery. This condition is sometimes called Saturday night palsy or honeymooner's palsy (use your imagination). I touch Juan's upper arm where the radial nerve is easily compressed against the humerus.

"Oh," he says. "It get better? I start job at the window factory."

"You won't be able to work for a while." We'd have a hard time explaining this one to Workers Compensation. "Your arm will work again when the nerve heals, but it may take weeks or even months." I apply a splint to keep Juan's wrist and fingers in a neutral position. "I'll give you a requisition for physiotherapy, you know, exercises? Come and see me at the clinic in two weeks and we'll see how it's coming along."

"I can't work?" Juan asks. He gestures with his good arm. "No money."

"Well, I don't really know what to tell you," I say. "I guess you have to see your boss, explain the problem, and hope the company will hire you back once your arm is healed. You have no family here? Are you living with some people in town?"

"Yeah, Friesens on Barkman street over there. Cousin, my father."

"Let's hope they're understanding enough to let you stay there until you can work again. If nothing else, we can try for social assistance. And, Juan – try and stay out of trouble."

The neuropathy healed, though it took the better part of four months, with no residual loss of function. Juan found another job hanging chickens at Granny's Poultry eviscerating plant. In the meantime, he had outlived his welcome at the Friesens, and now shared lodging with a friend he met at his workplace.

It's late July, summer holidays are moving swiftly, and we need to get away for a break. It had been a hectic spring and summer. Full-time jobs, end-of-school functions, baseball windups, high school graduations. Rose and I are charter members of the Rat Race. A vacation is long overdue.

Friday arrives, the last day before our planned vacation. I had hoped for a routine, no-surprises day. There are so many last minute things to look after before a holiday. Thursday, I had completed all the EKG reports, and assigned my hospital patients to two of the other physicians. Dan Morgan agreed to look after all the lab and x-ray reports and referral letters that couldn't wait until I got back. Any prenatal that went into labor would be looked after by the on-call physician.

I'm still shaving when I get the first phone call of the day from Resthaven nursing home about a patient with a cough and shortness of breath. Would I come have a look? "Can it wait until a little later," I ask. "I have to be in the operating room in twenty minutes. I'll try to get there over the lunch hour."

After half a dozen interruptions and minor emergencies, I arrive at the nursing home after seven that evening. "Tina Neufeld is sick," Hilda says. "Could you check her lungs – she has a bit of a fever and cough. She hasn't been eating that well."

Tina Neufeld is a frail, desiccated woman, slowly fading into the sunset. She's ninety and has lost her mobility along with her appetite. She still has all her mental faculties, which gives her enormous credibility in a place where everyone is waiting to depart this mortal coil and many have lost their marbles. Fortunately, she only has a chest cold, with no evidence of pneumonia.

"Let's just watch her for now," I tell the RN. "Call Dr. Kroeker if she isn't doing well. He'll be on call if there are any problems while I'm gone. Everything else is okay? Everyone is pooping abundantly?" In a nursing home, timely bowel function is the criterion of good health. A resident may have a barely perceptible pulse and no blood pressure, but if they have satisfactory droppings, everyone is happy.

"Sometimes I wonder if holidays are worth the hassle," I say to Rose at the end of the day as we are packing. "We have to scramble like mad before we go, and then it takes a week to catch up when we get back." Medicine is rewarding, but a callous taskmaster. Besides the usual office hours and anesthesia, I take my regular shift in ER, deliver babies at any hour of the day or night, take my turn at weekend hospital rounds, look after my nursing home patients, and do anesthesia emergency call every other week. That means doubling shifts before and after going away. We don't take enough holidays, and the ones we do take, are often combined with educational (school board) conferences or medical refresher courses.

"Well, you still have to get away for a break," Rose admonishes. "You are going to have to cut something out of your schedule, like ER."

I did, in fact, soon thereafter stop taking ER rotations, and after an extensive guilt trip, quit obstetrics. It was a difficult decision. There was mild resentment among my colleagues – family practitioners were expected to do their share, particularly when it came to ER and obstetrics, the most onerous of our many duties. Seniority was no excuse – they might let you off the hook if you broke your hip after a fall with your second stroke.

All four of us enjoyed baseball and Scott and Jodi played the game, so we had decided to take a driving holiday to Minneapolis, St Louis, Milwaukee, and Chicago for major league baseball. I was inclined toward science museums, live theater, and history. The kids inherited half their DNA from me and would like the same stuff, right? Actually, no, it turns out. So it was baseball. This was to be a genuine family holiday tuned to the interests of the two youngest.

Scott had had a knee injury suffered sliding into second during a baseball game. The wound had developed into a nasty abscess that had to be opened and drained. He spent several days in hospital for intravenous antibiotics in the care of one of my colleagues. A hospital stay is no big deal for a patient, but it's different when it's your own flesh and blood. Scott said little, and I knew he felt abandoned in this strange, hostile environment, but he endured the indignities of the hospital without a whimper.

Unfortunately, the abscess left a gaping hole near his knee, which would take a long time to heal and needed to be cleansed and repacked every day. Rose, mother and nurse, was appointed to the position. We prepared a medical kit with antibiotics, antiseptic, tapes, and half a kilometer of gauze packing.

Finally, everything is ready and we set off in great anticipation. Mozart had been sent to Rose's sister for the duration. As usual, Rose had packed a lunch for our first meal, which is gone by the time we reached Highway 59, twelve miles from home.

We drive to Minneapolis, and then on to Chicago. I'm not particularly interested in going to the windy city. Besides the art and architecture, Chicago had a reputation for crowded streets, ghettos, and crime. We determine to avoid all of that. My researched strategy is to stick to one freeway, drive to Wrigley Field in plenty of time for the game, and then hightail it out of there, avoiding the city altogether. I had checked the maps closely – take Interstate 94 to West Irving Park Road, then the south turnoff to Wrigley Field. As fate or inattention would have it, we missed the turnoff, and suddenly the shining waters of Lake Michigan lay before us.

"Oh, shoot, now what?" I wonder aloud. "We missed the exit." I scan the green signs overhead. North to the concrete canyons of downtown Chicago, which is the last place I want to go during rush hour. "Let's take the off ramp. If we make a right turn, and then go west parallel to Irving Park Road, that should take us to Wrigley sooner or later, right?" Hope and bravado.

"I have no idea where we are," says Rose. "Let me see the map. Aren't we going to get lost if we do that? Maybe we should stop and ask for directions."

"Who are we going to ask?" I reply.

"We're bound to run into a service station or some people on the street."

"There's nobody around here to ask." Rose shoots me that patented look of exasperation.

"Okay, okay, I know – men don't ask for directions. Christopher Columbus didn't need to stop for directions and I don't either. Listen, if we come across something promising, I'll stop. We're going west, so we should run right into the stadium, right?" I'm asking a woman who spent two weeks in the same hotel room in Hawaii and still headed down the wrong hallway. "We could try getting back to the freeway, but we might miss our exit again."

"Dad," says Scott, "this doesn't look very good." The streets are narrow and dirty, derelict houses and tenements on both sides. Everyone stares as we passed. Even the air seems oppressive and heavy with danger. We don't belong here. I feel targeted, like Chevy Chase in Vacation. There seems to be an unusual number of youths loitering at the street corners. A late-model Lincoln with Manitoba license plates is in stark contrast to the battered jalopies that growl past, sans muffler.

"This is scary," says Jodi, "let's go back."

"We can't go back now," I reply. "Maybe we should stop and ask for directions. How bad can it be?" I slow to a stop and rolled down the window. Several youths from both sides of the street start converging on the car.

"Dennis! Don't stop!" cries Rose, panic in her voice. "Close your window! Just drive!"

I gun the engine and we take off, tires squealing. I have visions of being pulled from our vehicle, robbed and left for dead on the street. We barrel straight ahead, ignoring stop signs, and five blocks later, there's Wrigley Field – as majestic as the Taj Mahal, and as welcoming as the lights of Steinbach.

We arrive in time to get good seats behind first base, and watch batting practice. First order of business is to order Pepsi and bratwurst, with gobs of mustard and ketchup – cuisine fit for a king. Andre Dawson is in batting practice. This is life at its finest.

After the game, we make our way back to the I94. It's dark by this time. "Okay, let's just stick to the freeway." I say. "It's only ten, so we should be able to find a motel. There were a bunch of them about fifteen or twenty miles back the way we came."

"I hope we find something soon," Rose says. "I'm really tired and so are the kids."

"Okay, we'll stop at the first decent place we see."

We pass a Howard Johnson with a NO VACANCY sign. We pass a Ramada Inn. "Let's try that," Rose says. "Get off at the next exit." The sign also indicates no vacancy. "Why don't we ask anyway? Maybe they can tell us where we can find a room."

The clerk is a paradigm of customer service. "We're full," she says as I walk into the motel lobby.

"Any motels around here that might have room?"

"Nah."

"Well, are there any places I could phone?"

"Don't know."

"Is there a town anywhere near here?"

"Nah, don't know nothin' about this stretch."

We stop at a Hampton Inn, a Roadway, and an Americinn without success. It's now eleven thirty and a strange alarm sets in – we may not find anything, and we may have to keep driving all night, or park in a Wal-Mart lot until morning.

"I suppose we can just keep driving," I say. "The kids can sleep. Eventually we should find something."

"There," says Rose, pointing to a sign that says simply MOTEL in large red neon letters. "Stop there. Maybe they have something."

We drive up to the lobby. There's a wide ribbon of cigarette butts, paper cups, and weeds around the entrance. The place has peeling paint and a broken concrete pad at the door. Some of the second floor balcony railings are missing. This is not the New York Ritz-Carleton.

"Are you sure we want to stay here?" I frown and look at Rose. "It looks pretty seedy."

"Well, its twelve o'clock, and I'm ready for almost anything."

"Okay, I'll see what they have."

There is a room with two beds available. The bathroom is ancient, but the cockroaches are away at a convention, and there's hot water. The bed is an old metal four-poster, but the sheets are clean. Inside a small fridge is a small container of yogurt growing new life forms. The room will have to do. We settle in for the night.

"Sorry, Scott," says Rose, "but we have to change your dressing before you go to bed. It's been over twenty-four hours." She cuts the old dressing, pulls out several feet of purulent gauze packing, and cleanses the wound with water and hydrogen peroxide.

"Ew, that's gross!" says Jodi, wrinkling her nose.

"Well, you don't have to watch," says Scott. He winces as Rose uses the forceps to fold fresh packing into the wound. He takes his antibiotics and the kids are off to sleep in short order. I venture to the lobby to ask where the pop machine is located. The clerk is sitting at the desk with a beer and a cigarette. She's on the telephone.

"Yeah, right – there was this guy murdered in one of our rooms last night." She takes another drag on her cigarette and blows the smoke over her shoulder. "What? Oh yeah, I'm okay. It was kinda creepy with the cops all over the place. Nah, I didn't know the guy – I guess he was pushing drugs or somethin'. I gotta go – there's a guy at the desk. Talk to ya later."

I find the drink machine, grab a few cans, walk back to the room, and bolt the door. I tell Rose about the conversation I overheard.

"Oh, brother," she says. "Do you think it's safe to stay here?"

"It's a dive, but what choice do we have? Are we going to pack up the kids again and drive? It's midnight. Anyway, what are the chances, those things usually involve drugs or dealers. I'm sure we'll be okay."

We sleep fitfully, expecting someone to burst through the door and stab us in our beds. With the early light of dawn, we are packed and on our way. Our trip continues without incident with baseball games in Kansas City, St. Louis, Minneapolis, and then back to Steinbach.

Once home, our first priority is to retrieve Mozart. As Rose opens the door to let him in, he begins his frantic buzz, ecstatic to be home, pausing briefly at intervals to sniff, making sure everything is as he had left it. With that assurance, he proceeds to ignore us. He won't look us in the eye, and even snubs Rose, whom he usually follows about every minute of the day. He's offended – we had abandoned him and he is not about to forgive us. The sulking continues for several days. Mozart had been easy to train and hadn't had an accident in a year, but for several mornings we have small brown peace offerings on the living room rug. He has made his point, and by the turd day, as Mr. Gudreau would have said, he was back to his old self.

I hadn't seen Juan for some eight or nine months until he showed up at the clinic, complaining of stomach pain, shortness of breath and fatigue. He looked like warmed-over death.

"Juan, you don't look so good," I say. "You're in trouble again. What have you done to yourself this time? Have you had some bleeding anywhere? Nosebleeds?"

"Nosebleeds, no."

"Are your stools black, like tar?"

"What is stools?" he asks.

"Stools. Um, bowel movement. Number two." He has a quizzical look. "Kack," I say in Plautdietsch.

"Oh," says Juan. "Shit. Yeah, it's sometimes black."

Juan's hemoglobin is nine, about sixty percent of normal.

"How much are you drinking, Juan?" I ask.

233

He fidgets and tugs at his ear. "Ah… some beer," he says.

"Juan, just tell me the truth. How much is some? You drink every day?"

"Six, seven beer and some whiskey."

"Whoa, that's a lot," I whistle.

I ask him to lie down and palpate his abdomen. He is exquisitely tender in the epigastrium, the area just under the sternum. "You probably have a bleeding ulcer. It has a lot to do with the alcohol. I'll give you some Losec to take every day, and the ulcer should heal. I'll talk to Dr. Sanderson about getting a gastroscopy done – you know, look into your stomach with a telescope? – to see if the ulcer is healing and make sure there are no other problems."

I find Juan enough samples of the medication to last three weeks.

"Here, take one of these every twelve hours. You have to stop drinking, Juan." I pause to let this news search for a few receptive neurons. "Are you still on cocaine or some other drugs?" Juan is silent. He gets up to go.

"Juan," I say. "Please sit down for a few more minutes." He sinks back into his chair. He looks like a beaten cur. "You're only twenty-two years old – what's going to happen in ten or fifteen years if you keep this up? Before this stomach problem, it was cocaine and prison, and then your arm, and who knows what's next. You come to Canada from Mexico, and you keep expecting people to bail you out. If you're doing drugs or selling them, sooner or later it will get you into prison again. You have to stop doing that. I'd like you to come back in a week, and we'll see what we can do. You should go to AA, or I can get some other help for you. You have serious problems, but you can't get your psychiatry out of a bottle. You have to want to change. I can't do it for you and neither can anybody else."

"Yeah, I know," he says. He avoids my eyes. He shuffles his feet and hums tunelessly. I send him on his way with a reminder to return in a week.

He does not show for his follow-up visit, nor does he keep his appointment with Jim Sanderson.

Juan was the dark side of the Mennonite journey. Many of those who had fled Manitoba in the thirties to escape compulsory education in Manitoba public schools and a perceived invasion into their way of life and worship had emigrated to Mexico. Their conservative religion was based on a prescribed formula as a shield from the world's evils, but it contained a shallow personal faith. It told them that television and fashionable dress were wrong, but failed to show them how to live positively. Their beliefs proved inadequate as a moral foundation to keep the youth away from drugs, alcohol, and a life of crime. Many who returned to Canada were assimilated in some fashion into the prevailing Mennonite faith and culture. Some, like Juan, were not.

Breakdowns like Juan happened too often. I mused about our failure as a community to reach out in a meaningful way. We were smug in the conviction we had gotten it right, but were often unwilling to get dirty and share our lives with people less fortunate. While the church was an important part of faith, in reality it too often interfered with God's work. The Christian community sometimes found it easy to prejudge habits and lifestyle, and shun the individual within.

Juan was seen once more by the ER staff after our last encounter. He had received the worst end of the transaction in an alcohol-fueled tête-à-tête. He suffered a broken jaw, and the loss of a few teeth. He was sent to Winnipeg for repairs. The last I heard of him, the long arm of the law had encircled him with its own special brand of love, giving him a home with a barred steel door and three square meals a day.

## Chapter 19

# A DOG'S DINNER

TGIF. That means tomorrow is Saturday – no surgery or clinic hours, no meetings, a day like no other. Weekends are a wonderful innovation, but Saturday is like a precious sapphire. John Keats could have written *An Ode to Saturday*. A nightingale or a Grecian urn does not rank with a pure, unadulterated, golden-as-a-tropical-beach Saturday. Saturday is personal time, gardening, golf, dining out with friends or family. Adrenalin levels are barely detectable. Would that life was a perpetual Saturday. Sunday is okay, but being the day before Monday, it loses some of its luster.

Anyway, it's Friday – I'm getting ahead of myself, anticipating the weekend. We still have a job to do. It promises to be another ho-hum day of drug pushing, but you never know how the slate will go.

By this time, anesthesia had advanced considerably. Cardiac monitors had been in use for sometime, but now there were automatic blood pressure machines and oximeters. Oximeters are instruments that measure the oxygen saturation in the blood – an alarm would sound long before you noticed poor oxygenation by the patient's color. Nerve stimulators were used to determine the level of drug-induced paralysis so the surgeon can perform surgery on a patient whose abdominal muscles are relaxed.

We were perpetually short of medical manpower in town, and when a first-rate application arrived in response to our ads, we contacted him immediately. Dr. Andrew Rhodes-Seaford was born and educated in Great Britain. The name alone had the ring of blue-blood royalty. According to his curriculum vitae, he had experience in obstetrics, emergency medicine ,family practice, and anesthesia, and came highly recommended by the College of Physicians and Surgeons of Manitoba. He seemed too good to be true. I was pleased – it would mean relief, particularly for anesthesia call.

Andrew is a dapper young man with impeccable British manners. "Good morning," he says one morning soon after his arrival, and we are already on the morning's coffee break. "So sorry, I'm a tad late. I had such a beastly time with my hair. It can be such a difficult thing, don't you agree?" He flips his head in a gesture of exasperation.

"Good morning," I put down my coffee cup. "I wouldn't know about the hair. I don't really fuss very much with mine." One has to be anal to obsess over a crew cut.

"Yes, yes, I do see that," he says. "My hair is a dog's dinner. I shall have to try again later."

Andrew has great hair – perfect, in fact. It flows back from his generous forehead in sumptuous waves, a glossy dark brown with an absolutely dead-straight part on the left. His face is finely chiseled with flawlessly trimmed eyebrows, an aristocratic nose, and steel-blue eyes. He wears beige trousers with a knife-edge crease and a navy double-breasted jacket with nary a speck of lint or a hint of wrinkle. An ascot is tied around his neck.

"My, don't you look elegant," I say. "The ladies are going to swoon."

"Why thank you," he replies with a condescending nod. "How very kind of you to say so."

Andrew was something of an anomaly in our town –
coming from Britain, single, patrician manners, and a flare for
style. It was odd that that Andrew would settle in one of the
colonies, particularly a staid Mennonite town in Manitoba. He
piqued the curiosity of the female contingent of our office staff,
who endeavored without much success to find out more about
his personal life. He was knowledgeable, but his arrogance and
condescending manner were hard to stomach.

A bowel resection has been scheduled for the morning.
I had seen Martha Bonds preoperatively and was certain she
would do well. But she was extremely apprehensive – she had
already postponed her surgery several times out of intense fear,
but now seemed determined to see it through. The surgeon and
anesthetist are expected to discuss all the risks with the patient
preoperatively. The goal is to reassure patients and answer their
concerns, without dwelling on all the possible adverse outcomes. There are hundreds of possible problems – postoperative nausea, strokes or heart attacks, even temporary dementia.
The trick is to inform the patient with sensitivity, particularly
someone already coming unglued. I was careful to explain the
unquestionably higher risks to people who are obese or have
underlying heart disease.

Martha is fifty-two with no prior history of heart or lung
disease. However, she does have several concerns. One is nausea
and vomiting after a previous hysterectomy. I assure her the
problem can be minimized by administering Stemetil (pro-
chlorperazine). We had not yet come to the modern class of
drugs like Kytril (granisatron) a drug that has proven its worth
for patients undergoing cancer chemotherapy and radiation,
also useful in the postoperative period.

I would also limit the inhaled gases, especially nitrous oxide
(laughing gas). Nitrous oxide is used a great deal in anesthesia.
It has been around since its discovery in 1775; people realized
the gas dulled the sensation of pain considerably, and soon it

was used widely in surgery and dentistry. Laughing gas gained appeal as a recreational drug – it causes euphoria and mild hallucinations – an early "turn on, tune in, drop out," psychedelic drug. Although the effect is short, two to five minutes, it can be addicting, and very dangerous if used over a longer period in combination with other drugs or without additional oxygen. Its discoverer, Sir Humphrey Davy used it on himself and tried it on a few friends like the poet Samuel Coleridge. It is still used in combination with oxygen (Entonox) as an analgesic in dentistry, childbirth, and emergency medicine. Nitrous oxide is also used as a propellant in cooking sprays and whipping cream canisters.

A nagging concern for me is Martha's past history of a dislocated jaw and a stiff temperomandibular (jaw) joint that had caused a problem with intubation (placing a tube in the windpipe to aid breathing) in a previous anesthetic. For easy intubation, the patient's mouth needs to open wide, and the neck must be supple enough to extend the head to expose the vocal cords. This problem is more common in obese people with short necks, where the head seems to emerge straight out of their shoulders. Martha Bond's mouth opens no more than three centimeters and she had limited movement of her neck. She isn't overweight, and with the relaxation of anesthesia, I anticipate that we will be able to intubate. In any case, the surgery needs to be done, so we decide to go ahead.

"Okay, Martha," I say, "The sandman is here – are you ready? They'll be wheeling you into the operating room any minute."

"Sure. What are you using – Pentothal? That's what I had last time."

"No, actually I'm using Propofol – it's a newer drug and has fewer side effects. What flavor would you like? We're out of chocolate."

She is in no frame of mind for lame humor. "Dr. Giesbrecht, do you ever pray before surgery?" Martha grasps my hand.

"Yes, we do. This is scary, isn't it? Would you like me to pray with you?" She nods.

"Father God," I pray, "thank you for your loving care in all circumstances. Thank you for loving Martha. Please give her comfort and assurance at this time. Guide the surgeon's hands as he operates. Amen."

"Thank you," she whispers.

Martha is wheeled into the operating theater, and the nurses begin buzzing around connecting blood pressure cuffs, monitors, and cautery pads, like an astronaut being suited up. I connect the syringes and pump to the IV lines. "My word," Martha exclaims. "All we need yet is a hairdresser and a mani-curist." Her words trail away as the Propofol works its magic. I push 120 mg of succinyl choline into her line to paralyze her larynx. A size seven endotracheal tube lies ready on the table. Candace places the mask over her face and ventilates her lungs with pure oxygen for several minutes. Martha's limbs twitch slightly as the drug paralyzes her muscles. I insert the curved laryngoscope blade, but can see nothing except the back of her tongue. Normally the epiglottis flips up nicely to reveal the white, glistening vocal chords, and the tube is easily positioned between them. Her jaw won't open further, and all I can find is the tip of the epiglottis. I attempt to extend the head a little more, and reposition the scope for another look. It's no better.

"Give me a six with a stylet." I say. The endotracheal tubes are flexible, and with a metal insert, the tube may be curved enough to do a 'blind' intubation. The tube slides in. I place a stethoscope on her chest and listen as we attempt to ventilate her lungs . There is a harsh rasping sound – the tube is in the esophagus. "This light is terrible, get me another laryngoscope."

Meanwhile, Candace places the mask back on Martha's face for several minutes. I try again. The light is a little better, but I still can see nothing of the essential anatomy.

"Find a straight blade, and the fibreoptic introducer, and I'll try again," I say quietly. Sometimes a straight blade will push the tongue out of the way and the larynx can be seen. It doesn't work. Martha's lips are taking on a dark tinge.

"Her O2 sats (oxygen saturation) are dropping," says Candace, with a frown. "She's down to 68. She looks…"

"Put the mask back and bag her," I interrupt. Martha moves a little – the previous dose of succinylcholine is beginning to wear off. I quickly give Martha another 100 mg. Her color is much better with ventilation and an airway. The oximeter reads 99 percent.

I try again with the fibreoptic introducer. Fiber optics was another thing we had never heard of in medical school, but had spawned many noteworthy improvements in diagnostic tools. "Give me some cricoid pressure, please." Candace pushes down on the windpipe to push the larynx into view. I can see a bit more, so I attempt another intubation. I thread the tube over the fibreoptic light into place. "I don't know. I can't see a thing. Let's try it – I may be in the esophagus again."

We attach the anesthetic hoses to ventilate her lungs. Her chest doesn't move and with the stethoscope, I can hear the telltale rattle of air going into her stomach.

"Her O2 is dropping again," Candace says, urgently.

I pull out the tube and put the mask back on her face to ventilate. I'm not easily ruffled in emergencies, but I'm having a few palpitations of my own. Take it easy, I tell myself, I've been here before. What do we try next? I could use a laryngeal mask, another airway device, as a last resort, but this is not very satisfactory with a procedure requiring mechanical ventilation for hours. There's another technique available, but that would involve introducing a wire from the outside through the trachea into the mouth and threading the tube over it. That would be the last resort only in a dire emergency.

Jim Sanderson has arrived and sizes up the problem. "Have we still got that bronchoscope?" he asks.

"Didn't we get rid of it?" says Candace. "It wasn't being used much."

The bronchoscope is still available and functional. We slide the endotracheal tube over the thin fibreoptic bronchoscope. Jim struggles to find the larynx.

"Where's the suction?" I say, "Let's get rid of the secretions – that should help."

"Ok, where is the light?" asks Jim. We watch for the telltale glow on her neck from the bronchoscope in her throat.

"It's off to the right. Ok, now you're centered – try it now."

Again, the tube is in the esophagus. We ventilate again. Another attempt. "Hallelujah, I think you got it!" I inflate the cuff on the tube and turn on the ventilator. Martha's chest moves rhythmically with the bellows. There's a collective sigh of relief, as Martha's skin turns a beautiful pink.

Martha still has the rattle in her throat. "Do we have those small-bore suction catheters?" There are secretions and blood in the trachea from the repeated attempts at intubation. I slide the catheter through the tube into the trachea and suction. After that, all is well. Martha's oximeter reading is 100, her blood pressure and heart rate normal.

The rest of the procedure is uneventful, and "the patient was transferred to the recovery room in good condition" is recorded on the operative report.

I walk back to the change room and slump onto the vinyl couch that occupies one wall. The couch is ancient – it likely had been brought in by oxcart. It's uncomfortable and hideous, but still in perfect condition. If I come back in thirty years, it will likely still be here. I look around me. I have entered this room a thousand times before – it's tiny, about eight by seven, woefully inadequate, with a small desk, a clothes rack, and a shelf for OR clothing. Every seven or eight years, talk of OR renovations would surface, only to disappear into the depths of a yawning bureaucracy. Other priorities always seemed to take center stage, like replacing the hospital's brick siding that seemed perfectly adequate or adding to an already hugely bloated head office.

Dr. Rhodes-Seaford was scheduled for the next anesthetic. He arrives just as Jim comes back from the recovery room.

"Boy, I'm glad that's over," I sigh. I take off my glasses and rub my eyes. "That was pretty nerve-racking. I think I aged a few years."

"Bit of a sticky wicket, was it?" says Andrew.

I tell him about Martha's anesthetic.

"You might call me when you have a beastly case like that. I am quite proficient, you know. I have never had a problem with intubation."

Jim rolls his eyes, but keeps his peace. Andrew has a fondness for self-aggrandizement, boasting of his expertise in many fields of medicine. Every anesthetist will have trouble intubating some patients – it's simply a matter of time

"Why, thank you," I rejoin, "Kind of you to offer your services."

Andrew has changed and proceeds to the operating room.

"What an insufferable gasbag." Jim shakes his head. "That reminds me – what is the normal amount of intraoperative fluid a patient should get?"

"Why do you ask? It depends on the age of the patient, how long the person has been fasting, how long the procedure is… For an average adult who has had preop IV fluids, let's say with a hysterectomy – probably eight or nine hundred ccs?"

Jim nods. "That's about what I thought. Our prima donna, Dr. Andrew Rhodes-Seaford, has been giving two or three liters, and some of my elderly patients have been going into heart failure postoperatively because of fluid overload. Do you think you could speak to him? He tells me I should mind my own business and stick to cutting."

"I suppose I could, but our esteemed colleague doesn't take advice too graciously."

"Yes, well," Andrew says when I broach the subject, "I do pour in a jolly good lot of fluid. I don't mean to be cheeky, but it's none of your bloody business – I'm the anesthesiologist. I did some research on intraoperative IV fluid, you know. And I have the experience of thousands of cases."

"You are the anesthesiologist (I'm thinking *pompous ass*), but you have to individualize. Some people are going into failure with all that fluid. A young, healthy person can handle two or three liters, but not an elderly patient with a compromised heart."

"Thank you ever so much for your concern, but my patients will be fine." He throws a disdainful scowl in my direction.

I stand up and face him squarely. I consciously unclench my hand and lower my voice. "Well, Sir Andrew," I snap, "You seem to be a legend in your own mind, but I have done a lot more anesthesia than you. You are new to Canada, and you are still subject to our assessment of your competency. I wouldn't be quite so sure of your position here."

Andrew turns abruptly and yanks the change-room door. "Bloody colonial upstarts."

Herman Penner is my next case. "Hi, Doc. How are you?"

"I'm just fine. How are you? Ready for *Meddachschlop*, after-dinner nap?"

"*Gaunss je'wes*, absolutely. I hear you've done a few of these before, so you should know what you're doing."

"Yes, twenty or twenty-five thousand by now. Besides, I have a regular subscription to Reader's Digest, so I keep up."

"That's very comforting," Herman says. "By the way, I found out why the operating room is always so cold."

"Okay," I say. "I'll bite, tell me why?"

"To keep the meat fresh."

Herman laughs so hard the table shakes. I start the pump. This guy doesn't need laughing gas. "Okay, Herman, here we go."

"What are you giving me?"

"It's called propofol – here, this white fluid in the syringe. We call it milk of amnesia."

"Milk of amnesia. Good one. Oh...this is really nice stuff. Where can I buy some?"

"Well, they wouldn't sell you any, but for a small fee, I might make a house call."

The Fentanyl is in and the propofol is flowing. Herman loses any lingering inhibitions, and begins singing loudly in several keys at once, "When the moon hits your eye, like a big pizza pie, its amore..." Herman is a big man and requires mega-doses to bring his musical flair under control.

# Chapter 20
# SNAKEOIL

"I finally found out what was wrong with me," Elizabeth Goosen says triumphantly.

"So what is wrong with you?" I ask.

"I went to the iridologist, and she showed me right on the chart what my problem was," she sniffs. "I guess you doctors don't know everything."

I had now been practicing medicine for thirty-some years and had looked after Elizabeth for the last five of those. I had been under the impression that I had acquired some expertise, but apparently I was wrong. I had not acquitted myself in a fashion worthy of my profession. It was difficult to impress Mrs. Goosen.

"Well, you're absolutely right," I say, "we don't." However, we can usually pretend in a convincing fashion. "So you went to an iridologist? I'm curious. What did you find out?"

I'm not sure I had ever really helped Elizabeth, but she came at regular intervals, perhaps to consolidate her own theories. Or as insurance just in case her own remedies bombed. Every part of her body had contributed something to her personal lexicon of ailments, *a* through *z*: arthritis, athlete's foot, bad breath, back pain, cold sores, constipation, dandruff, diarrhea, all the way to yeast infection, zits and zero energy. (She had nothing for $x$. I could have given her one – xantholasma, small harmless cholesterol lumps that she had in the skin of her eyelids.)

It's not that Elizabeth is unhappy. On the contrary – her medical inventory is a first-rate hobby, and gives her endless pleasure and prestige at family gatherings and the *Neiferein*, church sewing circle. It is also a great forum for one-upmanship, confounding the doctor who can't seem to get it right, and comparing his advice with what the reflexologist, iridologist, or quack-of-the-month has told her. An entertaining variant of the game is comparing advice from another doctor. Many of Elizabeth's symptoms are vague and nonspecific, and if I don't have an immediate black-and-white answer, it's great sport to let me flounder, then tell me what the previous doctor has recommended.

In the first few decades of my career, there was little quackery to rail against other than the home-style, self-trained chiropractor, a true pillar of Mennonite society. Now there were literally hundreds of varieties of snake-oil salesmen, with new ones cropping up almost daily, each more bizarre than the last. Some therapies like chiropractic and acupuncture have some value; others like reflexology, colon cleansing, magnets, and stem cell medicine are patently absurd and of no worth except for the placebo effect.

There is some quack medical treatment to suit everybody's whim or temperament. These practitioners produce a slick brochure with just enough science thrown in to make them seem plausible, and with testimonials from suffering individuals who have been miraculously healed. They develop a nice-looking website and advertise their training school with names (American College of Iridology, Canadian Institute of Neuro-optic Research, etc.) that sound prestigious and scientific, and another profitable scam is born. Trainees can become a member of the healing arts in as little as two weeks. The age of consumerism, more public awareness, and more science and technology has also brought about a whole cornucopia of phony health care. 'A little knowledge is a dangerous thing' was never more true than today.

"The iridologist asked about my medical history," Elizabeth replies. "She knew I had my appendix out. She showed me a little white triangle on the eye chart where I had had appendicitis, and a little black speck that meant the appendix had been removed. She explained that I had a brown-eyed constitution and had trouble with gas, constipation, indigestion, even arthritis. She was right about everything." Her voice runs on, but she is in no hurry to tell me why she has come. I begin to wonder what color my constitution is – likely black. I don't ask.

"And she gave you some pills, right?" I inquire. "How much did that cost you?"

"Only seventy dollars a month, with a money-back guarantee."

"Mrs. Goosen, don't throw your money away. Those people can't tell you what is wrong with you. Iridology is basically nonsense."

She waves her hand, dismissing my counsel. "No, Dr. Giesbrecht, she was right. She also said that I will probably get diabetes. She showed me on the chart."

"You may very well get diabetes, but that's because you have a strong family history and you are overweight. Mrs. Goosen, the pattern of your iris has absolutely nothing to do with the parts of your body. It has been shown that people who practice this stuff don't have any idea what's wrong with a patient unless they find out about your health and history first. They become very good at guessing and picking up on subtle clues."

It takes another herculean mental effort, but with that little exchange I abandon my rant. After many years, I had acquired a small measure of immunity. I felt less indignation at being told an iridologist or chelationist was being consulted. I was a professional, but it wasn't necessary to win every argument. Really. Even though I *was* right. Early in my career, I thought it was part of my mandate to correct all misinformation. Okay, it's still not always easy to keep quiet – but with age and experience comes a bit of wisdom. The real danger lay in having the patient delay necessary diagnosis and treatment.

"Anyway, Mrs. Goosen, why did you come to see me today?"

"Well, my periods quit a few years ago. I was forty-nine then. Last week I had a little bit of spotting, so I was worried."

"Just a few drops of blood?"

"It wasn't even really blood – some mucus with red streaks."

I'm sorely tempted to ask what the iridologist thought about this. "We should check and see what's going on," I say. "Please take off your clothes, put on the gown, and I'll do a pelvic exam."

It's difficult to feel her pelvic organs through a thick abdominal wall. I have the impression of an enlarged uterus, perhaps fibroids. I take a routine Pap test. I explain that any postmenopausal bleeding should be investigated, and will order routine blood tests and an ultrasound to check for an enlarged uterus or ovaries. She also needs a referral to Jim Sanderson for a D&C. She uncharacteristically agrees to return once the ultrasound results are back.

Summer is short. It's already mid August. I needed to take a bit more time off, although I find that hard to do. The bills pile up every month, and we have no idea how to budget or put away money. Fiscal wisdom for me is paying off Visa with MasterCard. And what if most of my patients have left for another doctor while I'm gone?

Dr. Mike Nesbitt called me about doing a locum in Grand Beach for a couple of weeks. The community's population explodes in summer with cottagers, campers, and beach-goers. Mike is in charge of medical services for the summer months.

"You have the use of the cottage free. You just need to open the clinic for two hours or so every afternoon, and take call the rest of the time. You charge fee for service just like at home. You just have to keep a record of everything." In a moment of weakness, I agree to take one week – I'll have most of the day to read and explore, and the kids will have a holiday at the beach.

We arrive on Saturday, throw the suitcases into the cabin, and head for the beach. The weather is gorgeous – clear skies, a warm breeze, and a mile of sandy beach. This is going to be a great week!

We find an umbrella, spread out our blankets, and watch Jodi, Scott, and Greg, Scott's friend, explore the beach. We have just opened our books and are beginning to feel the tension dissipate. "What is that?" Rose says. "It kind of sounds like thunder, but the sky is clear." The noise becomes louder and more ominous. It sounds like a tornado approaching or a low-flying aircraft. I walk toward the parking lot to investigate. Wave after wave of Harleys appear out of a swirling cloud of dust.

Hell's Angels! They line up their bikes row after row, and gather in a growing knot of people. Some are solo, some with biker chicks, all with their emblem emblazoned on their black leather jackets. There are some sixty bikes.

I go back to Rose and the kids. Hundreds of people have lined up to watch the spectacle. "Hell's Angels," I say. "Just what we need to make our week complete."

"I hope they don't cause trouble," Rose counters. "This is supposed to be a holiday."

"I hope they're all healthy," I say. There is a palpable edge to the buzz of conversations around the beach. Not that we really expect trouble from the bikers – they probably couldn't care less about us. On the other hand, these are not Girl Guides selling oatmeal cookies. Before very long, a number of RCMP arrive in town, just to keep an eye on our guests and to reassure the beach-goers that things are under control.

Sunday morning all the bikers have vanished, replaced by fish flies. These three-centimeter insects, also known as mayflies or sand flies, hatch by the millions almost overnight, fly about for several days and mate. Then, exhausted by the orgies and egg laying, they die almost on signal, leaving everything covered in little dead carcasses. We venture outdoors, the ground squishy, crunchy, and slippery as ice.

"Ew..." Jodi says, "They're so gross. I'm staying indoors." We try sweeping them up into large trash bags, but they are everywhere. We are more or less confined to the cabin. The bonus came on Tuesday when the bodies began to rot and permeate everything with a putrid fishy bouquet, adding to our holiday mood.

Wednesday, it rains all day. No beach and the masses of fish flies are now putrid, slippery, *and* soggy.

I run the afternoon clinics with a supply of antihistamines, Tylenol and sunburn lotions, and an occasional week's worth of Amoxicillin for ear infections or strep throat. Things settle down toward the end of the week – the wind sweeps the beach relatively free of decaying flies, and in the evenings, we play Masterpiece and Rummy with Scott, Jodi, and Greg.

Friday arrives, and with it, a small army of teenagers from Winnipeg for a weekend of revelry away from parental control. Things are quiet until 2:30 A.M. There's a loud knock at the cabin door. I grab my housecoat and stumble to the front door.

"Are you the doc?" asks the first teen, his hands bloody, and his shirt torn. "Einstein here isn't doing so well." Tom has obviously partied with great gusto. Dried blood streaks down the left side of his face from a gash on the temple, and the eye is swollen shut. He has no shirt and his pants are caked with blood, vomit, and mud. He's supported by a third lad in only slightly better shape.

"Yeah guys, I'm the doc," I say wearily. "Come around to the clinic door at the back. You'll need some stitches."

I let them in, pull out a suture tray and proceed to clean up Tom's face. "So what happened? It's three in the morning!"

"Oh, some of the guys got into a fight. That's from a broken beer bottle."

"And the other guy got the girl? You guys are behaving like a couple of rutting moose."

The lids have to be pried open for inspection, but Tom's eye was okay. I pull away the matted hair and cleanse the area gently. I fill a large syringe with lidocaine, put a sterile drape around the wound, and insert the fine needle to freeze the edge of the wound.

With the prick of the needle, Tom rouses with a blood-curdling yell, flinging his arms wildly. The needle, drape, and instrument tray spray over the clinic floor.

"Tom, listen! I'm not enjoying this, either. I'm just trying to freeze the area and put in a few stitches. You'll have to hold still."

I gather some new supplies, enlist the help of his marginally helpful friends, and manage to close the wound.

The next evening, more parties, more displays of male gallantry, more blood, one broken arm which has to be sent to Winnipeg for proper care, one young woman with a huge guilt trip after the weekend activities had included carnal knowledge. She realized the straight and narrow has no place to park.

Bring back the Hell's Angels!

Sunday evening we pack our things, clean the interior of the cabin, and head back to Steinbach, thankful for the end of our vacation.

Mrs. Goosen's co-operative behavior is short-lived. Her appointment date comes, but she does not. I asked Carolyn to phone her with another appointment to discuss the ultrasound. That date came and went. I decided to phone her myself. She agreed to come in and talk about her problem.

"Hi, Mrs. Goosen." The fact she shows up is a good sign. "How are you doing? I was a little concerned when you didn't keep your appointments. I wanted to give you the results of your ultrasound – it shows an enlarged uterus. It could just be fibroids, but we can't be sure. You need the D&C to make an accurate diagnosis. Carolyn tells me you didn't keep your appointment with Dr. Sanderson, either."

"I don't think I need the D&C," she says slowly. "I don't have any more spotting."

"Well, just because the bleeding has stopped for now doesn't mean the problem is gone."

"A friend of mine told me about chelation," Elizabeth replies without looking up. "So I went to this doctor in Winnipeg. He told me my body was full of toxins. I have been going for treatments and it's cleaning my system. I feel great and no more spotting."

"You're getting IV chelation therapy?"

"Yes, I go in three times a week. I'm going to have forty treatments altogether."

I wince. People will go to great lengths to preserve their ignorance.

My blood pressure remains stable. I smile philosophically. Proverbs says: "He who has knowledge spares his words and a man of understanding is of a calm spirit." I'm not going to win this one, but I have to give it a shot.

"Mrs. Goosen, you're throwing your money away again," I say calmly. "What's that going to cost you – three or four thousand dollars? Chelation is not going to help you no matter what your diagnosis is. Bleeding from the uterus will often be intermittent, and you might not have any for weeks at a time. We still need to make sure there isn't anything serious. Nobody likes to have surgery, but a D&C is a simple, short procedure and hopefully we can rule out anything serious."

"They told me that I will be cured in four or five months, so I'll see when the treatments are finished."

"Mrs. Goosen, don't do this. It could be very dangerous to neglect proper treatment." In spite of myself, my voice is taking on a sharp edge. "What if there is a cancer – you need to have that checked."

"I appreciate your concern, Dr. Giesbrecht, but I'm feeling good and the bleeding has stopped, so I'm going to continue with the treatment."

"All right," I say in a conciliatory tone. What more can I say? "I hope things go well. If you have any more bleeding, please come and see me."

The blind leading the blind. Chelation had become a popular therapy, particularly since it was very lucrative for its practitioners. EDTA, the basic drug used in chelation, was originally proposed as a binding agent that would remove arterial plaque and improve general circulation, and specifically help people suffering from angina and coronary artery disease. It had been touted as a substitute for bypass surgery, but chelationists have also made claims that they can cure arthritis, diabetes, anemia, bleeding problems, and probably unrequited love. There have been numerous well-designed studies that have shown no health benefits whatsoever from chelation.

Mrs. Goosen's chances of having endometrial (lining of the womb) cancer were high. She had many of the associated risk factors: late menopause, obesity, gallbladder disease, and a family history of uterine cancer.

I meet Jim in the hospital on one of those 'corridor consultations' before heading off for home. I briefly explain Mrs. Goosen's case. "I guess there is nothing we can do, is there?"

"Not really," he responds. "It sounds like she really needs the investigation. You can't force anybody if they are determined not to have treatment. As they say, it's a free country."

"It's a shame that scams like that are allowed to continue. I guess people have to find out for themselves."

"How does the public know what's legit and what's not?" Jim says. "There is enough proof to outlaw some harmful practices, but there are some that are helpful, so you can't ban everything that isn't mainstream medicine."

"Exactly," I agree. "There are a number of alternative medical therapies that have some scientific validity and benefits. And a patient who doesn't have any serious ailment will likely not be harmed by chelation or reflexology, either."

"The problem is that people seek out these snake-oil salesmen and delay proper diagnosis and treatment," Jim says. "Anyway, let me know if she decides to come back."

I appreciated Jim. A skilled surgeon, honest and compassionate, but he had no time for playing games. If people didn't want his help, that was okay. Tell them what they need to do, then it's up to them. His answer was usually black or white, rarely gray, take it or leave it. Asking him for a consultation was like money in the bank – it was safe, secure, and I had the confidence it was the best option.

Mrs. Goosen returned eight months after her last visit. She had had a hemorrhage at home. She looked ill and had lost weight. She had pelvic pain, and pain with urination. She agreed to a D&C, which produced white friable tissue, unusual at her age. A bad sign. Pathology confirmed uterine cancer and a liver scan showed probable metastases. A hysterectomy was slated on an urgent basis, although we knew that the chances of a cure were slim.

It was a difficult surgical procedure – the cancer had eroded into nearby pelvic structures and bowel. The mass had to be painstakingly dissected off the pelvic floor, and part of the vagina and a small section of bowel were removed. A nodule in the liver was biopsied. It was not a happy picture – stage IV endometrial (lining of the uterus) cancer, an advanced stage. Staging gives the oncologist some idea as to treatment and prognosis.

Elizabeth was started on hormone and chemotherapy. Most patients with advanced endometrial cancer live only a year or two, even with aggressive treatment. She defied the odds and lived three.

## Chapter 21
# FOOT AND MOUTH DISEASE

The Kornelsons were deliriously happy after the birth of a daughter, adding to their family of two boys. Her birth was uneventful, as we say in medicine, which is good – the baby arrived headfirst, there was no tear or excessive bleeding, and the placenta emerged dutifully after the birth. George Jamieson had actually been there for the delivery. He assured John and Gladys everything was fine and that the baby had all the standard equipment.

The Kornelsons were casual, once-or-twice-a-year friends of ours. I dropped in after completing morning rounds to offer my congratulations. The baby was asleep in a basinet and I didn't have to make the required cooing noises, which was okay – there is nothing like a newborn to make a babbling dufus out of an otherwise normal adult.

A month after bringing their baby home, John and Gladys invite us for evening coffee.

"Congratulations," Rose says, as we arrive at the door. She gives Gladys a hug. "How are you doing? You're looking good."

"Oh, fine, thanks." Gladys invites us into the living room. "I'm a little tired, but mothers are supposed to be tired, right?

Please sit down." The house is orderly and meticulously clean. A wooden rocker sits beside the fireplace, an afghan draped over one arm. Several family photos stand proudly on the wooden mantelpiece. The accoutrements for a new arrival can be seen through the doorway, a bassinet and a heap of cloth diapers on the kitchen table.

"So, let's see your little bundle," says Rose.

Gladys brings the baby. She's tiny, pale, and her eyes are closed.

"Oh…she's cute," coos Rose. "Geraldine, right? What color are her eyes?"

Women think every newborn is cute. Estrogen and a few maternally oriented genes make them that way. I had by this time helped a fair number of newborns into the world, and many were somewhat less than adorable. I recall one infant in our nursery that would have done Jimmy Durante proud. His poor mother likely had an episiotomy just to get his proboscis through. Still, every newborn is God's opinion that life should go on.

"I think her eyes are blue," says Gladys. "She doesn't open them much. She's a bit slow with nursing, and hasn't gained much weight so far. But Dr. Jamieson says she's fine – just give her a little time."

Contrary to parenting experts, looking after a newborn is quite simple – keep the top end wet and the bottom end dry. Unfortunately, men aren't physically equipped for the first function, nor do they have the mental capacity for the second. I learned this in medical school.

Gladys and John serve coffee and cake. I glance at the baby with male indifference – I'm neither a parent nor their doctor, though I had a fleeting disquiet that didn't develop into conscious thought until some time later.

After an hour at the Kornelsons, we had compared our precocious offspring, our flourishing gardens, and Alberta's flamboyant premier, Ralph Klein. John thinks he great, I say it's a wonder he beat out millions of other sperm. All that remained was our appraisal of the elementary school principal. Rose said he had wonderful manners, Gladys said he was charming, and John wondered about his abilities as a disciplinarian. Once we have sorted that out, we thank our hosts and say goodnight.

Rose and I drive home. We walk to the patio and sit in silence, thinking about our conversation. I scan the flowerbeds and the lawn, mentally surveying the yard. The garden is doing well this year – the beds are a riot of color, orange marigolds, white daisies, with white morning glory and purple clematis falling in long cascades from the trellis. The resident humming-bird hovers briefly at the slender honeysuckle trumpets around the lamppost, and then heads for the feeder. Another hummer suddenly appears out of nowhere, and a fencing match ensues; tiny rapier bills thrust and parry. Just as suddenly, the interloper gives up the battle and vanishes in a whir of wings. A bumblebee buzzes in to sample the nectar, meets the diminutive combatant, and leaves without a sip.

"You're very quiet," Rose says.

"You know, honey," I say pensively. "Something is not right with that baby. I'm not sure what it is, but she isn't normal. Her eyes look funny and nobody can tell us what color they are. She has those jerky movements, and her head looks smaller than normal to me. Isn't that a bit strange?"

"I had the same feeling," Rose replies. "Gladys told me the baby has gained only a pound in the last month, and has trouble nursing."

"Well, it's still early. Maybe Geraldine is just a slow baby and needs a little time."

"Let's hope so," Rose says. "Anyway, don't say anything to the Kornelsons."

"Oh no, absolutely not ... but it makes you thankful for our kids doesn't it?

Several months later Rose and I are in Safeway. Yes, both of us. I adhere to the International Married Male Protocol, which includes putting down the toilet lid and squashing spiders. Another is not to darken the door of a supermarket. A grocery store should remain a woman's domain – nothing good can come of husbands being in these places. Not that shopping for frozen peas can't be vital and fulfilling; it's just that we are forever bumping into acquaintances and stopping to chat. I suggest that Rose doesn't need me – I will just be in the way – but she thinks we need to do some of these important tasks together.

So here I am, a sensitive male, sharing household chores. These are things you learn only after many years of marriage and your brain starts to get a little pulpy. My second problem is that the acquaintances we meet are often patients. You're trapped in a grocery store aisle with your cart, unable to turn and flee. Sure enough, I spot a short, stout individual bearing down on us from the meat counter, waving a kielbasa in one hand, and guiding her cart with the other.

"Hi, Dr. Geesebritch. So nice to see you. You shop for groceries too, eh? Is your wife?"

"Yes, Mrs. Fedoruk, this is Rose." I turn to Rose. "Mrs. Fedoruk has been a patient for many years."

"Pleased to meet you, Mrs. Rose. Your husband such a nice man."

"See, what have I been telling you, honey?" I say smugly.

Mrs. Fedoruk continues undeterred. "My husband is bum – you so lucky. My husband never shop with me. He should be married to TV." She takes Rose's arm as if they are long-time comrades in the marriage wars. She turns to me. "I phone for appointment, but I can't get for a week. I got stomach trouble, and so much gas. What you think could be?"

"I don't know, Mrs. Fedoruk. Take off your clothes, and I'll check it out."

Her eyes widen in astonishment, then she waggles her finger at me and grins. "Oh, Dr. Geesebritch, you so funny. Maybe we shouldn't talk about such in grocery store."

"It's probably nothing serious. You look fine. If you still have trouble on Monday, come to the clinic, and we'll see what the problem is. If you are really sick over the week-end, go see the emergency doctor at the hospital."

"Okay," she smiles benevolently. "Thank you, I wait. Mrs. Rose, take care of husband – he nice man." She maneuvers her cart around a few shoppers and lurches down the aisle.

"There you are," I say. "I'm a precious commodity and you're supposed to look after me."

We negotiate the next aisle safely, but hit pay dirt on the third.

"Hi, Gladys, how are you?" says Rose. "How's the baby? Growing like a weed, I suppose?" Geraldine is sleeping soundly in a lounge in the shopping cart.

"Oh, fine," says Gladys. "She's gained another pound, and she's eating a little better. The doctor says just give her time. Everything is fine." It sounds rehearsed, as if she knows something is not quite right, but can't allow herself to think it. She bends down to pull the coverlet from Geraldine's face.

"Great," says Rose. "Have you had time to check your calendar? Remember, I phoned you a few weeks ago? We still need a few ladies to help with the refreshments for the women's fellowship meeting next Tuesday evening."

"Well, I'm kind of busy with the new baby and next week is my mom and dad's thirty-fifth wedding anniversary. The family is planning a big shindig."

"Oh, really?" replies Rose. "I didn't realize your parents have been married that long. What are you planning?"

I look at the baby. Geraldine is awake now, but her eyelids are droopy and only the whites of her eyes are visible. She's tiny for five months. The tongue is protruding and she has barely discernable muscle twitches.

I listen to the conversation until my eyes start to mist and I feel my brain slowly descending into gridlock. I think about the school board minutes I should be reading, and the thistles and quack grass that are threatening to ambush our yard. I slowly drift to the next aisle looking for New Bothwell cheese. Rose catches up with me.

"Honey, there is something terribly wrong with that baby," I say in a low voice. "And George Jamieson keeps telling her the baby is fine. I think there are serious developmental delays – probably mental retardation."

"Yes, there is definitely something wrong. I hadn't thought of retardation."

"That's likely only part of it. The head is small for the age. The baby is five months old and far from sitting up – she can't even hold her head properly. Did you notice the jerky movements? Do you think I should say something to them? I hate to see what's happening and they don't know."

"No, don't say anything. They'll be very upset. And you're not their doctor."

A shopper saunters past and our conversation halts for a few moments.

"You're right. But they are friends, and they really should know what's going on."

"Well, let's just wait," Rose cautions. "If we meddle, we may not be friends for long. Maybe George will smarten up and tell them." Another pause "Hi, Diane."

"That's the problem. I don't think he even knows there is a problem."

"Let's wait and see."

I wasn't sure what the problem was, but I vaguely remembered a syndrome from medical school. As soon as we got home and put the groceries away, I dusted off my pediatric textbook, and flipped the pages until I came across something: *Small baby, small head, protruding tongue, feeding problems.* It could be Down's, but the facial features and hyperactivity did not match. I continue the search. Suddenly, there it is – Angelman syndrome. That must be it! I show Rose the page.

"Angelman syndrome? I never even heard of it."

"Well, I heard of it in medical school," I say "but I've never seen a case. Look here: *nursing difficulties, hyperactive movements, small head, and protruding tongue.* The long-term outlook isn't good – *severe mental retardation, seizures, balance problems, strabismus* (crossed eyes). That's it! It also says that in spite of the mental problems, these kids smile and laugh a lot, often inappropriately."

"It certainly does seem to fit," Rose says slowly. "I still say we don't get involved."

Another month goes by and from what we hear, the Kornelsons still seem oblivious to the looming tragedy in their family. As for the diagnosis, I may have missed the bus once or twice in the past, but I'm certain about this one.

"Maybe you should talk to them," Rose says after a few more discussions.

"I wish I knew what was best," I muse. "I just don't know. They should get an accurate diagnosis – see a specialist. It might be something else."

This was the '90s, just past the midpoint of my career. As family practitioners, we relied heavily on the clinical expertise of specialists when faced with obscure conditions. Angelman syndrome was first recognized in 1965, and discovered to be a genetic defect in approximately one in 12,000 births. Now, scientists know the precise location of the mutation on chromosome 15.

I still had occasional delusions of invincibility, although it may not have been so much invincibility as idealism that needed to right wrongs and correct misinformation wherever it reared its ugly head. I didn't always correctly discern the time to speak up, and the time to shut up.

I telephone John and Gladys to ask if I can talk to them. I drive over to their house with a good deal of trepidation. I tell the Kornelson's what my fears are, and suggest they ask Dr. Jamieson to make an appointment with a specialist. The two of them sit there in stunned silence for a few moments. Gladys starts to cry, and at that moment I grasp the fact that I'm an idiot. I mutter a few soothing words, promise that we will keep in touch, and beat a hasty retreat.

Several days later, John and Gladys call back to ask if they can come over for a few moments.

"Oh, oh," I say to Rose. "I wonder if they took Geraldine to the specialist. That was fast. Gladys sounded quite happy, though – I wonder what that means."

"We wanted to talk to you about Geraldine," John says immediately.

"Please come in and sit down. Did you see a specialist?" I query. "That was quick."

"Thanks, we'll just stay a minute. No, we didn't see a specialist," says Gladys quickly.. "We took Geraldine back to Dr. Jamieson and he said we didn't need to see any specialist. He checked her over, and told us she was fine. We just need a little patience."

I bite my lip and hang my head. We stand awkwardly in the hallway. I'm at a loss for words.

John continued, "Dr. Jamieson said the baby is a little slow in her development, but she'll catch up. He said you meant well, but you aren't as experienced as he is, and probably don't know much about babies. He has delivered so many, you know. Anyway, we want you to know we aren't angry and we don't hold anything against you. We're just very relieved that Geraldine is okay."

"I'm terribly sorry for butting in," I say lamely. "I hope everything will work out." They turn to leave. There is an uncomfortable silence as they open the front door. "Thanks for coming. I'm really sorry about the whole thing."

"That was interesting," says Rose as we walk back to the kitchen. "I guess we really blew that one."

"Yeah, mind my own business." I sit down at the kitchen table. I cover my face with trembling hands. "I have an advanced case of foot-in-mouth disease. I should know better – don't get involved with another doctor's patients, especially if they're friends." I get up and look out the window at a bleak, grey sky. "But that baby is not normal. It has serious mental and physical abnormalities. George Jamieson is a cretin – I don't know how he made it through medical school."

"Well, they're going to find out the truth sooner or later."

"George is wrong, but he's god to his patients. That is so unbelievably infuriating. Even so, I should have stayed out of it."

I feet terrible. We avoid the Kornelsons. I can't avoid George. We meet the next day in the hospital. "I'm sorry I got involved with the Kornelsons," I blurt out at the first private moment that presents itself. "That was none of my business."

"You'll learn," he says condescendingly. "When you've looked after as many kids as I have, you'll be able to tell what is normal and what is not."

"Okay, George." I swallow and feel a flush rising in my face. My resolve to keep my mouth shut crumbles. "Hold it right there. I shouldn't have gotten involved, I know that, they are your patients. I apologize – that was stupid of me. But the baby is not normal – it has serious developmental problems, and ..."

"There's nothing wrong with that baby."

"Yes, there is! It's obvious, and you're totally incompetent if you can't see that." After the frustrations of this affair, my umbrage knew no bounds. "Your medical knowledge is bush-league. You're doing John and Gladys a terrible disservice by not sending Geraldine for a specialist opinion. You've probably never heard of it, but look up Angelman syndrome in a textbook, if you have one – you might learn something." George's face darkens several shades of crimson and lavender like the western sky before a prairie storm. The veins stand out on his temples and his eyes narrow.

"You're an asshole," he sputters. His mustache quivers with rage. There are a few more choice words any sailor would proudly display in his vocabulary. "You don't know what you're talking about. Just stay the hell away from my patients." He turns on his heel and walks away.

That George and I were not bosom buddies for the next month or two is an understatement. We hardly spoke except for the necessities of running a practice.

Rose and I began to hear via the grapevine that the Kornelsons had a mentally challenged child. We were told they were going through a terrible emotional upheaval. They had finally taken Geraldine to a pediatrician, it seems, and were given the bad news.

"What do we do now?" asks Rose. "Should we talk to them again? We haven't spoken to each other since they were here. I met Gladys in the mall the other day – she just said hi and kept walking."

"I don't know what's best. We should probably just wait and let a few wounds heal. Let them make the first move. Otherwise, it will look like we're trying to seek vindication. We don't want to add fuel to the fire."

The Kornelsons never did get in touch with us. It was awkward – we avoided each other for some time, but eventually drifted back to casual chitchat. George Jamieson was never mentioned. They shared their frustrations and problems parenting Geraldine with others, but never with us. Geraldine, it turned out with further consultation, had a variant of Angelman syndrome. She learned only a few dozen words in her lifetime, and required constant care. Seizures began at about age three, and over the years necessitated many hospital admissions in spite of daily medication.

If George was chastened by the experience, I wasn't aware of it. We never discussed Geraldine, although I looked after her on a number of occasions when George was away. As for me... I had learned another lesson. There are times to keep one's mouth firmly shut. One may be right, but wrong in attempting to correct all misinformation.

# Chapter 22
# BOVINE BABIES

I pull up to our ocean-side mansion in my new Maserati. The stunning brunette in the passenger seat is Rose (of course). Our staff is everywhere, manicuring the grounds, pouring the new helicopter pad, washing down the yacht rocking gently in the ocean swells. The valet is just about to park the car when the grating jangle of the phone shatters my castle in the sky.

I pick up the receiver, and squint blearily at the alarm – 6 AM – not my finest hour. A call at that time can only bring unwelcome news. My mind starts racing through the possibilities – a woman about to deliver, a motor vehicle accident, someone with a heart attack.

"Hello," I grunt.

There's a long pause. I can hear the measured rhythm of an ancient alarm clock.

"*Docta Giesbrecht?*"

I switch over to Plattdietsch. "*Ekj sie Docta Giesbrecht.* I'm Dr. Giesbrecht. *Wäa es dit.* Who is this?"

Another long pause. I hitch myself up in bed. "*Dit es Kloasse.* This is Klassen," he drawls.

We continue in Low German. "Klassen? Which Klassen?"

"Klassen," he says. "You know me yet. Johan Klassen."

"Oh, yes, I remember," I say, shaking off the cobwebs. "What is the problem?"

"I was there yesterday by you. You said I had too much fat in my blood and my blood-veins were clogging. Can I once have fried eggs for breakfast?" His speech was slow and halting with a long hiatus between thoughts.

"Sure, Mr. Klassen, once in a while is okay."

"*Nah jo.*"

He hangs up. I turn over in bed and snuggle under the covers. Try as I might, I can't get back to my yacht on the ocean. The best I can manage was a rowboat on the Red.

It all started with an office visit the previous day. Johann Klassen was an unschooled eighty-year-old with a worn, wrinkled face, a man of few words and simple wants. He had spent his entire life on the farm working from sunup to sundown to earn a hardscrabble living, but moved into town after his wife of fifty-eight years passed away. He still made frequent trips to the family farm. He had never seen a doctor before.

Johann had worn a plaid shirt and patched coveralls. His boots were worn and sported large smudges of what looked like dung, with age vulcanized into a protective veneer. He still smelled faintly of pig manure. During the midpoint of my years in medicine, there were still many men like Johann Klassen – uneducated hardworking farmers and craftsmen who spent their lives in one spot. As medicine became more sophisticated, these folks with their simple wants and needs slowly disappeared.

"Are you more comfortable in Low German?" I had asked, knowing what the answer would be. Johann complained of shortness of breath and fatigue. He had gained three or four pounds. I placed the stethoscope on his chest – the air movement sounded like the crackling of tissue paper, a sign of fluid buildup. He had hypertension, mild heart failure and much evidence of aging. His blood tests showed early kidney failure, and high LDL, the 'bad' cholesterol. I suggested a diuretic to get rid the fluid and treat the hypertension. I also started digitalis tablets to give his heart a boost.

"*Doa ess toa fäl schmolt em Bloot.* There's too much cholesterol," I said. "*Met de teit woare deine Blootodre fe'schlekje.* In time, your arteries are going to plug up."

"*Oba waut kaun en oolla Knacks soos eck doone.* What can an old codger like me do?"

"Perhaps you could cut down on your salt and reduce the saturated fats and cholesterol in your diet." He struggled with the concept of his heart failing and the arteries clogging with plaque. "It's like a water pump clogging with rust and debris." His face brightened with comprehension.

The telephone calls had begun the next morning.

The second day, the phone explodes in my ear again while I'm still under the soothing spell of Morpheus. I feel more like the worm than the early bird. The previous morning comes back to me.

"Can I have cracklings today?"

I recognize the alarm clock clanking in the background, like an old Rumley tractor. "Mr. Klassen?" I ask wearily.

"Yes, this is Klassen. Can I have cracklings once for breakfast?"

"Yes, yes, that's fine," I say. "Don't you have any *Howajrett,* oatmeal? That's better for you."

"I'll buy some." He hangs up.

"You know," says Rose at our breakfast of whole-wheat toast and orange juice, "He'll probably want to know what he can have for breakfast every morning. You're going to have to tell him to quit phoning. Either that or give him his menu the night before."

"You're right. But I hate doing that. He's uneducated and a bit slow, but he's a nice old man and he's trying. I'll think of something."

"Oh yeah, Dad," says Jodi that evening. "Some old guy phoned here and wanted to talk to you. He was trying to tell me about his plugged blood oda or something?"

"*Blootoda*, artery. That probably was Mr. Klassen."

"Why do people tell me stuff like that? Just because I'm a doctor's kid, they think I'll know what they're talking about."

The phone shrills the next morning at the same immoral hour. I groan as I pick up the phone, "Mr. Klassen. What would you like to have for breakfast this morning?"

"Can I have fried potatoes and ham?"

"Don't tell me that's him again," Rose groans from the far side of the comforter.

"Sure, that's okay," I say. This type of patient care does not have much of a future. "You know, Mr. Klassen, I checked your blood tests again. I made a mistake, your blood is fine. You can eat anything you want. Come and see me at the clinic in a couple of weeks."

"*Nah jo*," he says, and hangs up.

I saw Johan Klassen three or four times after that. His heart failure was getting worse – he was weak and still short of breath. Any advice would have to be very basic. I encouraged him to try some fruit and vegetables, but anything more would have been a mental pole vault for him. I asked him if he was enjoying his cracklings and fried eggs. He said he liked them very much.

One weekend Mr. Klassen arrives at the hospital, pale, very weak, and vomiting blood. His stools had been black and tarry, a sign of gastrointestinal bleeding. His hemoglobin (blood count), is down to eight, just over half of the normal level. Jim Sanderson does an emergency gastroscopy. There's diffuse bleeding from the stomach lining, but no ulcer or perforation. Mr. Klassen is given several transfusions and started on omeprazole to reduce the acid production in his stomach. The gastric problem is likely a result of the daily low-dose aspirin I had suggested in view of his heart disease, plus the anti-inflammatories I had prescribed for his arthritis.

"No more aspirin, Mr. Klassen," I say as I discharge him from hospital a few days later. "Get this prescription (omeprazole) and come to the clinic in a couple of weeks to check your blood count."

When he comes back, his hemoglobin is thirteen, he has stopped the aspirin and anti-inflammatories, and he's eating whatever he wants.

His family found him dead in bed three months later. He had likely been felled by a blood clot to his heart or brain. His relatives asked that no autopsy be done, and I honored that request – there was little to be discovered that we didn't already know.

I had learned another lesson. I had sought to give John Klassen good preventative medical advice for his advancing heart disease – altering his diet, prescribing aspirin, and controlling his heart failure with medication. I had coaxed him to try some gentle daily exercise. He tried for a time, but his knees were painful and he couldn't grasp the concept of exercise being therapeutic. He had worked hard all his life, and now it was time to take it easy. All my good advice had been making him miserable. Mr. Klassen did not live very long, but he enjoyed his cracklings right up to his very last day.

I always felt an affinity for farmers. Mennonites had after all, been people of the soil for hundreds of years; most of my extended family had been farmers, as was my father for many years until the teaching profession lured him back. I spent the first eighteen years of my life on the farm, and had surely earned some of the blessings of the good earth. The soil Mennonites worked had something of a spiritual quality for them. I knew a few things about farming, myself – I could spot a crop of sunflowers, or a John Deere combine every time.

Perhaps it was the social strata that linked farmers and doctors. I liked to quote a survey to my farming patients that determined which professions people most trusted. Politicians and used car salesmen were in the dung heap at nineteen and thirteen percent. Farmers were at ninety percent and doctors at eighty-nine. My farmer friends liked that – we were equally virtuous and trustworthy.

Over the years there were many calls in the wee hours. One night at 5:30 AM, I am once again wakened by an urgent voice on the telephone.

"Dr. Giesbrecht? This is Jake Penner. Uh ... Dr. Giesbrecht?"

"Yes, hello, this is Dr. Giesbrecht."

"Doc, can you please help me? She's been laboring for hours, but just can't deliver."

Now I'm fully awake. Babies do pop up at the most inopportune times, and this sounds serious. "Who can't deliver? Your wife is having a baby? Why haven't you taken her to the hospital?"

"No, no... not my wife, she's been tied off. No, one of my cows. I've been trying to help her, but the calf is stuck or some ..."

"What?" I sit bolt upright in bed. I regain my voice. "Jake, you've got to be kidding! You want me to come to your farm and deliver a calf?"

"Yeah, sure, can you come and see what's wrong? You've delivered lots of babies, right?"

"Well, of course I've delivered human babies. I really don't know anything about cows."

"Yeah, but animals are the same, right? Same equipment? I can't afford to lose that calf. I stuck my arm in there, but I can't tell what part is coming first. You'll know what to do."

I can't believe we are having this conversation. "Cows are a lot different than humans and a lot bigger," I protest. In any case, I have no burning desire to shove my arm up a cow's vagina. "I don't think I'm qualified to handle this. Shouldn't you call the vet? He would know what to ..."

"We have to do something soon, Doc. I thought I would call you first. The vet doesn't like to come out at night."

I hop out of bed and walk down the hall. My blood pressure is starting to climb. The only thing that keeps me from a cerebral hemorrhage is the pure absurdity of the situation. "Jake, let me get this straight. You don't want to bother the vet at night, but it's okay to call me?"

"Well, the vet costs a lot of money."

"Jake," I say. I'm close to a boil. My brain has just pulled a hamstring. "Listen to me. This is ridiculous. I don't think Manitoba Health covers livestock. I understand you have a problem, but that isn't my line of work. I think you had better call the vet. He's the expert."

"Okay," he says, "Sorry to bother you."

It has been another unwelcome infringement on my REM time. Night work comes with the territory, but it's never easy. It's just as difficult the twentieth year as it was the first. In fact, my body protests more vigorously with each passing year. My body seemed to be engaged in subversive behavior. I knew that at age 55, people expected things to wear out, fall out, or spread out – I just didn't think it was going to happen to me. I turn over and close my eyes, but my mind is churning, and I know sleep will not come.

Daylight is breaking, I may as well get up. I dress and walk out onto the yard, the morning air cool and fragrant. There's not a breath of wind, and the dew on the grass is heavy. The light is soft and low with a red flush in the east, like a flower bud unfolding, promise of another sunrise. There's serenity at this time of day, before the roar of traffic signals another frantic day.

I could go to the hospital and look after some of the discharge summaries that are stacked on the shelf with my name. The row of charts gets longer and longer until my conscience has a meltdown, or I get a letter from medical records, and I reluctantly start on this thankless task. No, the charts haven't yet reached critical mass; medical records they will have to wait.

It's annoying the way medicine and the yard get in the way of a tranquil moment. There is too much to do. The rush of the world has a tenacious grip on me, and I find it difficult to relax – guilt and an overdeveloped work ethic see to that. Ah, well, when I retire… I should review some recent literature on heart disease. Instead, I lie down on the basement couch with some easy reading by James Herriot.

These things happen so often in the middle of the night, after I've had three or four hours slumber – just enough to keep me from nodding off again when I get back to bed. I'd often read for an hour or so, something sufficiently boring to eventually lull me to sleep – perhaps a journal article about Aspartylglucosaminuria (a rare genetic inborn error of metabolism), or Cockayne Syndrome (a form of dwarfism, also very rare), both of which I had never seen and likely never would. Even with that, it's usually another hour before I find myself trying to read through my eyelids, and I shut off the light.

I wake up at 7 AM every day without an alarm, the habit of many years. I bath, shave, and get dressed. I'll have a quick breakfast, probably orange juice and toast or cereal – not dietary wisdom, but it's the only thing that can be prepared and eaten in four minutes. Frequently I'm late getting up, and so I'd tried eating a bowl of cereal and shaving at the same time. I stopped doing that when I realized the sprinkles on my corn flakes were probably not supposed to be there.

## Chapter 23
# TANTRUMS

This week has had enough Hippocratic struggles. Now I have one of those rare, wonderful weekends when I'm not on anesthesia or ward call. An equally rare Saturday off. I change into grubbies after lunch and go outdoors. Rose comes out to transplant some perennials.

September has faded into October. Autumn is a delightful time of year, the air cool and invigorating. The days are shorter, the nights cooler. Long rivers of Canada geese navigate the sky between farmer's grain fields and the Heritage Village pond. Thousands of them gather nightly like troops training before a battle. The silver maples are turning a brilliant yellow and the sumac a deep wine. Most of the flowers are dry and spent, except for stonecrop and chrysanthemums. It's dry, no rain for weeks now, and the neighbors' honeybees buzz about the fishpond and fountain, the only nearby source of water. Things are dying and need little care, and the grass has stopped growing.

The autumn light is mellow and warm. The leaves rustle and crunch underfoot as I walk to the garden to retrieve the last of the tomatoes and cucumbers. There's a heart-stopping flurry of wings as a covey of Sharptail grouse suddenly take flight.

Just a few more chores and we can put the yard to bed for the winter – spray Scoot on the trunks of the young trees, especially cherry and apple, which often become part of the larder for winter mice and rabbits. Lower the water lilies to the bottom of the pond to winter, and do one last mowing. The fall-germinated dandelions will have to wait until spring. We won't clean up the flowerbeds – the dead stalks trap snow cover for the perennials. Cleanup will have to wait for spring when we're more motivated.

Rose and I work until it's too dark to continue. I change into pajamas and housecoat, my favorite attire for the last few hours of the day. I wander into the library and absent-mindedly flip through the stack of medical journals I should be reading to keep up to date: *New Therapies in the Treatment of Heart Failure, Eating Disorders: Raising Awareness*. I put them down again. I've had enough medicine for one week. There are times when one needs something easy and mindless. I sit down in the easy chair beside the fireplace with *Life with Jeeves*. Jodi wanders down from her room and I give her a playful nudge. She turns and smacks my arm, and the wrestling begins. She struggles to get free and slides over the arm of the chair straight onto a brass unicorn that adorns the hearth. She lets out a yelp of pain as the ornament skids across the floor.

"Jodi! Are you okay?" I jump out of the chair and kneel at her side. "Where did you get hurt?"

She gets up slowly with my help. "Ow, my back," she moans.

"Here, let me have a look." I turn her around and kneel to check her back. I'm horrified! Most of the three-and-a-half inch horn is buried in her back.

"Oh my God!" gasps Rose. "That thing could be right in her spinal column."

"Jodi, do you have any pain or tingling in your legs?" I ask.

"No, just my back." She winces as she gingerly sits down.

"I don't know," I say, slowly. Think… what's the best thing to do? Cool objectivity has vanished. "Should I pull it out? I don't think anything serious has happened. You know what, let's leave it. We'll take you to the hospital. We'll get an x-ray, and have Jim Sanderson take a look."

An x-ray shows the horn has penetrated between her vertebrae, dead center – another millimeter or two would have punctured the ligament over the spinal cord. Jim Sanderson yanks the horn, leaving only a small puncture wound. Jodi returns home, shaken, but unharmed. The hole in her back heals in due time with no after-effects. However, I endure lingering side effects – ongoing commentary by friends and family on my abusive parenting style.

As for the unicorn, it continued its days as a horse, and finds a good home following a garage sale.

The weekend is over and Monday arrives. Two extra surgical cases are added to the slate. That happens so often it's almost the norm. A young woman has arrived in emergency with abdominal pain, and needs a diagnostic laparoscopy, and probably an appendectomy. It will be the keyhole surgery to look inside the abdomen to make a diagnosis, often including a tissue biopsy.

I quickly look over Marne's chart. No unusual health history, certainly nothing she would willingly divulge to anyone over seventeen. Marne is pretty, if you can see past the bright orange Mohawk, rings in her nose, eyebrows and ears, and an assortment of tattoos. Some of the artistry is Dali-esque with strange creatures and bright reds, purples and greens. Deprived of her boyfriend, her cigarettes, and the ring in her navel, she has become sullen and hostile.

"Hi, Marne," I say. "I'm Dr. Giesbrecht. I hear you are no longer on friendly terms with your appendix."

"Cut the crap! Just put me to sleep and get this damn thing over with!"

"Okay, I'm guessing there are other things you'd rather be doing right now. I'll start the anesthetic and we're on our way."

"Tell Dr. Sanderson not to mess with my tattoos," she snaps. She turns her head and closes her eyes, trying to shut out the unwanted scene around her. Marne's cortex is already steeped in propofol, and her antagonism is fading. She opens her eyes, but her lids are drooping. "What if you can't get me to sleep? I'm going to fight it, and you won't be able to do it."

"Go ahead and try," says Candace, cheerfully. "Dr. Giesbrecht has never lost yet."

"Well, I'm go… going to…" Marne yawns and closes her eyes.

"Why would anyone mess up their body like that," says Candace. She pulls back the blanket and gown to prep for the surgery. "Oh, wow, there's more." Marne also has rings in her nipples, pubic hair dyed bright lime green, and a little tattoo on her lower abdomen admonishing: "Keep off the grass."

Candace giggles. "Sorry, Marne, I'll have to do some mowing."

The appendix is hot, in medical lingo. There's inflammation and sepsis and it's about to blow. The surgery is done in short order, the one-centimeter cuts sutured, and band-aids applied.

The last case is Angela, a 14-year-old with acute abdominal pain, who has had a history of minor problems for almost a year. Jim has been called in by the ER physician to evaluate her.

"I think we have to take a look," Jim says to Candace. "She's been sick off and on for months, and her abdomen is very tender. Her white count is normal, so it's probably not a ruptured appendix or an abscess. I'm not sure what's going on."

"Okay," says Candace. "We'll add her to the end of the slate. Dr. Giesbrecht, you can stay?"

"Sure," I reply. "I have to make a living. My wife is shopping in Winnipeg. Need I say more?" I phone to tell Daphne it will be another hour and a half before I get to the clinic.

Angela is understandably anxious. "Am I going to be all right?" she asks. "I'm really scared."

"You're going to be fine," says Candace. "You're in good hands. This is all very scary, but it's a short procedure. You're young and healthy, and everything will go well."

"Oh, you know what?" Candace says quietly to Jim. "There is no brevindex (pregnancy test)."

"Why not? That's supposed to be routine. You can't be sure even about fourteen-year-olds."

"I know, I know," says Candace. "I don't know what happened. Someone in ER missed it."

"Well," Jim says, "We'll go ahead anyway. She hasn't menstruated yet, so she couldn't be pregnant." We watch the monitor. The laparoscope reveals blood and debris everywhere with a huge swollen fallopian tube. "What is that? It doesn't look like a tubal pregnancy. That's old blood. The ovaries are fine – it's not a ruptured ovarian cyst." He suctions the abdomen to clean up the blood and get a better view.

"You know," I say thoughtfully, looking at the screen. "I'm no surgeon, but I've seen something like this before. You should check her pelvis – I'll bet she has an intact hymen."

"Hmm… you could be right," says Jim. "I'll take a look and then scrub in again. Candace, can you get me a speculum, please."

He inserts the instrument into the vagina. "Sure enough," he says. "Give me a pair of forceps." He uses his left hand to guide the instrument and punctures the hymen. There's a gush of old dark fluid. "She has probably been menstruating for months, and it just accumulated."

"So the pressure forced the stuff out through the fallopian tube into the abdomen?" asks Candace. "Amazing. I'd never heard of that."

"Right," Jim says, "I hope she'll still be fertile. This will heal, but there's a lot of damage."

Jim scrubs and gowns again. "Get me lots of warm saline for irrigation," Jim says. He suctions out all the debris. "The left fallopian tube is completely mangled – we'll have to remove it."

The rest of the surgery proceeds normally. We wheel Angela back to the recovery room.

I change into my street clothing, and stop in the doctor's lounge to check my mail. There are a few x-ray reports, and a letter from Bethesda Hospital medical records:

*Dear Dr. Giesbrecht. We need to send in our monthly reports and require charts completed in order to update our statistics.*

*Charts incomplete over 30 days 12*

*Charts incomplete over 60 days 8*

*Charts requiring signatures only 13*

*In the event that charts are not completed promptly, we will notify the Chief of Staff, with possible suspension of privilege.*

Yeah, yeah. I crumple the letter and toss it into file thirteen. It's annoying, but hardly intimidating. No doctor has ever been suspended in our hospital. They can't afford to do that anyway, anesthetists are in short supply. Really, I wouldn't ever let things get that far, but I can safely ignore the charts for another day or two. Staff is just following protocol. The charts have to be done; they just don't seem very important when there are patients to see. Everyone has been indoctrinated with the fear of litigation. Good records are important, but the staff is neurotic when it comes to the paper chase: every period must be in place; every sheet must be dated and signed. Misspelled words or incorrect dates are an abomination and must be expunged from our lives at all cost. "We are just trying to protect you."

Every year brings more regulations, more directives from government health departments, hospital accreditation requirements, and the College of Physicians and Surgeons.

We have to write better admission histories, daily progress notes, discharge plans and summaries, death reviews, and consultations. We have to attend case conferences, drug review meeting with a pharmacist, nurses, social worker, and home care coordinator. There are audits, death reviews, chart completion deadlines, and countless committees.

Some of this is a good thing. Documenting treatment options and patient progress make you think about what you're doing, and provide better information for future patient care. The other side of the coin is that so much of the paper shuffling and hours in committees are patently useless and only serve an audit or accreditation requirements. It translates very poorly into better patient care. The major qualification for health administrators or academics is that they have never treated a patient.

Ah, well… Another of those 'might as well get used to it – it's not going to change' moments.

It's 1:15 – just time for quick rounds – visiting hours don't start until 2 PM, and if I'm lucky, I won't run into any family members. Patients are a walk in the park compared to some of their families. I'm innocently walking down the hall to the nurse's station when I hear Laura speaking to a woman at the desk, "Your mother is getting old, but she is doing quite well. Grace MacIntosh, the home care nurse is coming to see her again on Thursday to set up a meeting for discharge planning. Oh… you're in luck, Dr. Giesbrecht is just coming down the hall."

Too late, I'm trapped, like a deer caught in the headlights. This is about as welcome as a two-week case of Montezuma's revenge. Laura looks at me with pleading eyes. "Mrs. Poetker's daughter would like to speak to you."

"Dr. Giesbrecht?" A leviathan is bearing down on me, and I can feel the ocean swells, and churning in the pit of my stomach. "I'm Georgina Dufresne, Mrs. Poetker's daughter from Los Angeles. The nurses told me I might catch you here. I have some questions about my mother."

Mrs. Dufresne is a substantial woman, past middle age with graying hair pulled back in a severe bun so tight it pulls wrinkles around her eyes. Her face is dour and impassive, reinforced with a thick cosmetic accretion. She has pendulous jowls that jiggle as she speaks. A feeling of doom floods my soul. Laura's head is buried in a chart.

"Hello, Mrs. Dufresne." I smile weakly. The tuna from the hospital cafeteria sandwich is snarling in my gut. "How nice to meet you."

"I talked to you on the phone a week ago, remember?" Mrs. Dufresne continues. "When my sister told me Mom was in the hospital, I decided to come out and see for myself how she was doing. I was shocked. She is in terrible shape – she must have lost thirty pounds since I saw her last. What are those sores on her hips?"

"Um, those…"

"She says those weren't there when she came to the hospital. Mom says she is always cold and the nurses won't give her more blankets."

Laura looks up and gives me an apologetic smile. My little grey cells are beginning to overheat and self-destruct.

"Really, Mrs. Dufresne," I protest. "People get very good care here. The nursing staff is knowledgeable and they work hard. Your mother is failing and these changes have been coming on gradually over the past few…"

"They took her pills away and won't give her anything to help her sleep. My mother is not getting very good care." She impales me with her steely eyes, daring me to escape.

"She gets all the medications she got before," I say defensively, "although I changed the dosages a bit. She may not remember, but the pressure sores on her hips were there when she came in – they are actually healing quite well in hospital."

"My mother wasn't like that when I was here two years ago. She doesn't even remember who I am. I'm going to take her out of Bethesda Hospital and take her to Winnipeg – maybe she'll get decent care there."

"Mrs. Dufresne, the Personal Care Home is as good as any in the country." It's time to take the offensive. "That's where your mother will be going. People receive excellent care there. Have you talked to your brother and sisters about your mom? I have discussed her care with them, and they are happy. Besides, it's very difficult to move anybody. Hospitals and nursing homes are full everywhere and waiting lists are…"

"Well, my siblings obviously don't know what's going on. I'm in charge now – that's why I came."

"Are you planning to stay in Manitoba?"

"No, I have to go back in a week; I just took some vacation time."

"Then you are not in charge." I say emphatically. Her eyebrows rise over the top of her glasses, and her chins jiggle. "Discuss this with your family and if there are some things we can do to improve your mother's care, we are willing to listen."

"I want my mother moved!"

"Mrs. Dufresne, that's not going to happen." I'm gaining momentum as we speak. "And as long as you are living in California, we will plan your mom's care together with your siblings who live here. If you want some changes made, you will have to speak to them and come to a consensus."

I think I detect a few puffs of steam venting from a fissure.

"I'm going to talk to the hospital administrator and the Minister of Health. I'm very disappointed in you, Dr. Giesbrecht. You obviously don't care about my mother."

"I care about all my patients. Go ahead and talk to these people. If anyone has some good suggestions, I'll be happy to listen to them."

She huffs off to her mother's room. I sit down at the nurses' desk. I sighed. Sometimes I longed for the 'good old days' when the doctor's word was rarely questioned. "What a witch!" I say. "Isn't that typical, though? She waltzes in here every few years and has all the answers. She probably has a load of guilt about

287

her mother, and has to blame someone. Is her husband here, or isn't she married?"

"Apparently she is," says Laura. "But I've never seen him."

"I feel sorry for the poor guy." I reply. "He's probably some obsequious mousy little man who has to ask if he can go to the bathroom."

"Now you know what we've had to put up with for the last two days," Laura sighs. "Thanks for standing up for us."

"Oh, well, we have to stick together, don't we? If she has some reasonable requests, we can make changes. If she's far out in left field, just tell her I'll have to check with the rest of her mother's family. Anyway, now I'm late again."

I drive slowly to the clinic, thinking about Georgina Dufresne. The human body is made up of ten trillion cells. Georgina likely has a few billion she could donate somewhere. If indeed it is true that the molecules of every animal and plant are recycled, sometimes repeatedly, eventually they will resurface in another being. Georgina's may well have been in the snarling fangs of a hyena or the decaying tissues of a poison hemlock. It's an intriguing thought. However, this woman, too, has an eternal soul cherished by the Creator – a fact not to be trifled with. I hurry to the office, determined this will be my rubric for the afternoon.

"Good afternoon, constable" I say cheerily. Lloyd Wilson from the local RCMP was my first patient of the afternoon. "How are you?"

"Pretty good," he replies, "I need a physical."

"Any problems?"

"Not really. A few aches and pains, nothing much."

I feel a curious compulsion to be on my best behavior. I'm a (mostly) law-abiding citizen with no criminal record. I should have diplomatic immunity in my own office, but he probably knows that I was going 65 in a 50-Km zone this morning.

Constable Wilson has the usual physical, including a digital (finger) exam. (A woman once requested a digital exam, thinking this must be some new electronic wizardry.)

"Aren't you guys supposed to be fit?" I say boldly. I may live to regret this conversation. "You know, wrestle the bad guys to the ground? You're overweight and out of shape." This guy couldn't run half a block without an oxygen tank strapped to his back.

"You're absolutely right, doc," he says. "One of these days I'll have to get serious about some weight loss and exercise."

Encouraged, I add, "Your blood pressure is high – 150 over 100. We won't treat it just yet. Let's check it again in a couple of months. Apart from the blood pressure, and being overweight, your physical is normal. If it's okay with you, we'll get you an appointment with a dietician. Anyway, go to the hospital, and get your chest x-ray and ECG, and we'll check your blood sugar and cholesterol while we're at it." I find myself using the royal "we," as if someone else were sharing the blame. I hand him the requisitions as he leaves the office.

Hypertension is one of the most common conditions that we see in clinical practice – and there probably are an equal number of people, possibly three or four million in Canada, who have never seen a doctor and are unaware they have high blood pressure. The incidence of hypertension rises progressively with age and may eventually lead to an enlarged heart, heart failure, heart attacks, and strokes.

What do we recommend for high blood pressure? Well, this sounds like a broken record, but again it's about life-style – lack of exercise, obesity, smoking and all that other stuff nobody wants to hear about. Most people would much rather pop a pill.

Or perhaps people should talk to their barber. In a study conducted out of the University of Texas Southwestern Medical Centre, hypertensive men who were given pamphlets and counseling by their barbers, had their blood pressures drop significantly, especially if they were given incentives like free haircuts. This is almost full circle for a profession that was known back in the fourteenth century in England as the Worshipful Company of Barbers. In those times, barbers aided monks, who were the traditional practitioners of medicine because members of the religious orders were prohibited from spilling blood. Later, surgeons joined the barbers in the Company, and remained under their control for many years. It wasn't until 1745 that the surgeons broke away from the barbers. Perhaps barbers should be brought back into the healing arts. Bartenders might also be useful.

In a recent study conducted in Florida, 35 percent of patients were able to achieve optimal blood pressure reductions (by an average systolic of 11 mm Hg and 6.4 mm Hg diastolic) with printed information, extensive counseling to improve exercise routines, an alteration to their diets, and loss of weight.

Our success rate in having patients change their lifestyle is wretched at best. In my experience, weight loss clubs or medical advice work in 5 to 10 percent of people. What does motivate people, at least for a while, is a brush with death – surviving a heart attack or stroke, anything that gets your attention. Too frequently, though, bad habits return. Smoking cessation has improved in the last few decades, but 60 Canadians stop smoking every day – by dying of its causes. Obesity rates, however, are still rising. Most people who feel like exercising, lie down (or turn on the TV) until the feeling passes.

I arrive home at 6:15. Rose is waiting at the door with her coat on. Scott and Jodi are sitting on the sofa with their violins in their laps.

"Did you forget about the practice in Winnipeg? The kids are supposed to be at the concert hall at seven."

"No, I didn't forget. I got a late start at the office because of an angry daughter at the hospital. It'll just take me five minutes to change."

"Okay," says Rose. "I've got a sandwich made – you can eat on the way. The kids and I have eaten." I change and we are on our way.

"So who was the patient that took so long?"

"Oh, a large unhappy woman. I won't say the name," I say, glancing at the back seat. Jodi is reading a book and Scott has earphones, listening to his Walkman. "People like her drive me nuts. She hasn't taken time for her mom, and when she does come from California every few years, she can't believe that her mother is aging and ill. We can't do anything right, although the family that lives here is happy with their mother's care"

"Makes you wonder, doesn't it?" says Rose.

"Why don't you tell her to smarten up?" says Jodi.

"Dennis, aren't we going a little fast?" says Rose, as we steam along the Trans-Canada. Too late. I spot the cruiser.

"Oh rats," I groan. "Wouldn't you know it – a cop."

"Are you getting a ticket, Dad?" Scott says. "Now we're going to be late for sure."

I slow down, pull over onto the shoulder of the highway, and stop. I watch the officer in the rear-view mirror, approaching. "It's Constable Wilson. I just saw him this afternoon. I'm doomed – this is pay back time." I roll down the window.

"Well, Doc, we meet again. Where's the emergency?"

"Uh, no emergency, the kids have a concert in Winnipeg, and we're running late."

"You were going pretty good there," he continues cheerfully. "Fifteen miles over the limit. I'll have to give you a ticket. Please bring your driver's license and registration to the cruiser."

There's nothing that curdles my cheese like a speeding ticket, but there's no way out of this one. I walk over to the police car and get in.

"Okay." I say with an exaggerated sigh. "I've had a lousy day – you might as well make it complete." He ignores the histrionics, and starts to write out the ticket, using the steering wheel as a desk. I'm thinking... there must be some other psychological warfare available to me. "By the way," I say, "Daphne got a dietician's appointment for you. And we need to check your blood pressure again in a couple of weeks." He hesitates a moment, and stops writing. His resolve is beginning to crack. "Your blood tests and chest x-ray will probably be normal, but I'll let you know."

Constable Wilson turns and studies me for a moment. "Oh, what the hell, forget the ticket," he says as he tears it up. "Just don't drive so fast."

"So you got a ticket, dad?" asks Scott. "Are they going to add that to your criminal record?"

"Nope, no ticket. And I don't have a criminal record! Although if you guys aren't careful, I might soon have one."

"So what did you tell him?"

"I told him I had a couple of batty kids on board who can get violent and urgently need to see a psychiatrist. Okay... we talked about some medical stuff, and he said don't drive so fast."

"I'm going to be a doctor, too, and throw my weight around," Jodi says. "I'll phone the hospital and tell the nurses to give everyone cocaine."

It's a thrill to watch twenty young musicians play with the Winnipeg Symphony. Our bosoms swell with pride at the prospect of someday having our accomplished offspring touring the world. Mrs. Dufresne and Constable Wilson never come to mind all evening.

## Chapter 24
# JACK AND MRS SPRAT

Merely seeing some patients' names on the day's list can trigger angst. Most people take several years to achieve that status, but the Schroeders had accomplished the feat in just four months. The trepidation was due to recurring frustration and a sense of futility – nothing I suggested made any impact. Someone has said you only perceive real beauty in a person as they grow older, but Adolf and Tina were single-mindedly defying that principle.

I stride resolutely into the examining room. My pain has already been eased by curiosity: what would it be today, the coprastasophobia (fear of constipation) or some new fixation? "So how are the Schroeders today?" I warble. I know it's a stupid question, but we might as well get started.

"I'm still constipated," gripes Adolf, "I haven't had a bowel movement for two days. It's almost three. It's always two or three days. I feel terrible."

Adolf and Tina Schroeder are dressed, as is their custom, as if they are on their way to a funeral. In fact, funerals are their main hobby (funerals and scatology), providing a social outlet and a free meal. Adolf and Tina looks like an upscale Jack Spratt and wife. Adolf is tall, thin, and craggy with bushy eyebrows shielding sad bloodhound eyes and a hooked beak, the overall effect not unlike a pterodactyl. He always wears a navy suit and tie. He is about seventy years of age and in good health other than the usual ravages of time. Tina "could eat no lean," and is a little more than half his height, even with the towering hat she's wearing. There are many bulges, as if she has been poured into her clothes and has forgotten to say when. She and Adolf have an equal amount of skin, but hers expands to the left and right in a grand vista.

"That's okay, Mr. Schroeder," I say, with oft-repeated advice. "For some people it's normal to go two or three times a day, for others it's two or three times a week."

"But I feel sick if I don't go twice a day. I only feel good for three or four hours after a bowel movement." He fumbles in the briefcase he brought with him and pulls out a small binder. He opens it to October, and shows me the page. Neat columns listing his blood pressure: morning, noon, and night, his bowel movements with size, color, and consistency; and the quantity and bouquet of his urine. There are other columns for sleep, medications, and diet. A diarist worthy of Samuel Pepys. "See," he jabs with a bony finger, "nothing since the day before yesterday."

I'm incredulous. I remove my glasses and wearily rub my eyes. I lean over to catch his attention. "Mr. Schroeder, why are you doing this?"

"Doing what?"

"This journal – writing down all this stuff."

"I'm trying to look after my health. All these things are important."

I feel my temples tightening, and wonder how many people I have to see this afternoon. "They're important, Adolf, but they are normal everyday things that will usually look after themselves. You're getting older, but your health is good. You should throw that little book away. You don't need to record all that stuff. All you are doing is making yourself anxious and ill.

Your bowels are on your mind all day, worrying you, and that just makes things worse. Work on some hobbies, go for coffee with your friends, go for walks, volunteer at Self-help. Enjoy life – these other things are not a problem unless you make them a problem. If you need to record stuff, write down what the weather is like each day, or how nice the sunset was, or the things you're thankful for."

I thought that was a trenchant argument, but it didn't make much of an impact.

"I can't do that when I'm not feeling good."

"Do them anyway, and you'll feel better. The point is, you have to stop this fixation and replace it with something more pleasant."

"The lady at the microanalysis place said I had toxins in my blood," Adolf says. "She said that was from constipation and not enough vitamins. She showed me my blood under the microscope – the cells were all crinkly with funny shapes."

"Mr. Schroeder, your blood is fine." I hear my voice rising with exasperation. I settle back in my chair to regroup. I look about the room, searching for inspiration. "We tested your blood count, the blood sugar, the white cells, and kidney function. They are all normal. I could take a little sample of your blood, and let it dry out, or put a drop of acid on it, and the cells will look crinkly like that, too. Those shapes don't tell you anything. And then she sold you some expensive pills, right?"

"Well… yes, I have to take twelve pills everyday."

I take a deep breath, and try again. "Believe me, you are in good health for your age," I say. "Certainly you're getting older and will have some aches and pains. Everybody does. I know you're being very careful about your diet – plenty of fluids, lots of fruits, vegetables, and cereals. Take some fiber supplements if you like. In addition, take a multivitamin every day just to cover the bases. Stop worrying about your blood pressure and your bowels. We need to use common sense and look after our bodies, but trust God to do the rest, right? Buy a Pepsi and a doughnut once in a while."

"Well, there must be something wrong; I just don't feel well."

"I checked everything, and so did the specialist. The CT scan, the colonoscopy, and all your blood tests were normal."

"So you can't help me?"

The conversation had come full circle. I shook my head and stood up. "I guess not, Adolf. You need to use common sense about your health. The main thing you should do is enjoy life. I can't really help you with that."

Adolf walks out of my office clutching his dung diary, Tina trudging silently behind him.

Like the common cold, hypochondriasis is very common. It afflicts people of every age. It is often difficult to diagnose, because it may mimic any symptom under the sun, from abdominal pain to dizziness to palpitations. The symptoms are real, but are not caused by any pathology.

I'm talking about symptoms that are produced by an over-anxious and over-active mind. Let me hasten to say that a bit of hypochondria is probably a good thing – it makes us take note of our body and gets us to seek help. However, it can also control our lives to the point where we are miserable and can't function because of constant irrational fears.

"Hi, honey," Rose says as I walked into the house. "If you want to change, supper will be ready in five minutes."

"Sure," I say. "What are we having?"

"Lasagna."

"Oh, lovely," I say. It isn't really that great. Lasagna is not one of my favorites.

We sit down to eat, and I glance over at Rose's plate. "What is that?" She had a bowl of gruel, or what looks like it – brown liquid with some flotsam, and two slices of dry toast.

"Mom's on another diet," says Jodi, without looking up. "This is number twenty-six."

"So what's this one?" I ask. "We've been through South Beach, Atkins, and Weight Watchers. What is it now, The Tibetan Monk diet, or The Self-inflicted Guilt-complex diet?"

"I know, I know," sighs Rose. "But this one is supposed to work. I've got to do it – If only I had more willpower. They can put a man on the moon, but can't come up with a low-cal double bacon cheeseburger?"

"Shakespeare said, 'Thou seest I have more flesh than another man, and therefore more frailty.' Why don't you hire a trainer to supervise an exercise program? She would weigh you every week, and help you with a diet. I know, I know... I missed another great opportunity to shut up. Thankfully the rest of us don't have to live on turnips."

"A trainer might be a good idea," Rose says. "But never mind Shakespeare. Erma Bombeck said, 'Think of those women on the Titanic who waved off the dessert cart.'"

I had a free evening at home, a rare event. I wasn't on call for anesthesia or ER. No school board meeting, no arts council, no clinic meeting.

"Why don't you spend a few hours with the kids tonight?" says my ever-sensible wife. "After the kids are in bed, we can sit on the patio and talk."

I hesitate. I should spend more time with the kids. Evenings and weekends with no medical or community responsibilities are rare. Personal time is like a keg of water on a desert island – not a drop to be squandered. "Okay. Scott, what would you like to do?'

"Let's play catch or something," he suggests.

"Sure," I say. "I'll get the gloves from the back closet."

We walk outdoors. It's early October, unusually mild. A warm evening breeze from the west caresses our faces. The goldenrod blazes from the unruly yard next door, and a congregation of robins fly off as we approach.

We toss the baseball back and forth. Scott throws the ball as hard as he was able – see if the old man can still handle a glove. Male bonding at its finest – two guys with a baseball.

Jodi arrives with her glove. "Can I play, too?"

"Sure," I say. "Why don't we play five hundred?"

"Okay," says Scott. "Dad, you can bat. You're better at that than we are."

I was passable at baseball – I started playing in first grade. It was nice to be able to do something better than the kids. I remembered tackling Lego when Scott was six. I studied the diagrams and proceeded methodically. Scott looked at the illustration and assembled the tank by the time I had gathered the blocks for my project. "Darn kid," I had said to Rose. "Is he too young to learn chess? I should be able to hold my own for a couple of years."

I hit a few flies, when Rose shouts from the door. "Dennis, the hospital is on the phone."

"Wouldn't you know it. Sorry, guys," I say. "You'll have to play by yourselves or wait 'til I get back. I shouldn't be too long."

That was optimism on a grand scale. It rarely worked out that way. Inevitably, things took much more time to sort out than one anticipated. For once I was out there, spending some quality time with the kids. It's probably some demanding, irresponsible patient who has no consideration for a doctor's private life. I resented that. Long and irregular hours and patient responsibilities caused stress and damage to personal life and morale. I know it's happening, but how do I go about changing that?

It's Myrna from ER on the phone, "Dr. Giesbrecht, I know you're not on call, but Mr. Adolf Schroeder is here with severe pain in his pelvic area. He insists that he won't see anyone else. He seems to be really sick." I hadn't seen the Schroeders for eight or nine months – Adolf may have had a remission of his hypochondria and actually listened to my advice. Maybe he was living life deeply and drinking Pepsi every day. More likely, he had moved on to a leech specialist.

Anyway, I was surprised – he still wanted to see me. Did he need vindication that he really had not been crying wolf?

"Hello, Mr. Schroeder," I say when I arrive at the examining room, "I haven't seen you for a while. How are you? What seems to be the problem?"

He's lying on the stretcher in one of the small examining rooms. No suit and tie. He's flushed and obviously in pain.

"Hello, Dr. Giesbrecht. I've got lots of pain down there," he said, pointing to his genitals. "It started this morning and it just won't stop."

"Anything else? Any falls? Any fever?"

"Yes, I feel feverish. No falls or anything like that."

"Have you had any diarrhea or vomiting?

"No diarrhea, some vomiting."

"Let's have a look," I say, suspicious – likely another bogus complaint. I pull back the sheet, and help him undo his pants. He has a large red area on the right upper thigh, swollen and tender. Nothing bogus about this! "This looks like cellulitis, an acute infection of the soft tissues. You said no injuries, cuts, anything like that?"

"Well, I was giving myself an enema yesterday and there was sharp pain on the right side and a little bleeding from the rectum."

Giving himself an enema! Nothing had changed. "Well, I don't know if the infection came from that, but it certainly could have," I say. "We'll have to get you admitted so we can watch this and start IV antibiotics."

"Okay, Dr. Giesbrecht. We have to do something. I feel terrible."

"He has a cellulitis," I tell Myrna. "Let's admit him to main floor. We should start an IV of normal saline, and give him two grams of cloxacillin stat." I write the usual orders for blood work, order further antibiotics, and morphine to control his pain.

I drive home. Even if this was self-inflicted, the infection would soon be under control. I would see him in the morning, likely with significant improvement.

The kids have gone to bed, so I settle down for an hour of reading before bedtime. The phone rings. I toss my book on the sofa and reluctantly get up to answer. Diane is calling from the medical ward.

"Dr. G, Mr. Schroeder is still having a lot of pain, and the infection seems to be spreading. I'm worried – he doesn't look very good. Now there are some dark blisters on the skin."

"Oh, brother! Okay, I'll come and have a look."

The cellulitis has spread, extending into the groin, down the scrotum, and around the rectum. Adolf has a temperature of 103. The white-cell count, usually elevated with acute infections, is high at 18,000, and the BUN, a sign of kidney failure or severe dehydration, is also up. Another ominous sign is the dark, blistering skin – not only is there infection, but tissue breakdown. This isn't a run-of-the-mill skin infection.

Necrotizing fasciitis. The dreaded flesh-eating disease.

That was somewhat unusual – it occurs more frequently in individuals with weak immune systems from HIV or cancer chemotherapy or with chronic heart, liver, or lung disease. The infection can spread like wildfire, and the toxins produced may cause severe systemic illness within hours. Fasciitis can cause death in about a quarter of cases. It is often caused by a common pathogenic bacterium, Group A streptococcus, the same family of bacteria that causes tonsillitis or strep throat.

I phone Jim Sanderson. "Mr. Schroeder is very ill. I thought this was just cellulitus, but I'm wondering if this is necrotizing fasciitis."

"I'll be right over."

I wait at the hospital. Jim takes one look at Adolf, "The infection could have started from a small rectal tear, but it could be many other things. We've got to operate right away, or we may lose him. At his age, his chances are not that great. I'll call the nurses for the OR."

Within thirty minutes we're operating. Jim begins to excise the infected tissue, and it is evident gangrene is spreading wildly in Mr. Schroeder's tissues. Jim cuts away large sections of his thigh up to his anus, some of the muscle, and one testicle, leaving behind healthy tissue. The wound is left open, and dressed with saline and gauze.

"Okay, let's hope that will halt the spread," Jim says, grimly, shaking his head. "We'll change the antibiotics to ampicillin and gentamycin, and send him to the city for further treatment. They may have to debride further, but this should do it for now. His chances are pretty slim. If he comes through this, he'll need extensive skin grafting."

It's eleven by the time I arrive back home. The kids had been in bed for several hours. Rose was waiting up. "You were gone a long time. What happened?"

I explain Mr. Schroeder's case. "He probably won't make it. We don't know for sure, of course, but if he hadn't had that confounded bowel fixation, this might not have happened. Anyway, there goes my evening off, but we had no choice."

Mr. Schroeder was sent to Health Sciences Centre in Winnipeg for further treatment. He succumbed the next day. Dr. Sommers, the surgery resident, phoned me. "Mr. Schroeder didn't make it. He had toxic shock and kidney failure from the fasciitis. There wasn't much we could do."

Sometimes hypochondria *can* be deadly.

## Chapter 25
# ED and ER

"Everything is looking good, Sam," I say. "The blood pressure is fine – we don't need to change your medications. When you come back in three months, it will be time for a complete physical."

My patient is Sam Wollman, a pleasant, middle-aged Hutterite who shows up two or three times a year, always thirty minutes late, to have his blood pressure checked and get medication refills. He is modestly attired in the prerequisite Hutterite black trousers with suspenders, a plaid shirt, and grey beard – the dress of traditionalist piety.

I hand him his prescription, and we say goodbye. At the door, he hesitates, turns around slowly, then sits down again. "Uh… I hear you're going to retire."

"You know, Sam," I respond "every six months or so, someone tells me they heard I was retiring. Are they trying to tell me something? Anyway, in ten or twelve years, perhaps, not just yet. I will be cutting back on my office practice in the near future, though. Too much hospital work. It's time to slow down a bit."

"Oh, you're not leaving yet. That's good – I don't want to find a new doctor." He gets up to leave. He turns at the door,

"So what are you going to do with your time?" He shuffles back to my desk and sits on the edge of the chair, rubbing his calloused hands.

"Oh, I have lots of projects I'm working on. I'm writing a book. My wife and I like to travel. And our family is growing like a patch of Russian thistle – they'll keep us busy."

"That's good. It's nice to have family." He makes another trip to the door. He turns again and sits down.

"Sam, there's something else bothering you, isn't there?"

"Yeah." He looks at the floor for a moment. He strokes his short beard, takes off his wide-brimmed hat, and begins. "I'm having some kinda trouble. It looks like when I'm with the wife, you know... it, well... doesn't work anymore. It just goes like this." He crooks his index finger. "Like a noodle. Can we do something?"

He summons enough courage to look me in the eye.

"Ah yes, I understand your problem – limp noodle syndrome. I'm kidding, Sam. But it's like trying to shoot pool with a rope, right?" Sam laughs, which was more than I expected from a staid middle-aged Hutterite. "It's called erectile dysfunction. It's common in older men, and it may be associated with heart disease, diabetes, or anxiety and depression. There are some things we can do. There are implants and pumps, but you wouldn't want any of that – they're cumbersome and don't always work very well."

It was the mid 90's now and there had been great strides in medicine, including new designer drugs. "The best bet for you would be Viagra – it just came on the market. It's quite safe and works well for most men. The main precaution is in men who have heart disease and use nitroglycerin." I explain some of the more common side effects of the drug – headaches, flushing, stomach upset, nasal congestion – nothing that would deter an amorous male.

Doctors used to hand out a prescription, tell the patient what it was for, and that was that. We rarely explained how the drug works, or compared the benefits and risks. The consumerism culture caused some adjustments in our thinking. Patients were now partners in their own health care. That certainly had benefits, but it had not been part of our training. Pharmacists were also beginning to hand out printouts of drug interactions and side effects, sometimes making our job more difficult. *This drug can cause dizziness, tinnitus, diarrhea, inter-cranial bleeding, leucocytosis, constipation, anemia, hepatitis, muscle weakness, taste disorder, allergic reactions, difficulty breathing, halitosis, nausea, headaches, cramps, hair loss, premature ejaculation, premature dementia, renal failure, heart failure, and death.* To name a few! "I'm supposed to *take* this?" Physicians were now expected to discuss the relevant side effects, the probability of any of them occurring, and convince the patient that the benefits would outweigh any possible side effects.

"Can I get Viagra without a prescription? How much does it cost?

"You need a prescription. It's like gold – about sixty bucks for four pills."

"Whew," he whistles, and shakes his head. "That's a lot of money. Fifteen dollars each time? That's too much. I don't need sex that bad."

I sense his predicament. He doesn't have sixty dollars, and all bills go through the colony's office for payment. There would be some explaining to do. A line for recreational sex was not likely on the annual budget.

"Sorry, we don't have any samples at the moment," I say. "Tell you what – I'll try to get you some the next time the drug rep comes around. Phone me in a month, so we don't have to go through the colony office. If you're having problems with erectile dysfunction, we should probably do some tests. Let's do your cholesterol, blood sugar, and a cardiogram. If there's any sign of a problem there, we might do a stress test. Here's a requisition – go to the hospital lab any morning next week, but you have to be fasting. And let's do the complete check-up in the next month or two."

He thanks me and this time makes it through the door.

I managed to acquire some Vitamin V from the Pfizer drug rep. When Viagra first arrived on the scene, it was such a solid success, we had to make special requests for samples. Why give it away when men would willingly pay fifteen dollars a shot. Sam phoned in a month's time and picked up the medication. No one in the colony was any the wiser.

"So how did the pills work?" I ask on his check-up appointment.

"Oh, good. A little headache from the pills, but they work good. It looks like now I have a different problem. I have pain when I piss. And my stomach is sore."

No more details about his love life? I couldn't really picture Hutterites frolicking in the cornfield, but it might be interesting. "Do you have to get up at night?"

"Yeah, several times a night, and every hour during the day. I guess it's infection in the bladder."

"It's more likely a prostate infection, prostatitis. We'll have to do a rectal exam to check the prostate. Please lie on your left side on the table and pull your knees up."

"Oh, the finger," he winces. "You have to do that?"

"I don't enjoy this any more than you." I enjoy golf more, but it doesn't pay me twenty-three bucks a hole. Being a doctor is supposedly an esteemed vocation, but I have my doubts whenever my index finger is thus occupied.

Sam's prostate is boggy and tender, certain signs of prostatitis. I ask him to lie on his back, to check for abdominal tenderness. "It's a prostate infection. Too much sex, Sam."

He looks at me quizzically, "Now too *much* sex? Have you seen my wife? She's a good woman, but…"

I had, in fact, seen his wife and she was, well…probably a good woman.

"I'm kidding, Sam," I interrupt. "I'm just repeating what my urologist friend used to tell me." Sam laughs. "Anyway, I'll give you some antibiotics. You have to take them for five or six weeks – the antibiotics don't penetrate prostate tissue very well, so make sure you take the full prescription, even if you feel better after a week. Come back in three weeks and I'll check the prostate again."

I repeat the rectal when Sam returns. There's much less prostatic swelling and tenderness. I routinely palpate his abdomen, too. No lower belly tenderness – everything seems okay. Wait… let's check that again – the upper abdomen seems unusually pulsatile, especially in the epigastric area just below the sternum. "Does that hurt there?" He nods. I check his groin and ankles – good pulses. "Sam, we need to check something else. It may be nothing, but we have to be sure you don't have a problem with the aorta, the main blood vessel coming from the heart. Go over to the hospital. I'll phone them and see if we can get an ultrasound to check for an aneurysm – that's a weakness in the vessel wall. I'll call you if there is anything to worry about. It's almost five, so Dr. Levitt won't be there to give us a report. I'll give you a call as soon as I get it, probably tomorrow morning."

Ultrasound was another diagnostic modality that had come to be such an essential procedure. When I first started in practice, we had not even heard of it.

Sam doesn't have all the predisposing factors for aortic aneurysm such as smoking or diabetes, but he is past the age of fifty-five and he had a brother who died from an aneurysm. He needs to be checked urgently.

The rest of the afternoon hums along in an orderly fashion, and I return home at a respectable hour. Friday on a Remembrance Day weekend – the kids are all home for dinner.

"So, Carla, another year in Saskatchewan," says Glenda. "Think you'll have a better year?"

"What do you mean, better?" she replies. "Last year was great. My grades were good, and all my projects went well."

"Oh yeah, but still no guy."

Carla laughs. "Well, if you must know, I'm working on that – there is a handsome young dude from California I met last term. I think he's the American dreamboat. I'm hoping he'll be back – you never know what could happen." Carla laughs and cries easily – life for her is ongoing theater – comedy, sometimes melodrama, and an occasional tragedy. Everything with great enthusiasm.

"An American!" says Jann. "Has he got money?"

"Give me a week or two, and I'll find out for you, Jann. But he's mine, so hands off."

"By the way," announces Brent, "did you see our new pup? He's downstairs in the basement."

We all crowd down the stairs. A black, white, and tan mass of fur stands up, wags his bushy tail, and looks at us quizzically. He stretches lazily, and wanders over to greet us.

"Oh, he's adorable," says Kim. "A Bernese Mountain dog, right? He's going to be big."

"Yeah," says Brent, "full grown, he could weigh 100 to 120 pounds."

"They're great dogs - affectionate and loyal," said Kim, admiringly.

Keena was a much-loved dog, and seemed a harbinger of a growing family, fortunately not canine. Not long after that, Brent and Glenda announced that I was going to be a grandfather. That event started an avalanche with the marriages of Kim, Carla, and Jan, bringing a generous sprinkling of grandchildren, soon numbering twelve. Once the kids discovered how it was done, there was no stopping the juggernaut.

We truly were a family. We had grown into a family, but it hadn't always been easy. The older kids naturally had other loyalties. Without their love and generous spirit, it would have been vastly more difficult. Rose organized innumerable meals and family functions, and in a thousand modest ways fostered love and respect.

Monday morning I arrive at the hospital ER for several outpatient procedures. Erna Reimer from the nursing home is first. She has a thick, unsightly big toenail that's giving her trouble. This common condition has an awe-inspiring name: onychogryposis. The nail becomes very hard and thick, and may cause pain with pressure from shoes. It happens mostly in elderly people with poor foot circulation and repeated minor trauma to the toes.

"Good morning, Mrs. Reimer, how are you? Are you ready for this? It's not pretty surgery. Taking the nail off may hurt, but I'll put in lots of freezing."

"That's okay," she says. "I'm tough, I can handle it. Something needs to done. I can hardly wear shoes any more."

I inject around the nail and the base of the toe to numb the digital nerves. I tie a rubber tourniquet around the toe to minimize bleeding. After allowing a few minutes for the xylocaine to work, I grab a sturdy pair of forceps, grasp one side of the nail, and twist it off. A Vaseline and gauze dressing, and the dastardly deed is done.

"That didn't even hurt," she says. "Thank you."

"You know that's not a permanent solution. The nail will grow back during the next year or so. A permanent job means a bigger operation. Anyway, the nurse at the nursing home will change the dressing every few days. I'll call and tell her what to do."

Myrna is waiting at the desk. "There's a Peter Bergen here. He says he's a patient of yours. He's a mechanic, and has something in his eye. He's in Room 2."

"Hi, Peter, you've got a foreign body in your eye?"

"Yeah, that's a lot worse than a local body" he says, laughing.

"Right, foreign body." I smile politely. "How did that happen?"

"I was using a hammer and something sharp hit my eye."

"Okay, let's have a look," I say. "We have to put some freezing in your eye first. That stings a bit at first. Please lie down on the table."

His eye is tearing and red. As a routine, I peer into the depths of that most magical and fascinating organ, the window to the soul. The optic nerve is normal and the delicate roadmap of fine vessels on the retina looks normal. I put several drops of Pontocaine on his lower eyelid, and take the opthalmoscope. "Look up at the ceiling, please." I hold his eyelids open, and examine his eye using the magnifying loupe. I can't see any foreign body at first, but using the beam obliquely to cast a tiny shadow, there's a minute black speck on his cornea. "I see it – it's likely a tiny steel chip." I use the point of a fine 25-gauge needle to tease out the fragment and lift it off the cornea with a Q-tip. I put some ophthalmic ointment in the eye, and immobilize the lid with an eye pad. "That eye pad has to stay in place for twenty-four hours to allow the abrasion on the cornea to heal. When the freezing comes out, it may be uncomfortable. If there's too much pain, come back later in the day for some more ointment and we'll change the eye pad."

"Dr. Giesbrecht," says Myrna, "can you see another patient who just came in? A lady with a sprained ankle."

Those were the garden-variety problems we dealt with on a daily basis. We had been told so little in medical school about the myriads of small, but important health issues. We learned about Ehlers-Danlos Syndrome and Subaortic Hypertrophic Cardiomyopathy, but little about treating ingrown toenails, fungal rashes, or slivers. Many of these bread-and-butter treatments I gleaned from experienced colleagues, periodicals, textbooks, and common sense.

There's a lull. I decide to grab a quick coffee, and then make my way to the medical ward to make rounds.

I walk blithely down the hall, unaware of the peril lurking around the corner. Too late, the drug rep had spots me. I know better – go down the stairway and back up at the far end of the hall. "Good morning, doctor. How are you? Got a minute?" I fervently dislike talking to drug reps, especially in the morning, when there are rounds to be made or medical records to look after.

"Good morning," I say cheerfully – I can be insincere with the best of them. "What have you got today?" The rep is an exceptionally attractive brunette, smartly dressed – this could be labeled unfair trade practices – and so affable, you'd have think she's my long-lost cousin on my mother's side.

"I'm Tanya with ShamPharma. You're Dr. Giesbrecht, right? So nice to see you again." I hadn't seen her before. I would have remembered. "Would you like a doughnut?"

"No, thanks, I'm trying to quit. Can't be seen eating doughnuts in a hospital hallway, you know. Bad example."

She ignores my attempt at humor and launches into her lecture. She has the mellifluous, come-hither voice of someone trolling in a singles' bar.

"We're really excited about our new product for flatulence. Gasbanex has proven to be more effective than all the other leading drugs in this class." She stoops to conquer and pulls some pamphlets from her case. "Here is a study done by Dr. Carruthers et al of the Cleveland Clinic showing the results of a three-year study on 9350 patients showing an average of seventeen percent decrease in abdominal distension, and a twenty-six percent decrease in flatus with our drug as compared with Deflatron, our nearest competitor." She flashes another pearly smile. "Here is a copy of the study you can read when you have time. And this is a handy guide and questionnaire you can give your patients while they're waiting in your office. It will help you diagnose their gas problem and it gives the patient helpful hints to alleviate their symptoms."

"I really don't have time to do all that with my patients," I say defensively. Let's just finish this so I can get on with my day.

"Well, okay, take the study, and read it when you have time. I'll drop off some patient guides and samples at your office. And don't forget about our other products, Lortace, the number one ace inhibitor for hypertension and Exalt, our new drug for ED, shown to be twice as effective as Viagra at two-thirds the daily price."

Twice as effective? What does that mean – twice the allotted time? Twice the encounters? I don't ask, that will just take more time. "If I have suitable cases, I may prescribe them," I reply.

"I really appreciate your support for our products," she says. "By the way, we're setting up a golf tournament at Twin Oaks next Friday. Think you can make it? We'd love to have you come. I'll call early next week and remind you. Thanks for stopping by."

"OK, thanks. I'll read this for evening devotions," I say, as I stuff the propaganda into my pocket.

In three minutes flat, I have been brought up to speed by a drug dealer.

Hyperbole aside (there are no such drugs), the vast majority of reps are wonderful individuals, but I tried to avoid them like the Ebola virus. Some reps thought I only listened to them when there was a free lunch or golf game involved, which wasn't true – entirely. Drug reps are first and foremost salespeople. There is rarely much to choose between similar products from different companies – some have slightly different side effects or efficacy, or there may be a minor price advantage. Should we prescribe based on the advice of someone who has no medical training, has never treated a patient, and whose goal is simply to advance the company's bottom line?

I duck into our opulent doctors' lounge to check my mail. At one time, we had a large room with a couch, table, five or six chairs for committee meetings, a telephone, and dictation equipment. Over the years, the lounge has shrunk down to the size of a large broom closet – a cabinet with mail slots, a small desk, and two chairs – room for two people who can handle invasion of their personal space. We lost room to the medical records department during the first renovation. The next reconstruction moved us across the hall to make room for – you guessed it – administration.

There is a second notice in my slot about overdue incomplete charts, but they will have to wait. No time for rounds, either. I run down to the cafeteria for a V8, and then back to the ER.

I begin reports on the patients I had seen earlier.

Dan Morgan stands in the doorway. "Hi, Dennis. I was working in ER last evening. Did you hear what happened to Sam Wollman?"

"No, what? Don't tell me he died! I sent him over here for an ultrasound yesterday."

"No, no, he's okay. But he was a few miles out of town after his ultrasound, when he had this massive pain in his gut, so he turned around and came back. Turned out he had a dissecting aneurysm." The wall of the aorta had bulged like a weak spot on a tire where the blood pressure forced a tear. If it had ruptured completely it would have been fatal. "We sent him right in to Health Sciences. He had emergency repair last night and apparently is doing well."

"Whew, he's lucky. I figured he must have an aneurysm – he had this pulsating mass in his abdomen, but I didn't think it was that critical."

I should have sent him off to the city that evening. Wouldn't it be nice to get it right every time? Even with years of experience, our judgment isn't always on the money. You don't want to alarm the patient needlessly and demand an immediate response from an already overloaded system when it might not be an emergency. Fortunately, this crisis had ended well.

Sam Wollman had part of his aorta resected and a Dacron prosthesis inserted. He came out of this episode in good shape. He had not suffered any of the complications of aortic dissection such as kidney failure or some dead bowel when the dissection interrupts blood flow to internal organs. After three months of follow-up with the cardiovascular surgeon, he continued his hypertension therapy with me.

Sam refused any more Viagra, although I assured him the drug would be safe.

"No," said Sam, "Maybe it wasn't those pills, but I'm nervous about that stuff. I think I'll stick to playing my harmonica."

# Chapter 26
# BETTY AND VIRGINIA

During my first two decades in practice, the prevailing custom and expectation was that every doctor looked after his own patients twenty-four hours a day. That included hospital admissions, deliveries, telephone advice, and emergency room visits. That was part of the deal no matter the cost to our families. We were, beyond a shadow of doubt, dedicated professionals. I didn't know any better. Just simply take a day off to golf or go shopping? No self-respecting doctor would do that!

The ER was used much less by the public in those days – people were less demanding and respected the time and private life of the doctor. Every few years we discussed a call schedule for ER and weekends but it was always vetoed by David Kroeker and George Jamieson. They firmly believed they would be derelict in their duty – their patients wanted to see *them*.

It was now the early 90's – the time of the collapse of the Soviet Union and the creation of the World Wide Web. Consumers had become more health-conscious, medical advances were daily fare on the news, and people had high expectations. What was once accepted as God's will, or "that's life," now required a doctor. As the practice grew, we finally developed an on-call rotation for ER. By this time we had twelve or more physicians in town. Call wasn't onerous; there were fewer ER patients in those days and many problems could be handled by telephone and a competent nurse. We didn't stay in the hospital except during the early evening or other busy times. Nights were comparatively peaceful and one might be required to get out of bed once or twice. It could also be frenetic. Whatever the case, it was always an inconvenience and interruption to family life.

It's my stint in ER.

An early evening patient is a middle-aged gentleman with paralysis on one side of his face. His left eyelid is fixed, and the left side of his face is sagging. His right eye blinks normally. He's frightened as he thinks this is a stroke.

"Hello, Mr. Tompkins."

"Hello, Dr. Giesbrecht." His speech is slurred, and he's drooling from the corner of his mouth.

"That looks like Bell's palsy. How long have you had that?"

"I woke up with it this morning. I thought it was a stroke."

"Everything else is functioning normally?" He nods, and attempts a lop-sided smile. "Headaches or other pain?

"No headaches, a little pain around the ear."

"Wrinkle your forehead. Show me your teeth." There is normal movement on the right, but virtually none on the left. "When the paralysis is nearly complete, but only on the face, that's Bell's palsy. Sometimes it's triggered by a recent viral illness, stress, or even tooth extractions. I gather you haven't had any of those." He shakes his head. "Since you've had it for only a short time, we can probably treat it. At least there's a good chance that cortisone will shorten the duration of symptoms. I'll give a prescription. And get some artificial tears for your left eye, and we'll cover it with an eye pad for the night, so you don't damage the cornea. Go see your own doctor in a couple of days to check on things."

There's another patient with a sinus infection, then a break in the action. I wander over to medical records to clean up a few charts. Medical Records is deserted at this time of the day. It's strategically located between the patient wards and ER. It can't be avoided, and the doctors hurry past two or three times a day, usually with repressed guilt.

I check some lab results and dictate a few discharge summaries. There's still no call from ER, so in a rare fit of devotion to duty, I move on to *Transfer Audits* – a record of all patients from the emergency department who were transferred to a tertiary care hospital in the city. The charts are reviewed periodically as to routine, urgent, or emergent status, and the appropriateness of the transfer.

I pull the first chart. MVA (motor vehicle accident). Forty-six year-old male, closed head injury, CT scan shows possible subdural hematoma. *Emergent. Transfer within guidelines. Approved.*

Fifty-two year-old male, acute coronary syndrome, ongoing angina. For immediate angiogram and possibly angioplasty. *Urgent. Transfer within guidelines. Approved.*

Ah, here's a beaut: Thirty-five year-old male with a potentially fatal case of stupidity. After a couple of hours in the local tonsil-washing emporium with Brad, Fred feels the need to prove his masculinity. He stands on the hood of his car, while Brad gets behind the wheel and puts the car in gear. Fred manages to stay on until they reach a speed of fifteen miles per hour, whereupon Brad slams on the brakes, Fred falls onto the pavement and breaks the tibia and fibula of his right leg, but has the good fortune not to damage what cerebral function remains.

This pair should be nominated for a Darwin Award for their heroic attempt at eliminating themselves from the gene pool. *Urgent. Transfer within guidelines. Approved.*

"Dr. Giesbrecht, please call 228." The emergency department – a welcome rescue from *Death Review,* next on the list.

A 56-year-old year old woman with her right arm in a splint and sling has arrived. She had fallen and injured her arm. Myrna has splinted the arm. "Possible fracture of the arm," she says.

"Hi, Mrs. Klassen. Let's see your arm." I remove the splint carefully, unwrapping the arm like a delicate piece of china – the wrist is exquisitely tender. The deformity is obvious. "It looks like a Colles fracture – the radius is broken. We'll get an x-ray to verify the position and make sure there's only one fracture. I'll see you after the x-ray and put on a cast. Myrna, please put the splint back on and give her something for pain if she needs it."

It has been an evening of routine ER problems. That's about to change.

It begins when Betty Doerksen walks in. She's a unique individual. Intellect-wise, she motored through life with a K-car when all around her, people drove Buicks, even a few Ferraris. Some drank deeply from the fountain of knowledge, she gargled and spat. She looked in the obituary page of the paper, and if her name wasn't there, she relaxed and carried on with her day. She had often provided comic relief to the medical community. She had the open, guileless face of a child, and was not shy about her health problems, even those details usually reserved for private consultations with health professionals. Her motto was: Say it like it is. Tact and genteel talk only lead to misunderstanding.

Betty is chubby bordering on obese. She has large curves like a slalom course on a ski hill, but compressed because of her short stature. Her blue sweater and green skirt alternately bulge and sag like an unmade bed. She has made a garish attempt at make-up, dark brown eyebrows drawn in with a marking pen, bright pink lipstick that strays well beyond her lips. Betty's pate shines through her thin mousy hair like a disco ball.

Betty strides briskly up to the reception desk, "I'm Betty Doerksen. Is Dr. Giesbrecht here? I need to see him right away."

"Yes, you're in luck," says Myrna "He's doing ER today. What seems to be the problem?"

"I've got this terrible itch in my virginia."

Myrna furrows her brow, and leans forward. "I'm sorry, Mrs. Doerksen. I didn't get that. Where is the itch?"

"In my virginia. You know, down there." She points without hesitation to her pubic area. "You're a nurse. You should know that."

Myrna falters for a moment, her face contorts with effort, but she manages to regain her composure. "Oh, the vagina. Well... okay, Betty. Have a seat in the waiting room. Dr. Giesbrecht will be with you shortly." She flees to the coffee room behind the desk and collapses in a chair, howling with laughter.

I walk across the corridor to the nursing station. Betty is pouring her personal problems into the ears of an elderly couple seated beside her. She's earnestly explaining her health woes and receiving rapt attention from three or four others in the waiting room.

"I have such terrible problems. The doctors told me I'm allergic to my husband's seed, you know what I mean? But he won't let me alone."

She leans over toward the woman as if sharing a confidence only a person of the same gender would understand. She continues, "You know these men, they have to have their fun. Now I have this terrible rash. My whole bottom feels like it's on fire."

The couple exchange looks somewhere between fascination and horror. The woman turns a deep crimson, and glances around the room as if searching for a crevice in which to hide. The other patients raise their magazines over their faces, shaking with silent laughter, waiting for more.

"We had better rescue those poor people in the waiting room," I say to Myrna, who is still disabled. "That lady sitting beside Mrs. Doerksen is going to have apoplexy. Why don't you show Betty into the procedure room? She can wait there."

After another case of sniffles and a sprained ankle, I get around to Betty. Myrna has placed her in the room with the gyne table for doing pelvic exams. Gynecology is an important, but awkward part of family practice. Pelvic exams and Pap tests are essential, but most women aren't fond of exposing their nether regions, especially to a male. It seems like the ultimate indignity, and I could sense their discomfort. Betty doesn't have this problem. She is already lying on the examining table, her feet fitted into the stirrups, her naughty bits aimed at the heavens.

"Hi, Betty," I say. I hastily take the sheet from her hand and drape the bottom half of her body. "The nurse tells me you have an itch in your vagina. Have you used anything for it?"

"Yeah, I took that salve, uh… from the drugstore. Mon something? But it didn't help."

"You mean Monistat?"

"Yeah, that one. Then I went to see Mrs. Hildebrand, and she put my womb back – she said that would fix the trouble, but it only helped for a couple of days. It feels like my whole insides are going to fall on the floor."

"Mrs. Hildebrand? Which Mrs. Hildebrand are you talking about?"

"Oh, you know – the *Trajchtmoaka,* chiropractor, from New Bothwell."

Ah, yes, Mrs. Hildebrand. In fact, she's a patient of mine. She had developed a busy practice as a self-taught chiropractor, because, she said, she had the gift in her hands. Very few people had that gift, she told me. Mennonites, having a direct link to God, would have a disproportionate share of these talents. After several years of practice, Mrs. Hildebrand had decided to become legit and took a comprehensive two-week course to add to her curriculum vitae. The exams were very hard, she told me, because they added reflexology to her program of studies. She proudly pulled out a diploma from the Beaumont College of Healing Arts. She offered to do a diagnostic run on me right then and there. She said I might have some hidden health problems, like *Nearesteen*, kidney stones or *Kjräft*, cancer. Maybe another time, I told her.

Mrs. Hildebrand had made it clear I was privileged to be her doctor. She was quite capable of diagnosing and treating her own hypertension and arthritis if only the pharmacist would honor her prescriptions.

"Mrs. Hildebrand got your womb back?" I ask Betty, tongue-in-cheek. "So where had it gone?"

"She said my womb had fallen out, and that was causing infections. I lay on the table and she did, you know, *strijche*, massage, and put it back."

"I'm glad your womb is back. There is nothing more annoying than a wandering womb." Betty's face is innocence – my attempt at humor hadn't made it past her auditory canal. I find a speculum and proceed to the pelvic exam. "I'm taking a swab to see what kind of infection you have. I'll give you a different prescription for vaginal crème and some tablets to take by mouth. You can see me at the clinic in a few days."

"Dr. Giesbrecht, can you sign a paper so my husband leaves me alone?"

I look at her sharply. She is utterly serious. "What? Betty, I can't do that. That's something you had better discuss with him. Besides, he might ask me for a note that says he needs sex for *his* health."

The ER is quiet after that, almost eerily so. I'm about to leave for home, when I get a call from Eleanor, the RN on call for surgery, "Dr. Giesbrecht, we need you up here right away. We have a lady who has just delivered and is hemorrhaging."

"Okay, I'll be right up."

The operating room is pandemonium. Dan Morgan had delivered the baby, but with the emergence of the placenta, the uterus had everted. There is blood everywhere. Helga is moaning in pain. Everyone seems to be shouting at once. Dan is attempting to put the uterus back in place without success.

If that can't be done, the open vessels in the uterine wall will continue to hemorrhage as much as a liter per minute. Many of our surgical emergencies are obstetrical cases because they usually involve blood loss. I have a fleeting moment of terror – severe hemorrhaging in a 110-kilo woman. I breathe a prayer as I tie my mask – this is potentially a life-and-death situation. I remember an illustration in an obstetrical textbook of an everted uterus – clinical, clean, and matter-of-fact – nothing like the chaotic scene I'm facing.

"Dr. Sanderson just arrived," says Eleanor. "You know Helga, our patient, is a G19, P11 (19 pregnancies, 11 live births)?"

"Oh wow," I respond. "Her uterus must be worn out. You have some Fentanyl ready? She has normal saline running? Okay, can you get someone to bring up the emergency O negative blood from the lab? And have them group and cross-match for four units."

"The blood is on its way up. Oh, apparently there is also a family history of malignant hyperthermia."

"Oh, great. She hasn't had a problem? No? Well, there's not much we can do about that now, anyway. We'll just have to deal with it, should something happen. Can you start another IV while I put her to sleep?"

Helga is pale and sweating. She's maintaining her blood pressure at 110/70, but that won't last long if the bleeding continues. I open up the IV to let it run as fast as possible. "Is Dr. Sanderson on his way? We'll lose her if we can't get the uterus back." I give her some Fentanyl and small increments of Ketamine, fondly known among anesthetists as Special K. Then, 140 mg of succinyl choline to intubate. I keep her paralyzed and titrate a low dose of propofol attempting to keep her from crashing.

Jim Sanderson is hurriedly putting on gown and gloves. "I'm glad you're here," he says quietly. "She's lost a lot of blood.

Just keep her alive for a few more minutes. We'll have to move fast if we're going to save her. Can I go ahead? I'll try to get the uterus back. If the bleeding doesn't stop, we'll have to do an emergency hysterectomy."

"Yeah, yeah, go ahead," I say, "We need Mrs. Hildebrand."

"What?" say Jim. "Who's Mrs. Hildebrand?"

"Oh, a local chiropractor. I'll tell you about it later."

"Okay, it's back," says Jim, breathless and red-faced after several minutes of struggle. "Run the syntocinon drip. I put a pack in her vagina. Let's hope the uterus stays."

I shut down the anesthetic completely. I take another blood pressure. "It's dropped to 60 over 30. Let's start the emergency blood," I say, "and get me the pressure pump." I open up the second IV to run as quickly as possible. I push the bag of blood into the pressure cuff and inflate it – a unit of blood can be infused in five or six minutes with the pump. I press the button for another blood pressure reading. "It's back up to 100 systolic," I take off my glasses and rub my forehead. "Thank God."

"She may have had some air emboli," says Jim. "That could be the reason for the sudden blood pressure drop." After a birth, there are large open veins, particularly in a uterine eversion. Air may get sucked into a vein, almost like a vapor lock in an automobile engine, travel up to brain or heart, and cause a disruption in blood flow, often with disastrous consequences.

"That's quite possible," I agree. "If it were only blood loss, the blood pressure wouldn't likely come back that fast."

Jim keeps massaging the uterus between his hands. As it begins to respond, slowly but surely the bleeding stops. A wave of relief sweeps over the room. We won't need the hysterectomy, but Helga will have to be watched closely. We take her to the recovery room with a normal blood pressure.

"Is everything good?" Helga mumbles.

"Yes, you're fine," says Gwen, the recovery room nurse. "Here is some oxygen for you to breathe. Hold up your arm so I can put the blood pressure cuff on."

I walk back to the change room, and sit down on the couch. I decide to change and go back to ER and see what is going on – hopefully it's quiet and I'll be able to go home.

Andrew walks in just as I finish dressing. "Nasty business there, I hear."

"Yeah, it was a little hairy there for a while."

"Family history of malignant hyperthermia?" Andrew asks. "I know a bit about that. I've had four cases, you know."

"Wow, that's amazing," I say. "Four cases. How many years have you been doing anesthesia?"

"Five."

Truly remarkable. I had done twenty-five years of anesthesia by this time, but had never seen a case. Why was I surprised? If I had dealt with two cases of pulmonary embolism during surgery, Andrew had seen six. If I'd had one cardiac arrest on the table, Andrew would have had seven and saved them all.

Malignant hyperthermia is a dreaded complication in anesthesia, which can be deadly if not recognized and treated immediately. It is a genetic abnormality in which a patient reacts to inhaled anesthetic agents and muscle relaxants with increased metabolism, body temperature, and muscle rigidity. It may lead to hemorrhage, cerebral edema, cardiac arrhythmias, and even death. We kept an adequate supply of dantrolene on hand in case we ever needed it. Fortunately, malignant hyperthermia is very rare. The closest encounters I had were a few patients with a family history of the condition.

Jim arrives, slumps into the desk chair, and rubs his eyes. "That could have been bad," he says. "She lost a lot of blood."

"I guess the P19, G11 could have had something to do with that. Her uterine ligaments are probably stretched and worn like an old inner tube."

"Could be," replies Jim, "But we might see her again – she's probably got another dozen or so left in her. What was that about Mrs. Hildebrand?" I relate the story about the self-taught healer and Betty's fallen womb. Jim laughs. "We'll have to give her surgical privileges so we can call on her expertise next time."

Large families like Helga's were the norm in generations past. Rose was one of eleven in her family, my mother was one of eighteen (though that required the assistance of both her father and stepfather), and my father was one of eleven. Mennonites and Catholics alike saw birth control as thwarting the Biblical injunction of populating the earth. Engaging in intimacy purely because of lust of the flesh, but avoiding parenthood, was seen as sinful and contrary to the will of God. In any case, natural birth control was a gamble, and required impossible measures of self-control and a huge dose of luck, so the result was large families. The vast majority of Steinbach's residents had become enlightened by this time and used birth control pills, vasectomies, and tubal ligations like the rest of the country. However, there were still conservative ideas around, particularly among the immigrants from Germany, Mexico, and South America.

# Chapter 27
# EUPHEMISMS

Obesity and associated health problems have always been a major headache for doctors, more so in the last 10 years as the obesity epidemic has really taken hold. We no longer call people fat or obese – we now have a euphemism: high BMI (body mass index). That sounds much better. And more clinical. However, it doesn't alter the fact that they are... well, fat. Every doctor spends a great deal of time attempting to motivate people to lose weight, exercise, and otherwise change their lifestyles. It's so easy to pop another pill or use a questionable therapy rather than work at the underlying cause.

I have tried information by the boatload, monitoring with frequent visits, enlisting dieticians and weight loss clubs, and scaring the daylights out of a few patients. No matter the tactic, I have been stunningly unsuccessful. Compliance is a huge issue for doctors, but it's about much more than taking prescribed medication. Even in patients who have had heart attacks or interventions like bypass surgery or angiograms with stents, only about ten percent make real lifestyle changes. Why are we so spectacularly ineffective at motivating people? Yet when health problems begin, patients find their way back to a doctor's office, though often at the point where we can no longer offer much help. That's the real frustration.

A titan on the operating table can make any anesthetist quake in his sneakers. On this particular day, I will be in the operating room for my usual five or six hours of anesthesia. Hilda has had a life-long infatuation with cheesecake. She is the opening act for TAH (total abdominal hysterectomy). She weighs in at a svelte 135 kilograms. I have been dreading this day. I would rather anesthetize a healthy eighty-five-year-old than an obese forty-year-old. Heavyweights require more anesthetic drugs, are difficult to intubate, and desaturate quickly (become low on oxygen). Jim Sanderson has been worried about this case, too. Hilda is enough to make even a battle-hardened surgeon like Jim contemplate a career change. Hilda lies on the operating table, her abdomen spread out before us like a Wal-Mart parking lot. Candace hauls out the paintbrush and sets to work sterilizing the skin with Betadine.

"Okay," says Jim. He gives a sigh of fatigue. "Let's do it. This is going to take a while." His scalpel exposes a wall of body fat five inches thick; the pelvis is a long way down. "We're going to need the long instruments. Tie a rope around my waist, I'm going in." Long instruments are scalpel handles, forceps, and needle drivers that are nine or ten centimeters longer than normal.

People like Hilda may already be on a slippery slope because of their bulk – the muscle power required to move their heavy chest outstrips the ability of the lungs to supply enough oxygen. This is known as Pickwickian syndrome, made famous by Charles Dickens in *The Pickwick Papers*, where he describes a fat boy, Joe – red-faced, bloated, and always falling asleep – part of the syndrome known as sleep apnea. Add to this the debilitating effect of drugs and the trauma of surgery, and you have a recipe for trouble. Because anesthetic drugs are often fat soluble, they accumulate in the patients' large reservoir, and slowly leach out during recovery, keeping them groggy for hours.

"This is like building a ship in a bottle," Jim says. "There's fat as far as the eye can see. We need another retractor – let's try a flat brass. Lois, can you help for a bit? Hang onto this retractor."

Candace, the circulating nurse, produces the retractor and refocuses the operating room lights.

"There are more and more of these massive people," I say from the other side of the sterile drapes. The number of these patients I see for anesthesia and stress tests is unbelievable – they are not just overweight, but morbidly obese (a term we use to mean the patient is more than just fat, but has, or will soon have, severe health problems as a result)."

"At least you get paid a bonus for over-size people," Jim retorts. "We don't get any more for a difficult procedure like this."

"They know where the really tough job is," I say, smirking behind my mask. "Unfortunately, they've done away with that bonus."

"Well, all you do is sit and watch your monitors, tweak the dials every once in a while, and dole out more poison."

"Ah, but the secret is knowing what the monitors are telling you, and how much poison to give. That's why they don't allow surgeons on this side of the drapes."

Jim and David struggle through the entire procedure. It's an exhausting job – in addition to the fat, there are adhesions from previous surgeries that have to be dissected before the real operation can begin. We are an hour overtime by the time the skin is stapled.

"Okay," says Candace, "We'll take a short coffee break. We should be ready to go with the next case in thirty minutes." We transfer Hilda to the recovery room, the wheels of the stretcher squealing in protest. She's starting to move about and all her vital signs are normal. I can breathe easy – mission accomplished.

The next case is another gargantuan young woman of 132 kilograms for cesarean section. I don't have to worry about intubation – cesareans are done with a spinal anesthetic, but I will have a tough time trying to find her spinous processes (the knobby projections of the spine) to use as a guide.

"Okay, Carrie, we're going to do the spinal now. How tall are you?"

"About five, five." Height is used as a guide for the dose of marcaine to be injected to anesthetize an adequate section of the spinal cord. It must be at the right level to provide anesthesia for the surgery, but not so high as to affect the breathing muscles.

"Some Betadine here to sterilize the skin. It's cold," I warn. I put the sterile drape in place, and begin probing. My heart sinks. As I feared, there are absolutely no landmarks to guide me. "Carrie, try to curl your back like an angry cat, knees up to your chest and head down – see if we can open up the spaces a bit." With her huge abdomen and legs, there's little improvement. I try another guide, the crest of the ilium (hipbone), but I can feel nothing through the thick layer of insulation. I make an educated guess. "Some freezing in the skin here, Carrie." I infiltrate with local, but it will numb only a small area. I make a few futile attempts, hitting bone each time. Carrie is tensing with pain in spite of the local.

"Sorry, Carrie," I say, gritting my teeth. Sweat starts to trickle down my back. Untamed gluttony, no self-control, I think in frustration, and then we're expected to perform miracles. "I just can't find the space between the vertebrae. I'll have to put in a little more local and try again. Candace, can you get me the five-inch 24 needle?"

I use some more local and probe several more times, a bit higher, and a bit lower. Fifteen minutes have gone by and Carrie is sobbing. The crowd in the operating room doesn't help – two surgeons, one student nurse, one "baby doctor," one scrub nurse, one circulating nurse, one RN at the neonatal resuscitation station, all watching anxiously. Finally, as I insert the needle for one more attempt, I can feel less resistance, and the extra-long needle pops through the ligament. I feel an enormous weight drop from my shoulders as the clear cerebrospinal fluid drips onto the drape. I attach the syringe and push in the mixture of Marcaine and Fentanyl.

My contribution to this event is done – just make certain Carrie's blood pressure remains stable and start up the oxytocin once the baby emerges from its watery cocoon.

"What is it, what is it?" exclaims Carrie. "Is everything okay?"

"Well, from the parts I can see, it's a girl," I say. "Everything looks fine, but Dr. Morgan will take the baby over to the Ohio (neonatal resuscitation table) and check it out."

After a few minutes, he gives the verdict, "Everything looks great. Apgar 10. Congratulations."

Carrie and Chris are deliriously happy that all has gone well.

Jake Martens, seventy-eight, also a severe case of Michelin syndrome (spare tire), is up next. He has had a heart attack, suffers from diabetes, and weighs 110 kilograms. He's an ASA 4, American Heart Association risk scoring system from 1 to 5, one being a perfectly healthy, normal-weight individual, and five being a patient with multiple system disease, and surgery needs to be done to save the patient's life. In a small rural hospital, we rarely venture past a 3. Mr. Martens has a perforated bowel from diverticulitis, so we have no choice.

The anesthetic is a juggling act. Too much propofol for induction, or a bit too much sevoflurane gas, and his blood pressure plummets. The heart rate is high at 110, and his BP has fallen to 80/50. I turn the halothane down, and gingerly increase the IV rate to expand his blood volume (too much, and he may go into heart failure). I use small doses of fentanyl for analgesia, and small increments of ephedrine, a vasoconstricting agent, to shore up his blood pressure.

Jake Martens, Carrie, and Hilda all had good surgical outcomes. They are fortunate – their risks were high, and the results could have been different.

Three or four times a week my office case load would include anesthesia consults – people who had been slated for surgery, and who had specific risk factors for anesthesia, usually heart disease, asthma, or obesity.

Tim Osborne is sitting beside my office desk. There's a chair under him somewhere, but I can't see it. He weighs in at 375 pounds.

"Hi, Doc," he says cheerily.

"Hi, Tim," I reply, "I'm Dr. Giesbrecht. They call me the gas-passer, you know, the guy who gives the anesthetic for surgery. Dr. Brighton, the orthopedic surgeon, sent you here?"

"Yeah, I'm supposed to have an arthroscopy of my right knee. I'm having a lot of pain in my knees and ankles."

"Right. I understand you have a few other health problems – sleep apnea and asthma. Are you using any puffers?" I leaf through the voluminous chart to refresh my memory.

"Yeah, I use Ventolin and Flovent every day."

"Tell me about the sleep apnea."

"Well, I have a real bad case. I lost my driver's license after I fell asleep at the wheel and had an accident. They did a tonsillectomy, removed part of the palate, and that, um… that thing that hangs down the back of your throat."

"The uvula," I say. He nods. "Did the surgery help? Do you have CPAP at home?"

"No, it didn't help much. And the CPAP doesn't help much, either. I'm supposed to go to Vancouver to another sleep lab in September."

"You're taking furosemide (diuretic), too?"

"Yeah, it helps for my breathing."

"But you still smoke. In addition, you're very much overweight. You'll have to tackle those problems if you want to improve your health and lower your risks."

He nods. "Yeah, doc, I know. I've heard it all many times. They're talking about stomach stapling to help me lose weight."

"In the meantime you need the arthroscopy for your bad knee. I'm sure you realize that your joint problems are probably a result of your weight. You can't support a semi on bicycle wheels, Tim. With your weight, the smoking, asthma, and the sleep apnea, your risk is considerably higher, even though you're only 44." I leafed through the chart once more to be sure I haven't missed anything.

"We'll see what we can do. We'll give you a Ventolin inhalation preop with a facemask – that's our standard procedure in asthmatics. I'll administer a little sedation, and Dr. Brighton will use some local for the knee."

Tim dozes off while I talk, as if to prove his problem with sleep apnea, and my skill in anesthesia. Maybe it's true – a friend assures me I'm so good at my job that people fall asleep as soon as I begin talking.

Tim starts to snore, and his face becomes ruddy with a tinge of cyanosis. I shake his arm.

"Tim!" I say, "Wake up. Sorry, I guess I'm boring you."

He wakes with a start, "Oh, sorry, Doc."

"I guess you really do have a problem. Tim, please pull up your shirt and bend over," I say. I feel for his spine, the bony processes we use as landmarks. Again, there is nothing.

"I was thinking about a spinal, if the local anesthetic doesn't do the trick, but that would be very difficult." I put the stethoscope on his chest – reasonable air movement, but there are a few crepitations. The diuretic probably had been prescribed for early heart failure.

I muse on the countless ways people manage to sabotage their lives. Here's a man under fifty, unemployed, without a driver's license, and with a host of medical issues, none of which have an easy solution. Surely there is some way he could lose weight and reverse the downward spiral in his life. I look at his chart again. His blood sugars are high, and he has been started on metformin for diabetes. There's also a note under *social history* – he's taking paroxetine, an antidepressant. His wife had left him several years ago because of abuse.

"Boy, has this guy got problems," I remark to Eleanor, who is doing preoperative clinic that week. "Tim is morbidly obese, with asthma, sleep apnea, and smoking, among other things."

"Are you going to do him here?" she asks. "He must be very high risk."

"Well, he is high risk, but he wants very badly to have the arthroscopy, and it's a short procedure. I think he'll be okay, as long as we watch him closely in recovery. If necessary, we can keep him overnight and monitor his respiratory status. He's from Winnipeg, right? Does he have any social supports?"

"I talked to him about that. He's on welfare, and he's been through the gamut – psychiatry, mental health, you name it. He refuses any more counseling."

As it turned out, Timothy did well with sedation and a local anesthetic. I watched carefully for any compromise of his airway and his tissue oxygen level. I was enormously relieved – as we wheeled him to the recovery room, he was breathing well, and beginning to stir.

I lost all contact with Tim after that procedure. Then two years later, glancing through the obituary section of the *Free Press*, I was startled to see Tim's picture. He was 46.

We are told that at present 66 percent of American adults and 50 percent of adults in the rest of the industrialized world are considered overweight or obese. Canadians are not far behind. This is causing increasing health problems: hypertension, diabetes, heart disease, arthritis, and bowel diseases. There is worldwide panic when SARS hits several hundred people, but obesity is a vastly larger health problem. The irony is that obesity is something we can fix, or at least modify.

Most doctors struggle with obese patients. It's not just their medical problems. It's difficult to give them the respect every patient deserves, and a struggle to stifle the suspicion that they are indulgent, lazy, and deserving of their problems. We have stringent laws to deal with people who abuse illicit drugs or alcohol, and we endorse campaigns against tobacco use, but obesity with all the attendant health problems has become a much bigger public health issue.

From what they tell me, most of my patients have an unusual problem – their metabolism is different or they inherited their weight problem. And they eat virtually nothing!

Yes, we all have a different build and our work consumes varying numbers of calories. But weight is a straightforward formula of calories consumed versus calories burned. It's that simple. If you eat 2000 calories in a 24-hour period, and burn 1500, there are 500 extra calories looking for a permanent home on your derriere. This should not surprise anyone - our bodies can't manufacture fat out of air or water.

Here's the thing. It's true that some people use more energy doing the same task – some expend a lot of energy just fidgeting. And we can't pin the blame on our genes. What we do inherit, or more correctly, learn, is eating and exercise habits, and possibly a dissimilar cerebral appetite control mechanism. Some of the problem lies in simple things like taking the elevator instead of the stairs, or driving the car instead of walking three blocks. All those small habits may burn two or three hundred extra calories a day, which, over the course of a year can amount to twelve or fourteen pounds.

As if there weren't enough bad news for the overweight, recent studies of dementia using CT scans showed that the heaviest people were the ones most likely to suffer atrophy or wasting of the brain. For every one-point rise in BMI, the risk of temporal lobe atrophy increased between 13% and 16%. The temporal lobe, often affected early in Alzheimer's, plays a role in memory, verbal expression and language.

Ah, well – human frailty. George Bernard Shaw offered his take on a depressing subject: "No diet will remove all the fat from your body because the brain is entirely fat. Without a brain, you might look good, but all you can do is become a politician."

Chapter 28

# CLEAN COLONS

Just as suddenly as Andrew Rhodes-Seaford had arrived in our town and by turns dazzled and mystified us, he disappeared. He had survived this colonial backwater for a year, which was undoubtedly at the limit of his endurance. Andrew never did fit in. Steinbach's views and lifestyle were conservative and it didn't seem possible that he could become an integral part of the community. He returned to Britain where people were civilized and understood nobility. No one was surprised at his departure, but I rather missed his British pomp and eccentricities. Most of all, I missed his sharing anesthesia call – I was now the one and only sleepmeister.

I am pressed into service for an extra slate after Andrew's departure. Our first surgery is Diana Bradley, a tiny person so frail she's almost translucent, like one of those teaching mannequins. We can feel her spinal column and the aorta pulsating through her thin abdominal wall. A cantaloupe-sized firm mass is easily palpable in her abdomen. One can't help thinking cancer. She has a seven-month history of poor appetite, stomach pains, and constipation. She has already had an ultrasound and a CT scan, both of which show a tumor, possibly in the bowel.

Jim Sanderson has been consulted, and as he has no definitive diagnosis, decides diagnostic laparoscopy will be necessary.

"I have no idea what this is," Jim says, as he pushes the long instrument into the lower abdomen, and the image appears on the monitor. "It looks like a cancerous growth, but where is it coming from? It isn't ovarian; usually something that size would be cystic with fluid. What do you think?" he asks Dan Morgan, the assistant for the morning.

"I don't know," he says, craning for a better look at the screen. "It looks like an enlarged uterus with fibroids."

Jim keeps probing, pushing the bowel out of the way. "I can't get around the mass. Where is it coming from? We'll have to open her up."

The laparoscopic instruments are removed, and a six-inch incision is made through the abdominal wall. The tumor is brought into view.

"What in the world?" Jim asks. They pack and retract the bowel out of the way to get a better look. Jim answers his own question. "You know what this is? This is unbelievable. That's no tumor, it's large bowel filled with feces."

"What?" says Candace, "you've got to be kidding."

"I've never seen anything like it," Dan says.

"There must be five or six month's worth in there," Jim says. "This is incredible." They spend the next hour removing the offending 'tumor,' and irrigating the bowel. As much as possible is removed via the rectum, but the rest is removed through an incision in the bowel. Then the bowel is irrigated and sutured.

"This makes all my years in training worthwhile," Jim says. "And it keeps you humble."

"I've been telling my kids about the relentless glamour of being a doctor," I say. "It's all true." Every now and then I steal a glance, but I'm happy to remain on my side of the surgical drapes in the company of the sanitary anesthetic machine.

Diana is malnourished and weak, but she does well. We transfer her to the recovery room in good condition, down to 38 kilograms. On further questioning, she admits that she has not had a decent bowel movement in the previous seven or eight months (decent, not in the sense of honorable). With a little more attention to her diet and bowel habits, Diana Bradley remains well and gains back her appetite.

Coffee break. I go down to ER to see a woman with a radial fracture of three weeks ago. The follow-up x-ray shows good position and beginning callous (new bone around the break) formation. Return for removal of cast in three more weeks.

I hurry to the medical ward to make rounds. I manage to see two patients, when the call comes over the PA, "Dr. Giesbrecht, twenty-seven. Dr. Giesbrecht, twenty-seven, please." The next surgical patient is waiting on the table. We proceed through the surgical slate methodically, but I'm late again. I phone Daphne to let her know.

"Should I cancel some patients?" she asks.

"Yeah, I guess so. I have one more anesthetic consult to see. Cancel the first three, and I'll phone back if there are any more delays."

I race down to the basement cafeteria and grab one of their chicken-salad sandwiches – strictly self-preservation, a lifeline until the end of the day. It must take special training to make chicken and celery taste that bad. I wolf down the sandwich on the three-block drive to the clinic. By the time I turn into the parking lot, it's two-thirty.

This will be another late day – office hours were to have started at one-thirty. I hate keeping patients waiting as much as patients hate waiting for me. With unforeseen events like emergency surgery and deliveries, this is often unavoidable. Try as I might, I was never able to subscribe to the notion that because I was a doctor, my time was more valuable than everyone else's.

Some colleagues seemed to foster that attitude – I thought it was presumptuous, self-serving, and arrogant.

With the cancellations, I'm only half an hour behind – without too many longwinded patients and by ignoring coffee break, I may catch up. I walk into my corner of the building, where I share two examining rooms. I have my own office for phone calls and paper work – a haven for brief sanity breaks between patients.

"Hi, Daphne, what does it look like?"

"Well, not too bad, I guess," she answers. "We rebooked four people, but Mrs. Sawatzky insisted on waiting for you."

"Oh great," I groan, "Of all people. She's first?" I can see my afternoon stretching ahead like an abandoned highway.

Daphne nods sympathetically. I take Mrs. Sawatzky's inch-thick file and march resolutely into the examining room. Perhaps by some act of providence, she has a nice, easy problem – an ingrown toenail or a rash. I will tell her how to look after it, we'll have a nice little chat about her salt and pepper shaker collection, and she'll go home happy.

"Hi, Mrs. Sawatzky, how are you today? Nice to see you again."

"Terrible," she says

Okay, no salt and pepper chat. Most people manage to greet you with a smile or a friendly hello, even if they're frustrated or ill. Not Edith.

Edith's hair is graying, stringy, and in dire need of a hairdresser with magic hands. She wears a frayed navy suit jacket, much too large, over a blue cotton dress that hangs listlessly down to her ankles.

I glance over Edith's history – late-middle-aged woman with hypertension, depression, and life-threatening hypochondria. That's just the last visit. Charlie Brown summed it up: "Sometimes I'm awake at night and I ask, 'Where have I gone wrong?' Then a voice says to me, 'This is going to take more than one night." There's no doubt the world is a seriously messed-up planet. What with pestilence, HIV, and wars, now we have to deal with climate change and a pervasive influx of mindless reality TV shows. It's a wonder we're not all depressed.

"What's so terrible, Edith?" I ask with as much empathy as I can muster.

She opens her commodious purse and pulls out a folded sheet. I blanch when patients haul things out of pockets or purses – a long compendium of complaints, an article about a new wonder drug for falling hair. Or a jam jar with repulsive stuff from ears, bowel, or stomach. It's astounding the things people fished from toilet bowls, like something you'd find under a rock after a downpour. On the bright side, it isn't a summons from the RCMP or a tax audit.

Edith comes prepared with the libretto from an operatic tragedy. She unfolds the document and places it in front of me without a word. I summon courage from somewhere deep within and begin to read.

*Headaches. Always tired. Sore neck.*
*Bad stomach, gas, feel like vomiting after supper.*
*Hair is falling out. Dizzy spells. Can't sleep*
*Back pain. Constipation.*

The next three pages are a comprehensive organ recital spanning three decades and dating back to her marriage, condensed like a Reader's Digest Book-of-the-Month.

*October 15. 1965 Appendectomy. Winnipeg. Dr. Brock*
*September 3, 1967 Bladder repair. Winnipeg Dr. Vale*
*September 8 1967 St. Boniface Hospital six days -*
*Wound infection*
*April 13, 1970 High blood pressure. Started Furosemide*
*January 28, 1972 Exploratory surgery for stomach pain.*

*March 3, 1975 Nervous breakdown*
*I stop reading in the middle of page two.*

Martyrdom is hard to beat as a means of coping with a rotten life – that way you don't have to throw anything out or move on. Edith's life has become a tangle of illnesses – real or imagined – negativity, and dreadful circumstances. Frank has a starring role on the playbill as an unsupportive and verbally abusive husband. Edith is like Joe Btfsplk, the jinxed little man from L'il Abner, who has a permanent rain cloud over his head. (Edith is not alone – statistically, six out of seven dwarfs aren't Happy.)

Our Mennonite faith sometimes over-emphasized our unworthiness and sinfulness before God, sort of a 'worm theology" that contributed to a joyless existence. Life is an endless trial, but we will be rewarded in heaven. How could I possibly help her? She needed a massive infusion of joie de vivre. I didn't know what to say to her anymore. There was hardly an ember to fan into life. If I thought for a moment she would agree, I could ship her off to the local Freud squad, or give her a half-off coupon for shock therapy.

I feel a Freudian-size pang of guilt. I haven't even started and I'm ready to admit defeat. I can't do her any good like this. The first thing I need to do was to get rid of *my* negative attitude. This woman needs help. Where's my compassion? She's the author of much of her own misfortune, but she's as deserving as any other. Her husband is a bounder, but that's not her fault… entirely. In any case, she's looking to me as a professional, caring person to help her. I need to offer wisdom, patience, and respect. *I need to listen.* The practice of medicine is not so much brain as heart. That's not something you learned in medical school.

I take a deep breath and plunge in. "You know, Mrs. Sawatzky, I can't look at all those problems today, but let's see what we can do. What if we tackle two or three of them today and you can pick a few more for the next visit. What's bothering you the most?"

She folds her document and shoves it back into her purse. "Okay. Well, I'm very tired, but I can't sleep. I have lots of headaches. My back is so sore I can hardly get up. Oh, and I need more diazepam."

"You must be using a lot of those pills. How many do you take in a day?"

"Three a day and two for night."

"Edith, that's too much, you should take one only if things are really bad and you can't cope, and only one for bedtime."

She slams her purse on the desk. "I've told you this before! I can't sleep with just one pill."

"Okay, Edith, sorry." I change course. "You fall asleep, but wake up early?"

"Yes, I'm usually awake by four."

"Taking more sleeping pills isn't really the answer," I say kindly. "Do you get any exercise – go for walks or something like that? That would improve your frame of mind and help you sleep. And how about going for coffee, or visiting friends?"

"I'm just too tired. My husband doesn't want to go anywhere. He goes to Tim Horton's and drinks coffee with his buddies. He won't do anything with me. He complains that the house is dirty, and I spend too much money." She opens her purse and daubs her eyes with a tissue. "I'm not good enough for him. I can never do anything right." There are a few barely audible sobs – a hopeful sign – maybe she still cares.

"Do you feel sad a lot of the time, or feel like ending your life?"

"I've thought about it sometimes, but I wouldn't do it," she says without looking up.

I examine her back and legs and decide her pain is likely a mechanical problem. We'll do an x-ray, use a mild anti-inflammatory medication, and have her see physiotherapy. She also

has the symptoms of depression, with many of the predisposing factors: low socioeconomic status, excess worry, low self-
esteem, and social isolation.

I thought about giving her a placebo or a mild sedative and
lauding the beneficial qualities of the medication. I reject the
idea out of hand – it's dishonest and plays on a patient's trust.
Some would say if it works, why not? In any case, patients were
becoming more knowledgeable, and less willing to accept a pill
without question.

"Mrs. Sawatzky, you have a lot of reasons for being tired
and unable to sleep, but I think your problem is depression.
Antidepressants would help. They will lift your spirits and help
you cope. If you can cope better, you'll probably sleep better."

She shifts uneasily in her chair, her face mirrors resignation, as if the last ember has died out. "I don't want those pills
– I'm not crazy. I've tried antidepressants, they didn't help."

"Taking antidepressants doesn't mean you're crazy. When
did you take them?" I want to know. "For how long?"

"I took them for two weeks. That was a few years ago."

"The newer antidepressants are called SSRI's, they're more
effective and have fewer side-effects. I think some of your fatigue
is due to depression. You have to take the antidepressants for at
least three or four weeks before you know how well they work.
Excuse me, I'll be right back."

I go to my office, and pull out my Pharmaceutical
Compendium. I can't remember which antidepressant is the
least likely to cause insomnia. One's brain can't remember
everything, but it seems the librarian is getting on and having
trouble finding things – I may have to let her go. I don't want
to research something with Mrs. Sawatzky watching. She had
disdainfully told me about Dr. Vale, the urologist: "I didn't like
him. He can't be very good if he has to look up stuff in a book."

"Here is your prescription for Paxil," I continue. "We'll
start with half a tablet daily, and after ten days, take a whole

tablet. The bottle will have the directions. Any side effects will usually wear off after a few weeks, so give it time. Try to take less of the diazepam – use them only if things are really bad."

"Okay… I'll give it a try," she says, without looking up. She picks absentmindedly at a frayed cuff on her jacket.

"I'd also like you to get a few tests at the hospital – there are other things could make you tired and depressed. We'll check your blood count to rule out anemia or other problems, and a blood sugar and thyroid level." I hand her the requisitions. "Have you ever thought about the things in your life that might be causing depression?" She begins to sob quietly again. I wait patiently for a reply. "Have you discussed your problems with a counselor or a pastor? The antidepressants will help, but pills aren't really the answer. I'd like to refer you to someone in Community Mental Health – is that okay?"

"I don't want to see anybody like that," she says coldly, pursing her lips.

"The clouds are pretty dark right now, but we have to make a start. I know a counselor who would be able to help you sort through your problems. She's not preachy or condemning. You would feel very comfortable with her."

"Maybe later sometime."

"All right. We can talk about it next time. Make an appointment for three weeks. Ask the receptionist for the last appointment of the day, so we can talk a little longer and won't be so rushed."

I longed for some spiritual chemotherapy I could give her – laying on of hands, perhaps a purgative that would clean out all the bilge; a nostrum that would lift her depression, restore her self-esteem, and reformulate her husband into a sensitive, caring man. If pharmaceutical firms can produce designer drugs like Viagra, surely they could come up with something. (Edith needs an optorectotomy, cutting the nerve connecting the eyeball and the rectum – severing that would rid her of her shitty outlook on life).

Mrs. Sawatzky is back three weeks later. I'm encouraged she has returned.

"Hello, Mrs. Sawatzky," I say. "How are you doing? Are you feeling better?"

"No, I don't feel any better. I still can't sleep and my headaches are worse."

We go through her symptoms again. I listen to the litany of complaints about her life and her dead-beat husband. Her life will require UN intervention. A life without love is like a year without summer, and by that standard, Edith's is perpetual winter. She has a new list in her purse, but it differs little from earlier editions.

"You'll have to give the pills a little more time – sometimes it will take up to six weeks before you notice a difference. But I'm sure they will help."

"Um… I haven't taken the pills."

"What?" I say, eyebrows raised. I'm not really surprised. "Why not? I thought you had been taking them."

"Well, I had a dry mouth and some dizziness from the pills, and I thought I would try something else."

"Were the side effects that bad? They will usually wear off in several weeks."

"No, they weren't bad. I decided to see an herbalist. She gave me St. John's wort."

I'm tired and my temples are throbbing. I drum my fingers on the desk. "Okay, Mrs. Sawatzky, if you think that is helping, go ahead and use it. We can always go back to the Paxil later if you change your mind. But you know, studies have shown no real benefit from St. John's wort. The problem is that these products are not monitored, and you have no assurance about purity and the actual dosage you are getting. I still think you would benefit from some counseling to help you understand your problems, and give you some ideas on how to cope. Have you thought any more about seeing a counselor?"

"No. I don't want to see anyone!" Her voice takes on a hard edge and she crosses her arms.

"Okay, okay. Well, can you and I talk a bit more? I don't mean just medical things, but about your marriage, your life. If we pick out a few problems, maybe we can figure out some ways to deal with them."

"I don't want to talk. I just need some more diazepam."

"More diazepam is not the answer." There's no response. "Okay, Edith, I'll tell you what – I'll give you enough to tide you over for a couple of weeks, but we have to go in a different direction. I'll gladly see you again, but no more diazepam after this."

Edith Sawatzky needed someone to walk her through each day, help her change her thought patterns, and show her how to cope with the frustrations daily life was throwing her way. I didn't get another chance. Edith said nothing, got up and walked to the door. I knew I would not see her again.

I had tried, but hadn't been able to break through, even make it to base camp on her mountain of woes. I saw her occasionally in the waiting room. She had moved on to another doctor. I sincerely hoped someone would find a way to help her.

Chapter 29
# TRIPLE BYPASS

Paul and Helen Kraynyk came from the hinterlands of southeastern Manitoba, a devoted couple, married many years. They came for their bimonthly doctor's appointments together, bickering constantly, a time-honored means of conjugal communication. They were easy patients – jovial, undemanding, and untroubled in spite of their medical problems: overweight, heart disease, hypertension, and diabetes. Their intentions were honorable and they genuinely appreciated my concern for their health, but they were incapable of significant compliance.

Carolyn has already done the Kraynyks' blood sugars – his is fifteen, hers nineteen.

"Ha, yours higher than mine," Paul says in his thick Ukrainian accent. "I told you don't eat so much perogies. And my blood pressure is just as good as yours."

"Yeah?" she answers, and jabs him in the ribs. "What about that saskatoon pie? You eat the whole thing for supper day before yesterday. You eat like a pig. You know you shouldn't eat so much sugar." They chuckle at their clever repartee, a traveling vaudeville show, even if only for an audience of one. I often wondered if their squabbling would erupt into full-scale domestic violence, but it never did.

"You know," I interject. "Blood sugars of fifteen and nineteen are both much too high. One isn't really better than the other. And your blood pressures are higher than they should be, too. Let's see," looking at Paul, "you're 98 kilo, and Helen, you are 87. So neither of you has lost any weight. Are you trying to follow your diabetic diet? You did see the dietician, right?

"Yeah, we seen her last month," she answers, "but that's so hard. She told us measure everything. How can I measure everything? I buy lettuce and cucumber, but he won't eat. He says that's for rabbits." They both chortle, another thigh-slapper.

"I'm all the time hungry on that diet," Paul says. "Not enough food. No gravy, no sugar."

"You tried it one meal," Helen retorts. "Then you eat three doughnuts." More laughter.

"It will take a little effort," I say. "But that's the only way we're going to get your diabetes under control. Remember all those things we talked about – the complications of diabetes? You don't want to lose your eyesight or your feet. As they say, don't dig your grave with a knife and fork. What about the exercise I suggested?"

"I walk to the post-box every day," Paul says triumphantly, the usual wide grin showing craggy, uneven teeth.

"And how far is that?"

"About eighth of a mile."

"Well," I say, "that's better than nothing, but it's not really enough to do much good."

"I chase the wife around the house – that makes another half mile." They rock back and forth in their chairs, laughing uproariously. I smile.

I launch into my oft-repeated recital. "Diabetes contributes to heart disease, kidney failure, visual loss, and leg circulation problems. The better we can control your diabetes, the less chance of those things happening. You both have diabetes, high blood pressure, obesity, and heart disease – that's a dangerous combination. That's like driving a truck up a steep mountain road with a low tank, poor steering and no brakes. We'll have to start you on insulin if those counts don't improve. More exercise, less food. We'll increase the metformin to 850 mg twice a day, and I'll prescribe a newer drug, Avandia. I think we have some samples." For the Kraynyks, generous drug samples were essential for any hope of compliance.

"Okay," Mrs. Kraynyk says, looking at Paul for support. "We do better."

"Yeah," he says soberly. "I guess we got to."

I was not hopeful. I would have been willing to bet a six-month supply of holubtsi, that when they appeared again in two months, little would have changed. But they were such pleasant folks, and they brought me a pail of saskatoons every summer.

The afternoon slate drags on. It's three-thirty, time for coffee break. The staff lounge is safe, away from the inquisitive ears and eyes of patients, no need to be an authority figure, no professional deportment to maintain. As usual at this time of day, the room is full, all the women crowded to one end of the room, talking animatedly about difficult patients or their plans for the weekend. The doctors, all male, are ensconced at the other end, carping about interfering government bureaucrats.

George Jamieson is there, coffee cup in hand. "Can you believe it," he rants. "The Regional Health office added another financial analyst. That office is growing like a malignant fungus. Our ER is overcrowded, we need more equipment and nurses, while they keep adding paper jockeys."

"You're right. It's ridiculous," says Dan Morgan. "Remember when the RHAs were set up, the administrators were all moved out of the hospitals into head office. We were going to save huge dollars by having a central office. Now these positions have doubled, they're all back in the hospitals, plus they added a few dozen people to the RHA headquarters. What do they all do over there? The RHA concept isn't working. I've read the maxim: *when you discover you're riding a dead horse, the best strategy is to dismount,* but bureaucrats would say: *we'll buy a stronger whip or appoint a committee to study the horse."*

I chime in. "An organism like the RHA needs employees just to cater to its own needs. How all that administrivia is supposed to translate into better patient care, nobody knows. There should at the very least be some worthwhile preventive health programs coming out of that office."

"Meanwhile they find half a million bucks to spend for new windows and pavement," Jim Sanderson joins in. "How about a few more nurses? And they've been talking about a new OR for the past twenty-five years."

"Well," Dan replies, "They haven't got the leadership to stand up to the tall foreheads in the Health Department. But somehow there's always money for another administrator."

"Gentlemen," says David, who had just walked in the room. He pours a cup of coffee "Whining again. You guys sound like farmers."

"Oh, they're still way ahead," says Dan. "But then they've had many more years of practice."

The conversation drones on. David turns to me, "We're never going to solve that one. We can complain all we want, but nothing ever changes."

Andrea Goertzen, a young family physician who had recently joined the group, sits down next to me. "Good afternoon, gentlemen," she says with an exaggerated lilt. "I have a problem I'd like to ask you about. What do you do with a child of two who had a febrile convulsion? She is fine, but mom is worried she's developing epilepsy."

"Any family history of seizures?" I ask.

"No."

"Was it a generalized seizure? How long did it last?"

"Yes, mom said about three minutes."

"Well," David says, "some of these kids will have another seizure if they have a fever. Tell mom to use ibuprofen or Tylenol and sponge the child if she becomes febrile. And bring the girl in if there is another convulsion."

"I told her all that, but she thinks the child should be on medication."

I add, "Tell her that there is no brain damage with febrile seizures and they won't lead to epilepsy. Medication is not really recommended in this situation and may do more harm than good. The vast majority of these kids will grow out of this by five or six."

"I told her pretty much all that, but she isn't happy with my advice."

"Tell her you consulted with your older and wiser colleagues and they agreed with your advice," David counters with a grin.

Andrea laughs. "I'm sure that'll help. I feel better that you guys concur with me."

"That's enough shop talk," David said. "We'll have to make a rule there's no medical talk at coffee break. You'll have to learn to be hard-boiled and cynical like the rest of us."

"Okay," Andrea says, "I'll work at it. You mean forget the Hippocratic Oath?"

"At least for coffee break," I say. "Anyway, I've got to get back to work."

It was now a year later. Paul Kraynyk had been admitted to the hospital with acute chest pain. He had the typical crushing pain radiating into his jaw and left shoulder with sweating and shortness of breath. He had the ECG changes and increased blood enzyme levels of a heart attack. If the heart muscle is damaged, the enzymes leak into the bloodstream and can be tested to help make a diagnosis. The emergency physician, David Kroeker, had diagnosed an acute myocardial infarction (heart attack), and ordered streptokinase within thirty minutes of his arrival, early enough to be effective in dissolving the blockage in his coronary arteries. Along with many valuable new imaging modalities, medical progress has resulted in new drugs like streptokinase and tPA, used in heart attacks.

"Hi, Paul," I say when I arrived on the cardiac ward, "how are you feeling? Any chest pain now?"

"Oh, hello, doc," he says, almost in a whisper. "No pain now – they give me morphine or something. I'm very tired."

"Well, when your heart is damaged you will feel weak and tired. Some of that may be from the pain medication, too."

Helen is sitting by her husband's side, holding his hand. "He okay?" asks Helen earnestly. "Is it bad? I was so scared."

"He should be okay – he got the medication fairly early," I reply. "The blood test levels are quite high, though. That means that even with the clot-busting drug, he probably has heart muscle damage." I glance up at the monitor above Paul's bed. "Right now everything looks good – his heart rate and blood pressure are normal, and he has no pain."

"Thanks God," she says. She lowers her head. "You were right. We didn't listen so good."

"Well, let's hope he'll be okay. I'll be in again later today."

I check the chart. David Kroeker had ordered nitroglycerin and metoprolol, a beta-blocker that slows down the heart, lowers the blood pressure, and decreases the load on a damaged heart. The patient's blood sugar would also be monitored closely, and small doses of insulin given as required.

Next day was Sunday. I planned to drop in to see Mr. Kraynyk on our way to church, but before we were ready to leave, the phone rang.

"Dr. Giesbrecht," says Diane, "Mr. Kraynyk doesn't look too good. He has a pasty color, and he's having more chest pain. His blood pressure has dropped to 80/50."

"Oh shoot," I say, "That doesn't sound good. Okay, I'll be there in a few minutes. Get another cardiogram and enzymes."

Paul is a bit cyanotic, but his blood pressure has improved to 100/60. Morphine had dulled his pain and taken the edge off his anxiety. Intravenous nitroglycerin had been given to dilate his vital arteries and allow more blood flow to his heart muscle.

I pick up the ECG. "It looks like acute ischemia or another infarct," I tell Diane. "I think we'll have to send him to Winnipeg. He's stable right now, but he may not stay that way. We can't give him any more streptokinase." You develop a sixth sense about patients – who will do well and who will go over the precipice. Better to have him in a large city hospital with a high-powered intensive care unit and specialist support.

I dread the next task. I consult the list of Winnipeg hospitals and specialists' phone numbers. I make the first call to Health Sciences Center, "Could I speak to the intensive care resident, please."

"Yes, that would be Dr. Simmons. I'll page him for you."

I can hear the receptionist in her thirty-years-at-the-same-job drawl: "Dotrsimins, dotrsimins, twonefour, dotrsimins twonefour please." She had been there when I was an intern.

"Hello, Dr. Simmons here."

"Hi, I'm Dr. Giesbrecht from Bethesda hospital in Steinbach. I've got a sixty-two-year-old male in hospital who suffered an infarct yesterday. He got streptokinase, and was quite stable until this morning. His blood pressure dropped and he has more pain – I think he's having another infarct. We would like to send him in for intensive care."

"He's stable now? What are his enzymes?"

"Yeah, his blood pressure is a little better at the moment. I just ordered the blood work, so I don't have recent enzymes, but his symptoms are typical, and the ECG indicates an extension of his infarct."

"Why don't you monitor him a bit longer, and give him intravenous nitroglycerin and see what happens."

"This man is stable right now," I say patiently, hearing the familiar refrain. "But I don't think his cardiac event is complete. He is already on intravenous nitroglycerin, he's had one infarct and probably having another. In addition, he's diabetic. He needs intensive care – we just can't handle those cases here."

"Well, see how things go, and call me back. Sorry, we don't have any beds, anyway. Why don't you phone St. Boniface?"

"Okay, thanks," I sigh, "I'll try them." I lean back in the chair and rub my brow. The usual run-around. It never changes. I phone St. Boniface hospital, but fare no better. I call Concordia hospital – the resident isn't available and they have no beds, either. I decide to call Dr. Jeff Hamilton at home, the staff cardiologist at Health Sciences. I know him from medical training. He agrees this is urgent; he will call the hospital and find a bed.

"Okay," I say. "Let's go. Call the ambulance people. We're taking him to Health Sciences. I'll write a transfer history. Can you make a copy of his medications and lab results? I'll go in with him."

I explain the options to the Kraynyks, and that my advice is to take him to an intensive care unit in the city. They agree. The ambulance crew arrives, deftly move Paul to the stretcher, transfer the IV line, and hook the leads to the portable monitor, and we're on our way. Just as we're loading him into the ambulance, the resident from Health Sciences calls again, and speaks to Diane.

"Apparently, Dr. Hamilton called Dr. Simmons and told him that we were bringing Mr. Kraynyk, but Dr. Simmons says not to bring him, they have no beds," Diane says.

"Well, call him back and tell him the patient is on the way – he'll have to find a bed. We'll bring him through emergency if we need to." My mind's made up, there are no other options.

I don't like to force their hand, but when a patient's life is on the line...

I'm prepared to resuscitate Mr. Kraynyk on the trip to Winnipeg if necessary – I have the laryngoscope, intubation tubes, and emergency drugs to maintain blood pressure and stabilize the heart rate. I'm not looking forward to our arrival at Health Sciences. I know their facilities and staff are strained to the limit, and they're always under pressure, too. Paul Kraynyk is on the edge. We have been told by the cardiologists on more than one occasion: 'If you have a critical patient with a heart attack, you need to get them to an intensive care facility.'

"Are we going red?" asks Bert, the ambulance driver.

"No," I say. "Just get us there in one piece." The 150-kilometer-an-hour dash with ear-rattling sirens and flashing lights was mostly an adrenalin rush for the ambulance staff. A trip shortened by five minutes, with staff and patient flailing around in an ambulance, inviting an accident, rarely saved anyone's life. In some serious accidents, especially involving major loss of blood or a life-threatening head injury, speed was essential, but those cases were rare.

Paul remains stable throughout the journey. We wheel him into the emergency room. The charge nurse takes the envelope of medical records without a word. After perusing them for a few minutes, she comes over to me. "Are you Dr. Giesbrecht?" she asks. I nod. "Why wasn't he intubated? Patients like that are supposed to be intubated for transfer."

"Mr. Kraynyk was quite stable," I reply. "His blood pressure and oxygen saturation were normal, and he was awake and coherent. I do anesthesia and I'm prepared for intub... "

"Our protocol says patients like this should be intubated for transfer." She leans forward and crosses her arms.

"Yes, I know," I say, my coronaries beginning to knot. "My protocol says different. Transferring an intubated patient sixty kilometers in an ambulance isn't that easy. It's basically doing anesthesia in a cramped swaying vehicle with minimal equipment."

"If you're bringing a patient to our hospital, we want the patient as stable as possible, intubated and with two IV lines…"

"I'm sorry," I interrupt. I can feel the pulse in my temples. My throat tightens. "But every time we bring in a patient, we get this condescending attitude – we country bumpkins don't have a clue. I have been doing this for many years – I'm quite capable of transferring the patient safely and dealing with complications. In our hospital we have to deal with everything – heart attacks, motor vehicle accidents, obstetrical emergencies, pediatrics, everything. We don't have the luxury of all the equipment, and backup specialist expertise that you have here. Really, we practice good medicine under the circumstances. Anyway, do you need some more information about Mr. Kraynyk? If not, we can accompany him to the intensive care unit and I can talk to Dr. Simmons myself."

The nurse turns a pale shade of vermillion, as if she has been discovered dipping into the narcotics cupboard. She opens her mouth, her lips quivering, then closes it again. She turns on her heel, and strides to the nursing station. She picks up the telephone and dials. I can't hear the conversation.

Within a few minutes, Dr. Simmons arrives, "Hi, Dr. Giesbrecht, how are you? I'm Doug Simmons. Nice to meet you." He shakes my hand warmly as if we were long-lost friends. "If you want to accompany us, we can transfer Mr. Kraynyk to intensive care. Can you fill me in?" I give him Paul's history as the orderly wheels the stretcher through the halls and up the elevator to the intensive care unit. The staff treats us with the utmost courtesy and respect. At this point, I'm quite okay with profound insincerity.

It's 12 noon when we arrive back at the ambulance for the trip home. "I kind of enjoyed that little scene back there," says Bert as he starts the ambulance down the ramp, and eases into traffic.

"Yeah, well," I say, "Sometimes I get a bit steamed. I get so tired of that city attitude – you know... you're from the country, so you must be pinheads."

"Absolutely right. I'm glad you stood up to them. Don't you wonder what the nurses are talking about right now?"

"I can imagine. Anyway, let them talk. It would be nice to get a little more respect next time, although I doubt it. We'll likely run into another arrogant bunch. Do we want to stop at Robins? Coffee and donuts on me."

Monday morning I phone Dr. Hamilton to find out what had happened.

"Well, Mr. Kraynyk crashed (medical lingo for cashing it in) a few hours after he got here. We had to resuscitate him, and get an emergency angiogram. The team performed a triple bypass. He is doing well and pain free. We'll keep him for a few more days, and then transfer him back to Bethesda, if that's okay."

"Oh, wow," I say. "I kinda thought something like that was brewing. Anyway, have them phone our admitting office when he's ready to come back. We should have a bed for him."

"I hear you caused a bit of a stir in ER yesterday."

"Yeah, sorry, Jeff. I was a little frustrated, I guess. You know we are continually being told what is appropriate for us to handle, and what we should send to the city. But when we try to refer, we get this runaround."

"I know, I know," he replies. "The system doesn't always work the way it's supposed to. I know you guys are doing a good job and don't have the resources we have here. Anyway, our ward will likely call in a few days. I'll send you a summary of his hospital stay."

"Okay, thanks very much."

Mr. Kraynyk came back to our country hospital as promised. "Thanks, doc," he says. "I guess I was in bad shape. My wife didn't think I make it."

"Let's hope everything goes well," I reply. "We'll watch you here for a few more days, and if everything looks good, you can go home early next week. Your heart is in atrial fibrillation, so you will have to stay on blood thinners, and we have to check the level every day for a while."

"What is fib...what you said?"

"Atrial fibrillation happens when the normal pacemaker of the heart isn't working properly, and the electrical signal circulates around the heart muscle so the heart beats randomly. It often happens in older people, especially if you have some heart disease. If there is atrial fibrillation, the blood doesn't flow as it should, and there is a greater risk of blood clots that could cause a stroke. That's why you have to stay on warfarin, the blood thinner. Once you leave hospital, we have to check the level several times a week for a while. Later, testing once a month will be enough."

Paul Kraynyk did well. He was followed every few weeks in my office. His PT (prothrombin time – a measure of blood thinning) results came back regularly, and required only minor adjustments in his warfarin dosage. His blood sugars were reasonable as well. He had learned a hard lesson, and had become serious about his health. Or so I thought.

Six months later, I was called to the hospital to see Paul, again on a Saturday. Then I realized he had not been to the clinic for months, and I had not seen a PT test result either. Paul was in the hospital emergency room, awake, babbling incoherently, and unable to give a history. I noticed the drooping of the left side of his face, and soon discovered paralysis of his left arm and leg.

"What happened," I ask Helen, who is standing beside his stretcher.

"I don't know. We were eating lunch, and suddenly he get dizzy, and fall on the floor. Is he going to be okay?"

"He's had a stroke. It will take a few days before we know how much function he will recover. He will likely be quite disabled. Wasn't he taking the blood thinners?"

"He said he feels good, so he didn't take. I told him not to stop, but he wouldn't listen."

"That's really unfortunate – the blood thinners probably would have prevented the stroke."

Paul had a significant cerebrovascular accident, as if someone had pulled the circuit breaker for the right half of his brain. There was little movement of his left arm and leg, and he was unable to speak. I restarted the coumadin – it would not reverse the paralysis, it was too late for that, but it might prevent further episodes. We had made huge advances in medicine with clot-busting drugs, angioplasty with stents, bypass surgery, but that couldn't replace patient compliance. Paul spent several weeks in the active treatment hospital, and was then transferred to the rehabilitation wing for physio and speech therapy. He had regained some function in his limbs, and managed to walk slowly with a cane.

After several months, he's ready for a trial at home. "Thanks, doc," he says slowly, his words slurred. "I go to … place, ah … home. She … make … ah … food." He shakes his head in frustration. He has anomic aphasia, trouble recalling names or nouns. He also has a problem with reasoning and jumbles the sequence of events. More than one task at a time leaves him confused – all signs of right brain injury.

"Perogies," says Helen. "He wants perogies. Maybe he shouldn't have, but I make him some."

Paul is depressed, another common post-stroke problem. Physical and communication deficiencies make for a poor quality of life. Perogies are not textbook treatment, but they may help.

"Sure," I say. "Let him have perogies, but maybe not every day."

Chapter 30
# STRESS

L ate November. Cool days and frosty nights. The trees were
bare and forlorn, except for the willows whose brown and
cadaverous leaves clung tenaciously to the branches, determined not to yield to winter. On some nights, the aurora borea-
lis crackled and hissed across the sky in shimmering shades of
yellow, green, and blue. A light snowfall had covered the dreary
garden – an early warning of winter. A bone-chilling northwest
wind greeted me as I walked from the doctor's parking lot to the
back door of the hospital.

Many years back, I had become qualified to interpret car-
diograms, to which the hospital added stress testing. During the
latter part of my career, stress testing became a significant part
of my work. Colleagues referred patients for evaluation of possible heart disease, if they had chest pain, shortness of breath, or
palpitations. People with a family history of coronary disease,
diabetes, abnormal cholesterol profile and hypertension were
also referred. The Motor Vehicle Branch required stress tests for
truckers who wanted to retain their Class 1 driver's license after
a heart attack. These patients were, of course, a select population, but nowhere was the recent epidemic of obesity as evident
as in the stress-testing lab. Cardiac stress testing remains an

important screening test, with more sophisticated diagnostic tests such as angiograms, radioisotope scans, ultrasound, and MRIs available now.

Thursdays were my stress-full days. I looked over the slate of patients. Many stress-test patients were so unfit, often obese; they might pull a hamstring playing solitaire. Today would be no exception.

I enjoyed the cardiology part of family practice – reading EKG's, occasional consultations, and stress tests. The heart is the center of life, entwined in our notions of love and emotion. It beats an average of 100,000 times per day, pumping 7,500 litres of blood. Heart disease in its many forms affects 20% of North Americans, and is still the leading cause of death. The heart is a remarkable organ, and when it quits, death follows within minutes.

Gina, the lab technician, has already hooked up Norma Plouffe, and explained how the treadmill functions.

"Hi, Norma, I'm Dr. Giesbrecht," I say as I take out my stethoscope. "How are you?"

"Okay, I guess," she says. "I'm very nervous."

"There is nothing to be nervous about, Norma. It's really just walking. We won't make you do anything you can't handle. You were referred by Dr. Gregoire, right? The letter says you have had left-sided pain, not related to exertion, and some shortness of breath. How often do you get these pains – once or twice a day? How long do they last?"

"They come many times a day, but only last a couple of minutes."

"No pain in your jaw, shoulder, or arm?"

"No."

"What's the pain like – sharp, aching, pressure?"

"It's pressure, like a tight band around my chest."

"You're taking Lipitor for cholesterol, and vitamins. No other medications, right? No diabetes, high blood pressure, or asthma?"

"No, Dr. Gregoire said my blood sugar was a little high, but I don't need pills yet, just watch my diet."

"Family history of heart disease – parents or siblings?"

"No. One uncle had a heart attack, I think."

"Do you do anything for exercise?"

She shakes her head again. "We have a treadmill, but I haven't used it for years."

"Let me guess," I say. "You use it to hang laundry. Okay, let me check your heart and your blood pressure, and then you can get to work."

I make a note on her consultation form: *58-year-old female. Left-sided chest pain – possibly angina. Lipitor for hyperlidemia. BP 150/90 No specific family history of CAD (coronary artery disease). No history of hypertension. Early diabetic*

*Risk factors: Obesity –110 kilo*

*Inactivity*

*Hyperlipidemia (high cholesterol)*

*Smoking*

*Diabetic*

*Stress test to rule out/confirm coronary heart disease.*

Norma begins the first three-minute stage at 2.7 kph, a leisurely stroll in the park for most people. However, as I had anticipated, she's only one minute into the exercise and her heart rate is already 135. At two minutes, she has reached her target heart rate of 162, based on her age. She's flushed and gasping as if she had run the Boston marathon, hanging onto the bar for support.

"That's it," I say quickly. "Stop the treadmill." Norma slowly makes her way back to the bed with Gina supporting one arm.

"Are you okay?" I say. "Any chest pain?"

"Yeah, I'm okay," she wheezes, "I just have to catch my breath."

"We'll monitor your heart a few more minutes while you recover." I watch the screen, and run another monitor tracing. There it is. ST depression, part of the heart beat complex sags from the baseline – an indicator of ischemia, inadequate blood flow to the heart muscle.

I'm never quite certain what approach to take with people like this – a gentle, tactful word, which has likely been tried in the past, or hit her with both barrels. I decide to scare the daylights out of her… tactfully.

"Okay, Norma, here's the scoop – you don't need me to tell you this, but you are sadly out of shape – that level of exercise should bring your heart rate up to 110 perhaps, not 160. Your heart is struggling because you're very much overweight and unfit – like a Hummer with a Neon engine. You've likely heard all this before."

She laughs, then sighs. "Yeah, many times."

"Secondly, there are changes on the monitor that suggest the arteries that supply blood to the heart are plugging up with fatty plaque – you know, coronary heart disease. You're going to have to get serious about weight loss and exercise. These changes on the ECG are an early warning. You're not about to have a heart attack, but the risk is high. You have a few other risk factors – early diabetes, smoking, abnormal cholesterol. I'll send your doctor a report, and he'll take it from there. You should see him soon. Oh, and we should probably repeat the stress test in a year and see how your heart is doing."

"Okay, thanks, doctor. I know, I have to do better."

"What do you think her chances are?" asks Gina after Norma had left.

"Well, probably not that good. I see so many people who just can't seem to break out of those bad habits. Let's hope she can do it. I know one thing: if she doesn't, she won't be around for too many more stress tests."

I write the report while Gina readies the equipment for the next patient. I'm glad Gina is here. She's pleasant, efficient and makes the patient feel at ease. She loves people, and somehow makes them feel privileged to have her puncture their bodies for a blood test.

Our next patient is Brian, 42 years old and complaining of frequent episodes of chest pain.

"Is it really pain, or shortness of breath?" I want to know.

"Well, both, like it cuts off my air," he says.

"Do you have palpitations or a racing heart?"

"Yeah, racing heart, but that seems to come after the shortness of breath."

"Do you hyperventilate? You know what that means?"

"Yeah, I get panicky at times. The doctor gave me some lorazepam to calm me down. I only take it when I need it. There's lots of stress at work."

"I see from the referral that your blood pressure is normal, your blood sugars and lipids are normal, and you don't smoke. Your weight is normal, and you play hockey several times a week. You do have a strong family history of heart disease – your dad and a brother both had heart attacks starting in their early forties."

"Yeah, I think my grandfather died of a heart attack, too."

*42-year-old male with atypical chest pain, likely not angina*
*Panic attacks/anxiety*
*Good general health, no hypertension, diabetes, etc*
*Strong family history – no other risk factors*
*Stress test to rule out coronary heart disease*

Brian has no problem with the treadmill. He walks easily through stages one and two – heart rate 110.

"How long do I have to go?" he asks.

"Well, you're obviously quite fit. You'll probably have to go for twelve minutes or so. We have to push you a bit more, you don't look a bit stressed – we want this to be a memorable occasion for you."

Brian laughs. By the time he reaches his target heart rate of 156, he has been on the treadmill thirteen minutes. He's breathing hard, but looks comfortable. The ECG tracing is entirely normal.

"You passed with flying colors, Brian," I say. "There are no signs whatever of heart disease. We're looking for evidence of blocked arteries or abnormal heart rhythms. A stress test is not infallible, but I think your symptoms are most likely due to anxiety or stress. You do have a strong family history, so it's probably a good idea to have this done every few years. Keep up the exercise."

"That's great," says Brian. "Thank you very much."

It's nice to have someone do well – all they need is reassurance.

"Hi, Mr. Benson," I greet the next patient. "I'm Dr. Giesbrecht. How are you?"

"Oh, I'm okay. I think it's just indigestion, but my doctor insists I have a stress test. My wife is after me, too."

George Benson heads a thriving manufacturing business, and has up to that point successfully employed the head-in-the-sand technique. He probably knows there's something wrong with his health, but hopes it will somehow disappear if he ignores it. He isn't overweight, but he smokes ten packages of cigarettes per week, and doesn't take time to exercise. He has typical vise-like chest pain with exertion, which disappears after a few minutes rest. His doctor had already given him nitroglycerin spray for the angina, but he hasn't used it.

"I see from your history that your grandfather died of a stroke at 54," I continue, "and your father and an uncle died of heart attacks in their late forties – that's a pretty strong family history. You're on Altace for hypertension and your cholesterol is a bit high."

"Yeah, but the doctor said my blood pressure was normal now, and the cholesterol was nothing to worry about."

"Your blood pressure is 140/85 now, which is borderline even with the medication. Okay, time for you to get to work."

"You're not going to work me too hard, are you?" he asks as he steps on the belt.

"Well, no, but there is a certain heart rate we'd like to reach based on your age, actually it's 220 minus your age. If you don't walk fast enough, we get out the cattle prod."

"Okay, okay," George laughs. "I'll walk."

George has walked seven minutes when I see his face starting to tense. "I'm getting tightness right here," he says, placing his fist in the center of his chest. His face is florid and he's fighting for air.

"Here, take a couple of shots of nitroglycerin under your tongue. I'll take another blood pressure reading and then we'll stop the treadmill."

The blood pressure is 150/80 – a minor rise, and a bad omen. Normally, the blood pressure would go up to 190/80 or higher with exercise. Little or no rise may mean the heart has little reserve for increased demand.

The ST segment on the ECG plummets like a slalom run. George's angina has disappeared with nitroglycerin and rest, but the ECG changes lingered for another four or five minutes.

"Mr. Benson," I say. "The bad news is, your test is positive. That means there is likely blockage in the coronary arteries. In addition, you have quite a number of risk factors: family history, smoking, lack of exercise, high cholesterol, and hypertension. I don't want to scare you unduly, but you are a ticking time bomb. You can't do anything about your family history – I guess you should have chosen your ancestors more carefully. The good news is that you're a fixer-upper. You can do something about the other risk factors."

"So Dr. Morgan was right. I thought I was just working too hard, or maybe it was indigestion."

"Well, this is a fairly typical picture. The single most important thing you can do to help your heart is to quit smoking."

"I quit once for six months," George says pursing his lips. "I've tried a few times."

"Don't give up. Most people try three or four times before they succeed. Ask you doctor to help you with that."

"Okay, so what happens now?" George asks.

"The next step is up to your doctor. He'll probably send you for an angiogram. Dr. Morgan will have my report in a few days. His note says you have an appointment with him in two weeks."

My last patient for stress test that day is Warren Warkentin, a farmer who has retrosternal (behind the breastbone) chest pain. David Kroeker had already seen this man and had given him nitroglycerin and metoprolol. The metoprolol slows the heart and gives some protection against heart attacks.

"I'm sure Warren has cardiac disease although his ECGs are normal," David said in one of those corridor consultations. "He has typical exertional angina. The clincher is that he has had two episodes where he was walking across his farmyard when he suddenly collapsed and then came to after a minute or so. His wife witnessed one of these things. After he woke, he felt very tired, but had no pain. I think he will need an angiogram and perhaps surgery. Anyway, why don't you get him on the treadmill and see how he does?"

Warren manages the treadmill for three minutes, and appears to be doing well.

Suddenly the ST segment takes a nosedive and Warren begins to have mild chest pain. There are PVC's all over the map. PVC's are premature ventricular contractions – random contractions arising spontaneously from the muscle instead of the heart's own pacemaker, a sign of irritable muscle, probably from lack of oxygen.

"Gina, stop the treadmill!"

No sooner had I uttered those words than Warren's legs buckle under him and he slides across the belt. Gina manages to grab Warren and ease him to the floor. I hit the red panic button, and the treadmill stops abruptly. "Get the ER staff!" I glance at the monitor for a quick assessment – ventricular fibrillation – the cardiac muscle contracts at random, and there is no useful blood circulation to supply vital organs like kidney and brain. Death will occur within a few minutes.

We have to act fast.

I tear open Warren's shirt and thump his chest hard – sometimes a simple mechanical jolt will restart the normal rhythm in cardiac arrest. Without looking to see if it has the desired result, I grab the resuscitation ambubag with oxygen and ventilate his lungs. Mona and several other nurses have arrived with the crash cart.

"Dr. Morgan is coming," says Mona, as she kneels over the unconscious man.

"Okay, Mona, start chest compressions while I intubate. Get the defibrillator ready at one hundred joules."

Dan Morgan arrives. "Hi, Dan," I say. "Am I glad to see you! He's still in v fib (ventricular fibrillation), I'll keep ventilating him. Shock him as soon as you're ready. Remember the last one we did on the ward?"

"Yeah, I remember – that didn't turn out too well," he says as he readies the machine. "Let's hope this works. Everyone clear?" He presses the buttons on the paddles. Warren's body convulses with the charge. I resume ventilating his lungs. Almost immediately, a normal rhythm appears on the monitor screen. Within a minute or two, Warren begins breathing on his own and opens his eyes. Mona takes a blood pressure, 90/60. Warren begins fighting the endotracheal tube, so I deflate the cuff and remove it.

"What happened?" Warren says thickly, struggling to sit up, looking about wild-eyed. "Where am I?"

"Warren," I say, "Just stay where you are. You had a cardiac arrest. You're okay now. We'll get a stretcher and take you to ER. The nurse will call your wife." I turn to the ER staff, "Thanks, guys, that went well."

"I'll phone Dr. Hamilton," says Dan. "Someone call the ambulance crew."

Within half an hour, Warren is on his way to Health Sciences hospital. By the end of the day, he has had an angiogram and bypass surgery.

The fainting spells Warren had experienced at home were probably ventricular fibrillation. These episodes sometimes resolve spontaneously, fortunately for Warren, but the odds of surviving many more would have been slim at best.

"You saved my life," Warren says when we meet on the street about two months later. "St. Peter was already shaking my hand when you guys decided I couldn't leave yet."

"Well, Warren," I smile, "I guess God decided it wasn't your time. You're doing well?"

"I'm doing very well. I'm doing light chores on the farm. We've decided to sell, though. I want to find something easier."

Warren remained well many years after that incident.

There was absolutely nothing like Thursday's lineup of cellulite and self-inflicted physical abuse to motivate my own exercise program. I considered myself a lighthouse in a sea of physical neglect. A feeble body weakens the mind, it is said, and I wasn't about to let that happen – I still needed every grey cell I had. I could tell patients that yes, it was possible to become fit, and it was possible to lose weight – I had done it myself. Self-righteousness bestows enormous credibility.

Exercise is a health benefit that everybody knows about, but few people take seriously. It takes hard work and discipline. In the past, employment usually meant hard physical labor except for those with means. Therein lies the problem – today's jobs usually entail long hours, stress, and mental fatigue, but little muscular activity. Couple that with fast food and smoking, and you have a recipe for disaster. After a day's work, most of us relax on the sofa with the remote and a beer. In an ironic twist of our modern age, the average person has to expend extra time and effort to stay fit. For many people the most exercise they get is lifting another hamburger.

Thursday was my day to preach the gospel of lifestyle changes.

## Chapter 31

# A CHANGE OF PACE

It's the end of the afternoon office schedule. I have been called to the ER to see Jolene Gerbrandt. On my way, I drive downtown to the post office to pick up a package before closing hours. It's a frigid day in December just before Christmas. The trees on Main street are festooned with multi-coloured lights. The signs of Christmas glitter down every side street. The shops are busy and the windows beckon with last-minute gifts. People hurry down the snowy street trying to elude the cold, their breath hanging in the frosty air. Snow had fallen the day before, as it must for a proper Manitoba Christmas, and adds to the festive mood.

I stop at the hospital on my way home. Jolene looks as forlorn and wretched as ever. All she wants is a refill on her medications. I have no choice but to continue her narcotics, prescribed by her specialist in Winnipeg, and offer supportive care as best I can. She endures the rolling eyes and condescending looks of medical staff whenever she appears in ER. Having rehearsed her illnesses over and over, her miseries have produced deep mental grooves, and she knows no other behavior.

It all began when Jolene first came to see me twelve years previously. At the time, she worked as a filing clerk and

receptionist in a local lawyer's office. She was in her early thirties, an unclaimed blessing, as my aunt Anne used to say of those
getting on in years and unfettered by marriage. Jolene sat in the
chair beside my desk, her hands folded in her lap. She raised her
eyes as I walked into the room, her round face expressionless. I
immediate sensed melancholy, though I had seen her only once
before for a strep throat.

"Hi, Jolene," I say. "How are you? Cold, isn't it? Winter's
here to stay."

She doesn't return my greeting. "Dr. Giesbrecht," she says,
without emotion. "I've had so many headaches lately, and I'm
always tired."

"Tell me about your headaches," I begin, as we have already
dispensed with the small talk. "Are they throbbing or a steady
aching? Do they come at a certain time of the day? Both sides
of the head?"

"It's a steady pain across the front and back of my head.
Sometimes it throbs behind my eyes. It's usually worse at work."

"Do you sleep well? Are you under a lot of stress?" I ask.

"No, I don't sleep very well – I often have trouble falling
asleep and then wake up at five, and I can't get back to sleep.
There is stress at work, but it's not bad."

"Anything else bothering you?"

"I have trouble remembering things, like my brain is fuzzy."
She hardly moves, except for an occasional shift in her chair, as if
everything is too much of an effort.

"You mean you're dizzy?"

"No, not really dizzy – my head just doesn't feel right and I
can't concentrate on my work. And I'm so tired."

"Okay, Jolene, let's see what we can do. It may just be stress
or anxiety, perhaps a mild depression, but we'll check things out.
Let's start with a complete physical and get a few basic tests. Is
that okay?" She nods diffidently. "You can take off your clothes,
and put on the gown – the ties are at the back."

I word that directive carefully since I once told a patient to "tie the gown in the back," and Carolyn found him wandering in the staff room, trying to find the back of the building so he could tie his gown.

I complete the examination. "Your physical is completely normal, other than the fact that your blood pressure is on the high side of normal. We should do a few baseline tests, you know, make sure your hemoglobin is normal, check your liver and thyroid function, that sort of thing."

"What do you think is wrong?" she asks in a monotone.

"Well, I'm not sure. Your symptoms could be due to abnormal thyroid function, or perhaps diabetes or anemia. There are no definitive signs of any of those things, but we'll check. Why don't you come back in two weeks, and we'll see what's what."

I give Jolene the requisitions. I would have wagered a lifetime supply of rectal gloves the tests would all be normal. We had hardly begun, but I had a premonition that we were entering a long dark tunnel. However, medicine does have its surprises, and I couldn't absolutely rule out anything at this stage.

"Hi Jolene," I say at her next visit, "So how are you doing?"

"Not too good. I'm still tired, and I'm having a lot of pain in my back and legs. I had to quit my job."

"You quit your job? Things are that bad?" She nods, everything in slow motion, like a droid in need of a battery charge. "I'm sorry to hear that. You couldn't just take a leave or a holiday, or perhaps work part time?"

"No, I had to quit, I just couldn't handle it anymore. I'm still having memory problems and trouble concentrating. Sometimes I feel lightheaded."

"Well, all your tests were normal," I reply. "There is no sign of anemia, thyroid imbalance, diabetes, or infections." Everything is normal, so straighten up already, and get on with your life. If only it was that simple.

Jolene exhales slowly. Her shoulders sag. I can almost see hope draining away from her sad face. "There has to be something wrong." People want something to be wrong, or at least have a name for it –somehow that makes feel them better and relieves them of responsibility for their misery.

"There is something wrong. We just have to find out what it is. How is your mood? Are you feeling depressed?"

"Well, yes, I'm very discouraged – I'm so tired and I can't do anything. I moved in with my parents, I couldn't afford to live on my own anymore. Mom does most of the cooking and laundry."

"There are a few more things we should look at – your hormone levels for one. In addition, we'll get a CT scan of your head to make sure there is no problem. It may take four or five weeks to get the CT scan. Come back a couple of weeks after the tests are done. In the meantime, try to get some exercise – walking is good. Get out and socialize, don't just mope at home. Perhaps do a little more of the cooking and cleaning. Why don't we start with some mild anti-inflammatory medication like Advil. That should help for your muscle pains and headaches."

"Okay," she says, listlessly. "I hope we find something."

"Let's see how it goes for a couple of months."

Jolene is more despondent than ever when I see her next. An atmosphere of despair has descended on her like a cloud of noxious gas. Her gloom is contagious – I have seen her for only a few months, but feel this disquietude that we are on a slippery slope, and no matter what we do, it will only continue the downward trend. It's like reading Macbeth – you know you can't avert the tragedy about to happen. She recites the same litany of complaints. As I listen, I have a sudden surge of exasperation, but stifle the urge, "For crying out loud, Jolene, let's stop this and get on with life! There's nothing wrong with you!"

"Things aren't going too well, are they?" I say kindly. Jolene's CT scan is normal, as are tests of adrenal and other hormonal function. I decide that whatever else she has, she's also depressed. "So I still don't have any answers for you. It could be chronic fatigue syndrome or fibromyalgia, although those conditions are nonspecific and difficult to diagnose. There aren't any tests that definitively tell us you have it or don't have it. However, I do think you are depressed, and you should probably take antidepressants. I'll give you a prescription for paroxitine. Start with 10 mg a day, and increase to 20 mg after a week. You'll have to give it at least three or four weeks before you'll notice much difference."

"I don't think that will help," replies Jolene in a low voice. "But I guess we can try it."

"Good, let's give it a try for a month or two. In the meantime, I'll get you an appointment with Dr. Beasant in the city. He's an internal medicine specialist and has a particular interest in conditions like chronic fatigue."

A month later, I receive a letter from Dr. Beasant. He agrees that it could be chronic fatigue syndrome, and suggests Jolene continue with the antidepressants, but perhaps she could try some other therapies, like acupuncture.

We have a working diagnosis, even if it's grasping at straws. That's a relief. I'm also grateful someone else has a hand in her care – it's a faint hope, but perhaps Macbeth could be made into a comedy or love story with a happily-ever-after ending.

Jolene's symptoms range from GI complaints, musculoskeletal pain, depression, and neurological problems like memory loss – in other words, they are nonspecific and don't fit any particular disease entity. Chronic fatigue is a disease of the last decade or so. It is a diagnosis of exclusion; that is, everything else has been ruled out. Research has not yet found the cause or the cure for this baffling syndrome. Some physicians don't believe it is a genuine illness – some think chronic fatigue is simply depression in an unhappy, vulnerable person who has trouble coping with the stresses of everyday life.

We have not all been dealt the same hand. Some of us have been given an ace, some a joker. Everyone is born with about five percent defective genes, though some defects are more significant in terms of health. A remarkable example of defective genes was King Carlos II who came to the Spanish throne at age four. He was a walking medical experiment due to generations of inbreeding among the European royal houses. Carlos was deformed physically and mentally – he didn't speak until he was five, and couldn't walk before eight years of age. His lower jaw protruded to the extent he was unable to chew; his speech was barely intelligible and he drooled due to a tongue that was much too big for his mouth. He was married twice, but was unable to produce an heir because of impotence.

There are very few of us who have perfect bodies matched to perfect faces, superior abilities, and sparkling personalities. This is the unrealistic ideal that is flaunted everywhere around us, though there was no question Jolene could have used a little help from Revlon, and perhaps Dr. Phil. Our modern culture has created this problem – not only have we medicalized our lives, we have synthesized our bodies. Cosmetics, plastic surgery, even tooth whiteners and shampoos have become huge industries. And if we don't feel the need for all these enhancements, the industries will do their best to change our minds. Jolene had a poor self-image and everything around her seemed to prove her right.

Some people are born into poverty and neglect or a lifestyle of drugs and crime that lead to a ruined body. We may make thousands of less obvious, but harmful choices that over a lifetime have the same effect. Jolene had experienced her share of life's fender-benders, but I couldn't help wondering how many of these were due to her own choices. Good health is common sense, reinforced by an occasional expert opinion.

We have also lost the capacity to accept suffering and death as part of the human condition – it must be eradicated

at all costs. This mentality consumes our lives and our thinking, causes much unneeded stress, and costs astronomical sums
of money. Take repetitive stress injuries and whiplash – these
should in most cases be minor irritants – aches and pains of daily
life. We over-treat these ailments, use them for financial benefit
(insurance pain), and blow them into a major cause of pain and
disability. Not to say that we shouldn't ease suffering whenever
possible, but human suffering is ubiquitous and inevitable – no
medical treatment will ever end it.

I didn't see Jolene for several years. She had continued to
see Dr. Beasant and a number of other physicians in Winnipeg,
each of whom had a different take on her health problems.

"Hi, Jolene," I say the day she arrives unexpectedly in my
office. "Long time no see. How are you doing?"

Her straggly unkempt hair and melancholy face say it all.
The misery of earlier visits has been augmented by resignation.
Her wardrobe shouts Self-Help. She places a plastic bag with pill
bottles on my desk. There is an open book in her hand: *Living
with Chronic Fatigue.*

"Not that great," she replies in a voice barely audible. "But
I'm coping somehow. I need some pills, and I can't see my
doctor in Winnipeg until next week."

"What do you need?"

"Uh, I need some Demerol tablets and Fentanyl patches."

"You're having that much pain?"

"Yeah, I've been on these pain-killers for about a year and
a half."

"You realize those are narcotics, don't you?" She nods her
head and gazes vacantly at the wall poster of the circulatory
system. "Is there anything else I can help you with? Are you
back to work?"

"No, I just can't work. I still live with my mom. My dad
died about a year ago."

Jolene is further down the slope. Its three and a half years since her ordeal began; she's not working, and has become addicted to narcotics.

"I'm sorry to hear about your father," I say, gently. "You've had a lot to deal with. So what are you doing apart from family? Any social life, church, that sort of thing?"

"No, I'm just too tired. If I'm up too much, I have leg and chest pain."

I could simply hand her the prescription – it would be so easy. "Jolene," I say. "I know you've had a rough time. I understand you've seen many doctors in the past few years, and nobody has really been able to help you. And now you're addicted to narcotics. Even with chronic fatigue, though, things usually start to improve after several years. You have to make a choice to start on the road back. You can't spend your life picking at the scabs. Don't you think it would give you a boost if you found an easy part-time job, or volunteered somewhere? – there are so many organizations that need help. Phone someone to go for coffee, even if you don't feel like it. I'll gladly help where I can or get you some counseling. You also need some gentle exercise. Walk with a friend or try golf or some other sport that's not too strenuous."

I study her face for a glimmer of insight or the faint stirring of new life. I can hear the muffled voices of people at the reception desk. There's a screech of tires on the pavement on the parking lot.

She finally speaks. "You know, I've tried all that stuff, but I can't do it – I'm too tired. Can I have my pills?"

"Okay," I sigh. "But my advice is to throw that book away. All it does is reinforce your preoccupation with your problems. You are making this a way of life. You have to start thinking positively, and start moving."

She still doesn't get it. I need the kind of persuasive power that would convince Osama bin Laden to catch a Baptist service with George W. Bush. I take out the special triplicate prescription pad that is required for controlled narcotics – one copy for the pharmacist, one for the government, and one for my records. "I also think you have to reduce your dependence on these drugs – I'll give you enough to tide you over for a couple of weeks. I will gladly see you again if you wish. If you want to keep seeing your doctors in Winnipeg, that's fine, too. I would rather not give you narcotics in the future, unless it's an emergency." I have a feeling of inevitability, of swimming against the current; nothing I can do or say will break Jolene's cycle of dependency and misery.

Several months later, I'm called on a Sunday evening to give an anesthetic to a 'lady in her late thirties with an acute abdomen.' I go to the surgical floor; Jim Sanderson is already there.

"Apparently you know this lady, Jolene Gerbrandt," he says. "She seems genuinely ill, she has acute tenderness in her right lower quadrant, with some nausea and vomiting. Her white cell count is normal, but I guess we have to open her up, and see what is going on. Probably her appendix."

Jolene has the laparotomy, and although her appendix is normal, it is removed, which is the normal practice. Her bowel, ovaries, uterus, liver are pristine. Postoperatively, she is given narcotics for pain control and sent home after a few days.

A month goes by. I'm called at the office just before noon break.

"There's a thirty-eight-year-old lady here. She had her appendix out a month ago," says Mona. "Jolene Gerbrandt. She thinks she has a kidney stone."

Is it really kidney disease, or another attempt at feeding a narcotic habit? We have to give her the benefit of the doubt, even drug abusers and malingerers have a constitutional right to get sick.

Jolene is lying on a stretcher, clutching her left side, and writhing with pain. She looks as if she has a time-share in Chernobyl.

"Hi, Jolene," I say. "More problems, I see. When did the pain start?"

"A couple of hours ago. I tried to wait it out, but it kept getting worse."

"Do you have blood in your urine, or pain when you pee?"

"I don't know if there was blood, but it looked very dark."

There is no distension, no liver or spleen enlargement, and no masses, but when I palpate the left renal angle and the lower abdomen following the course of the kidney, ureter, and bladder, Jolene winces and draws back.

Myrna hands me a report. "Good, you already sent a urinalysis," I say. We walk slowly back to the desk. "The urine is normal, no blood or white cells – a bit unusual with a kidney stone. But she seems to have the real thing. Let's admit her. I'll write some orders."

Morphine for pain control, 5 to 10 mg. as required. Strain the urine (to catch any stones). White cell count (to check for infection), BUN, and creatinine (to check for kidney function). Repeat urinalysis AM. Ultrasound in AM. (Ultrasound had replaced the IVP, intravenous pyelogram, the standard investigative tool for decades. An IVP was an x-ray of the kidneys, ureters and the bladder, aided by an intravenous injection of a radio-opaque substance concentrated by the kidneys, so it would outline the collecting system and show any blockage from tumor or stone.)

I check Jolene's abdomen again next morning – same tender areas. I nod to Laura.

"So, Jolene," Laura says, "where did you get the lovely afghan you brought with you? Did you make it yourself? It's beautiful."

"Well, sort of," says Jolene. "Actually I helped my mom years ago. Mom still does a lot of that stuff."

Meanwhile, I continue prodding, but with little reaction from Jolene, as long as she's distracted. Jolene's x-rays, urinalysis, and blood tests are all normal. She hasn't passed any stones. She is observed in hospital until the next morning.

"All your tests and the IVP are normal," I say. "There is no infection or tumor, and no kidney stone. We'll let you go home today. Let's see what happens."

Jolene drops out of sight for two or three years. She has rightly determined after repeated visits to ER seeking drugs that our local medical community has become very skeptical about her illnesses. She has moved on to other rural centers and then back to Winnipeg. She has been referred to an addiction centre with no success. When she comes back to see me again, it is for narcotics. Only this time she has a central line, a synthetic catheter that runs into the atrium of the heart, and allows drugs to be mainlined into the bloodstream without the need for a pill or an IV needle. She has been taught how to keep the port sterile, and give herself a dose of Demerol three or four times a day. Oral medication is apparently no longer effective.

Her abdomen is now a roadmap of surgical scars – an oophorectomy, another exploratory procedure, and a hysterectomy. She has acquired Crohn's disease with diarrhea, abdominal pain, bloating and nutritional deficiencies. Because of the inflammatory bowel condition, she has developed a fistula (abnormal connection) between the bowel and her vagina, which has been surgically repaired. Jolene's quality of life is poor in the extreme, and virtually every system is failing.

Jolene had been treated in emergency departments for perfectly-mimicked symptoms of kidney stones and gallbladder attacks. She had learned to copycat myocardial infarct (heart attack), and was given morphine until blood tests and ECG invariably proved there was no cardiac condition. This bizarre behavior is sometimes known as Munchausen Syndrome, named after a German, Baron von Munchausen who went about Europe telling fantastic, but fabricated stories about his incredible military exploits. People with this condition simulate or worsen symptoms, even self-mutilate in order to obtain medical treatment. They are often eager for hospital admission, surgery, and invasive medical tests. They move from clinic to clinic and hospital to hospital when they have exhausted the investigations and treatment of one center.

Jolene was by now a walking medical experiment with symptoms and diseases of nearly every body system. Some of it was misfortune, much of it self-inflicted.

So it was that on this cold December evening, I was seeing Jolene for narcotics once more. Over three decades of experience and I was no more successful at changing Jolene's health than when I first saw her. It was Christmas – a time of joy and hope, but all I could seemingly offer her was more narcotics. I thought back to the time I had first met Jolene with her headaches and fatigue, and wondered what I might have done differently to prevent this terrible tragedy. Was this a matter of poor choices, was it her environment, or had the medical establishment failed her? It had undoubtedly been a combination of all of these things, and like the Shakespearean tragedy, moved inexorably to a destiny no one was able to alter.

I leave the hospital for the short drive home. The streets are busy with people going to concerts and family gatherings, and last minute shopping. The fresh snow lies like a white canvas on the boulevards and spins into powdery jets from the wheels of passing traffic.

I do as I have done before on occasion – I slowly drive a few miles of country roads to think. The lights of the city are a few miles to the north and I can see Jupiter glowing brightly just above the dark eastern horizon. It's 2003. I have made an important decision – I'm going to retire from office practice. I reflect on the past years as I drive. There is a moment of profound sadness when I realize that after 37 years, I will no longer walk into our clinic as a personal physician. That's difficult to comprehend. It has been an eventful time, to say the least. There have been more failures than I dare admit. Cases like Jolene's that have not gone well weigh heavily on my mind, though I couldn't fix them all, try as I might. I was feeling melancholy, or as early physicians would have diagnosed – too much black bile.

It is time to move on, time to devote energy to other pursuits and a growing family. I'm well past middle age – you finally know your way around, but don't feel like going. The years have taken their toll and I find the responsibility and demands of patient care more stressful. I will never heal the world, nor do I feel the need to – at least some of my compulsions have begun to fade. Life has a way of accelerating as we age. I need to listen to the music before the song is over.

My melancholy thoughts begin to evaporate as I think of the triumphs, and the warmth and friendship of many patients. I will still contribute in anesthesia and some cardiology. My heart is buoyed by gratitude and anticipation of a new phase of life.

I arrive at our long driveway. The windows of home beckon like a lighthouse in a savage storm. I enter the house – the magic of Christmas is everywhere, and my despondency has evaporated. Rose is never better than at Christmas time, and the house is swathed in garlands, lights, green pine boughs, and red poinsettia. The tree stands in its usual spot beside the fireplace, the bottom branches resting on a mountain of brightly trimmed gifts.

I walk over to the sunroom and gaze at the backyard, silent and forgotten. The white lights strung in the willow create shadowy silhouettes of trees and shrubs. The garden is dark and desolate, but there's promise of renewal and rebirth beneath the blanket of snow. I think about that. The garden provides us with diversion, creativity, and healing, but with the passage of time,

I understand that real healing and restoration comes from faith and family.

Everyone will be home for the holidays: Carla and Eric from California, Kim and John, Jan and Chris from Winnipeg, Brent and Glenda from Steinbach. Jodi and Scott are both at university in Winnipeg, and will join us for the festive season. We are blessed with seven grandchildren and more on the drawing boards. It will be a marvelous time with family and friends.

CPSIA information can be obtained at www.ICGtesting.com
Printed in the USA
LVOW11s0919301113

363243LV00001B/2/P